T0292574

Respiratory Medicine

Series Editor:
Sharon I.S. Rounds

More information about this series at http://www.springer.com/series/7665

Anna R. Hemnes

Editor

Gender, Sex Hormones and Respiratory Disease

A Comprehensive Guide

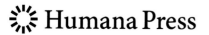 Humana Press

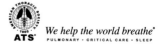

Editor
Anna R. Hemnes, MD
Vanderbilt University Medical Center
Nashville, TN, USA

ISSN 2197-7372   ISSN 2197-7380   (electronic)
Respiratory Medicine
ISBN 978-3-319-23996-5   ISBN 978-3-319-23998-9   (eBook)
DOI 10.1007/978-3-319-23998-9

Library of Congress Control Number: 2015958807

Springer Cham Heidelberg New York Dordrecht London

Printed on acid-free paper

Humana Press is a brand of Springer
Springer International Publishing AG Switzerland is part of Springer Science+Business Media (www.springer.com)

Preface

Men and women are not the same. Although somewhat of a truism, this simple fact was not seriously factored into medical research until relatively recently. Established in 1990, the National Institutes of Health's Office of Women's Health Research brought attention to the importance of research in women's health issues, ensured inclusion of women in health and behavioral science research, and also enhanced research related to diseases that primarily affect women. As a consequence of this and other efforts, there has been a tremendous explosion in studies of sex differences across all the health sciences. Although not traditionally thought of as asexually dimorphic structure, the lungs are, indeed, influenced by sex. This book on sex differences in lung disease is, at least in part, a product of this informative research.

In the past several decades, we have demonstrated that lung structure and function are different in men and women. We have discovered that men and women have different predispositions to developing various lung diseases. And, importantly, we are now beginning to understand on a molecular level how these sex differences occur. Sex-based differences in lung disease can be the result of many factors, not simply sex hormones. Environmental exposures may also be different in men and women, and cultural norms and shifts can influence sex-based differences in disease development, progression, and even response to therapy. In the future, there is hope that we can harness our understanding of these sex-based differences to meaningfully improve lung health for both men and women.

This book showcases some of the most important sex-based differences in lung structure and function in normal people and also the role that sex plays in lung diseases. The chapters highlight the successes in understanding why women have different pulmonary function testing results than men, how sex hormones may affect pulmonary vasculature, and why women have rising rates of smoking-related lung disease, to name just a few. But they also show the limits of our understanding: for instance, we don't know yet why women are more likely to get pulmonary arterial hypertension than men despite recognition for several decades that women are four times more likely to develop this disease than men. Finally, the chapters point to avenues of future research. In areas with greater understanding of the mechanisms that drive sex-based differences in lung disease, for example, we need to use this knowledge to improve treatment and outcomes for both men and women.

We hope that healthcare practitioners, researchers, members of industry, and any interested people will find this a useful reference on sex, gender, and lung disease. But, perhaps most importantly, the best possible outcome of this book is that it will stimulate young researchers to answer the important questions remaining about lung disease and sex to cure these devastating diseases and improve health for all people.

Nashville, TN   Anna Hemnes

Contents

Contributors

Eric D. Austin, MD, MSCI Department of Pediatrics, Division of Allergy, Immunology, and Pulmonary Medicine, Vanderbilt University School of Medicine, Nashville, TN, USA

Jeannette Zinggeler Berg, MD, PhD Division of Pulmonary and Critical Care Medicine, Vanderbilt University School of Medicine, Nashville, TN, USA

Andrew J. Bryant, MD Department of Medicine, Division of Pulmonary, Critical Care and Sleep Medicine, University of Florida, Gainesville, FL, USA

Timothy F. Burns, MD, PhD Department of Medicine, Division of Hematology-Oncology, University of Pittsburgh Cancer Institute, Hillman Cancer Center Research Pavilion, Pittsburgh, PA, USA

Xinping (Peter) Chen, PhD Department of Medicine, Division of Allergy, Pulmonary, and Critical Care Medicine, Vanderbilt University School of Medicine, Nashville, TN, USA

Andrea L. Frump, PhD Department of Medicine, Division of Pulmonary, Critical Care, Occupational and Sleep Medicine, Indiana University School of Medicine, Indianapolis, IN, USA

MeiLan K. Han, MD, MS Department of Internal Medicine, Medical Director, Women's Respiratory Health Program, University of Michigan, Ann Arbor, MI, USA

Craig A. Harms, PhD Department of Kinesiology, Kansas State University, Manhattan, KS, USA

Stephanie P. Kurti, MS Department of Kinesiology, Kansas State University, Manhattan, KS, USA

Tim Lahm, MD Department of Medicine, Division of Pulmonary, Critical Care, Occupational and Sleep Medicine, Indiana University School of Medicine, Indianapolis, IN, USA

Richard L. Roudebush VA Medical Center, Indianapolis, IN, USA

Catherine Meldrum, PhD, RN University of Michigan, Ann Arbor, MI, USA

Dawn C. Newcomb, PhD Division of Allergy, Pulmonary, and Critical Care Medicine, Department of Medicine, Vanderbilt University Medical Center, Nashville, TN, USA

Patricia Silveyra, PhD Department of Pediatrics, The Pennsylvania State University College of Medicine, Hershey, PA, USA

Joshua R. Smith, MS Department of Kinesiology, Kansas State University, Manhattan, KS, USA

Laura P. Stabile, PhD Department of Pharmacology & Chemical Biology, University of Pittsburgh Cancer Institute, Pittsburgh, PA, USA

Lisa Young, MD Division of Pulmonary Medicine, Department of Pediatrics, Vanderbilt University School of Medicine, Nashville, TN, USA

Chapter 1
Sex Differences in Normal Pulmonary Structure and Function at Rest and During Exercise

Craig A. Harms, Joshua R. Smith, and Stephanie P. Kurti

Introduction

There are important physiological sex differences that exist in most systems of the body. For example, it is known that there are important differences with regard to cardiovascular function, thermoregulation, substrate metabolism, and pulmonary function between men and women during exercise which may have important implications for exercise tolerance. Specific in regard to the pulmonary system, there has been considerable interest in defining sex-based differences in the pulmonary systems response to exercise. Changes in circulating hormones and structural changes generally account for the majority of the sex differences in the pulmonary system. These in turn might have an effect on the integrated ventilatory response, on respiratory muscle work, and on pulmonary gas exchange during exercise, which may in turn affect exercise capacity in health [124].

Normal Hormonal Fluctuations

Women experience a complex milieu of changes and fluctuations in female sex hormones, occurring primarily during the reproductive years. Hormonal variations are primarily due to estradiol, estrogen, and progesterone levels that fluctuate during the menstrual cycle. The menstrual cycle is depicted in Fig. 1.1. The ovarian cycle is composed of the follicular phase, ovulation, and the luteal phase, while the uterine cycle includes menstruation, proliferative phase, and secretory phase.

C.A. Harms, PhD (✉) • J.R. Smith, MS • S.P. Kurti, MS
Department of Kinesiology, Kansas State University, Manhattan, KS 66506, USA
e-mail: caharms@ksu.edu

© Springer International Publishing Switzerland 2016
A.R. Hemnes (ed.), *Gender, Sex Hormones and Respiratory Disease*,
Respiratory Medicine, DOI 10.1007/978-3-319-23998-9_1

1

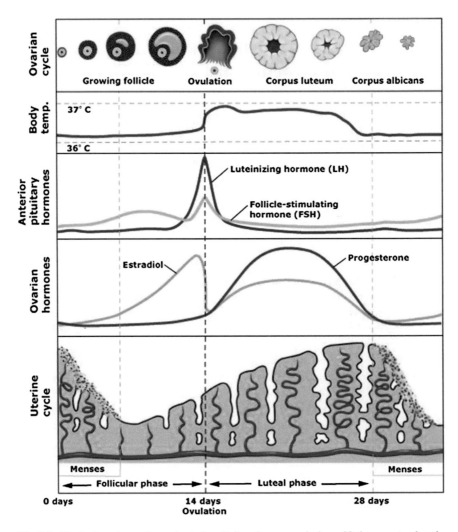

Fig. 1.1 Fluctuations in ovarian and anterior pituitary hormones during a 28-day menstrual cycle. During the follicular phase (day 0–14), estradiol increases. In the end of the follicular phase, estradiol drops while luteinizing hormone (LH) and follicle-stimulating hormone (FSH) rise. This is when ovulation occurs. The following phase is the luteal phase when anterior pituitary hormones (LH and FSH) drop; progesterone rises and then drops, starting the next cycle

Estrogen levels increase in the first half of the cycle (the follicular phase). Hormone levels [follicle-stimulating hormone (FSH) and luteinizing hormone (LH)] rise as ovulation occurs. The second phase of the females' menstrual cycle is the luteal phase. During this phase, FSH and LH drop and consequently the remaining parts of the stimulated follicle from ovulation produce progesterone, causing the adrenal glands to start producing estrogen. As the levels of FSH and LH drop even further, the drop in progesterone will eventually allow for the start of the next cycle.

Other physiological changes also occur during the various phases of the menstrual cycle. Body temperature is elevated mid-cycle primarily due to the action of progesterone, which increases body temperature approximately 0.2–0.3 °C [1]. Studies investigating how these physiological changes affect sports performance are sparse and inconclusive; however, Lebrun [1] reported variations in vascular volume dynamics, thermoregulation, substrate metabolism, and of primary focus in this chapter, pulmonary function [2].

It is well documented that circulating hormone levels affect pulmonary function. Progesterone may affect hyperventilation [3], partially compensated respiratory alkalosis [4], cause increases in hypercapnic and hypoxic ventilatory response [3, 5], and increase central ventilatory drive, all of which may affect breathing responsiveness during exercise [6]. Additionally, augmented ventilatory drive with reduced airway diameter contributes to expiratory flow limitation during exercise [7] (see section "Expiratory Flow Limitation"). Heightened ventilatory response to exercise may also be due to mast cells in the airways with progesterone and estrogen receptors, which may account for differences in ventilation (V_E) [8].

There are many discrepancies in the literature investigating resting ventilation (V_E) across the menstrual cycle. Several of these studies report resting V_E is elevated in the luteal cycle and tidal volume may be higher (by approximately 100 mL) and end-partial pressure of carbon dioxide (CO_2) lower (by about 2–3 mmHg) [4, 9, 10], albeit conflicting evidence suggests no difference in resting V_E [11]. As estrogen levels increase, fluid retention and subsequent increases in pulmonary capillary blood volume could affect gas exchange in the lung [12]. Previous work has suggested resting diffusion capacity (DLCO) is reduced during early follicular phase [13], although this finding is not consistent among studies.

Morphology

The structure of the pulmonary system (e.g., lung, airways, and chest wall) is generally considered overbuilt for the exercise demands at sea level [14], although differences in lung morphology exist between men and women. Demands placed on the pulmonary system include increases in minute ventilation and subsequent increases in flow rates, increasing lung volumes to maintain gas exchange of oxygen and carbon dioxide [14]. The structure of the lung is considered to be exceedingly capable of meeting these demands, albeit women are considered to be one of several exceptions. It is possible that the demands of the pulmonary system may exceed its total capacity. This is primarily due to morphological differences in lung size and airway size in females.

Women have smaller lungs and airways compared to men of the same sitting height [15, 16]. Additionally, women have decreased lung volumes and expiratory flow rates compared to height-matched men [17]. Women also have less alveolar surface area and smaller alveoli, consequently decreasing lung diffusion capacity compared to men [15–17]. There are also no sex differences in the recoil properties of the lung [18] or chest wall and pulmonary compliance [19]. Diameter of the trachea is also smaller in women compared to men [20]. In comparing airway size to lung size, women typically have smaller airways relative to lung size [15]. The comparison of airway size relative to lung size is called the dysanapsis ratio (DR) and is classified by Mead [15] using the following ratio:

$$\text{dysanapsis ratio} = \frac{FEF_{50}}{\left(FVC \times P_{st}(1)50\%\right)}$$

where FEF_{50} is forced expiratory flow at 50 %, FVC is forced vital capacity, and $P_{st}(1)_{50\%}$ is lung static recoil pressure at 50 %. Mead was the first to measure the DR of men and women. There was a lower DR in women compared to men, indicating the airways are smaller for a particular lung volume. This has been confirmed by Sheel and colleagues [22], who used tomographic imaging to measure absolute airway size in women. Researchers reported women had significantly smaller airways compared to male ex-smokers matched for lung size.

Pulmonary Function During Exercise

Pulmonary Gas Exchange

It has been previously believed that pulmonary gas exchange does not limit submaximal or maximal exercise at sea level. However, recent studies have shown that endurance-trained men and women experience pulmonary gas exchange impairments during exercise. Generally, healthy men do not experience significant reductions in pulmonary gas exchange during maximal exercise. On the other hand, women are more likely to exhibit pulmonary gas impairments because of morphological differences in pulmonary structures. The efficiency of pulmonary gas exchange is determined by the difference ($A\text{-}aDO_2$) between the partial pressure of oxygen in the alveoli (P_A) and the arterial blood (P_a). The widening of the $A\text{-}aDO_2$ is indicative of pulmonary gas exchange impairments. Mild gas exchange impairment is defined as a $A\text{-}aDO_2$ of 25–35 mmHg and a severe pulmonary gas exchange impairment is defined as a $A\text{-}aDO_2$ of >35–40 mmHg [23]. The $A\text{-}aDO_2$ can be widened by shunts, ventilation–perfusion mismatch (V/Q mismatch), and diffusion limitation (discussed below).

Gas Exchange at Rest and During Exercise

In resting conditions, there is a minor $A\text{-}aDO_2$ of ~5–10 mmHg due to V/Q mismatch and shunts. Figure 1.2 displays the arterial PO_2 (P_aO_2), arterial PCO_2 (P_aCO_2), and $A\text{-}aDO_2$ during an incremental exercise test. At rest and during submaximal exercise, P_aO_2 is maintained near resting values. P_aCO_2 is maintained near resting values as well until alveolar ventilation increases out of proportion to CO_2

Fig. 1.2 Pulmonary gas exchange during incremental exercise. Arterial PO_2 (P_aO_2) (*top panel*), arterial CO_2 (P_aCO_2) (*middle panel*), and alveolar–arterial PO_2 difference (A-aO_2) from rest to maximal exercise. With increasing exercise intensity, P_AO_2 and P_ACO_2 are maintained near resting values, but A-aO_2 increases linearly. At near maximal workloads, P_ACO_2 will decrease due to hyperventilation and P_AO_2 is generally maintained near resting values except for certain populations (e.g., endurance-trained men and women)

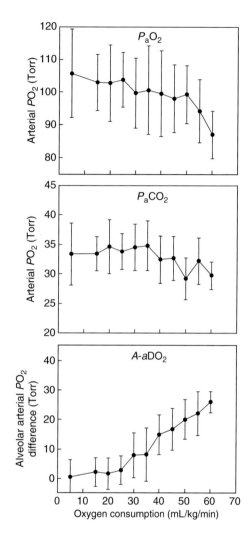

production to assist in acid–base balance which will lead to a hyperventilatory response and a reduced P_aCO_2 compared to resting levels. Because alveolar ventilation increases in proportion to exercise intensity, A-aDO_2 also increases with increasing exercise intensity. Although A-aDO_2 is increasing, P_aO_2 is maintained near resting levels and P_AO_2 will increase leading to a greater diffusion gradient between the alveoli and the pulmonary capillary. At maximal exercise, P_aCO_2 is lower than resting values and P_aO_2 is maintained near resting values despite the large widening of the A-aDO_2. However, in endurance-trained men and women, P_aO_2 can sometime decrease below resting values which reduces oxygen transport and exercise tolerance and increases exercise-induced peripheral fatigue [24–28].

Exercise-Induced Arterial Hypoxemia

Exercise-induced arterial hypoxemia (EIAH) is the reduction in P_aO_2 and/or oxygen saturated hemoglobin in the arterial circulation (SaO_2) during exercise. The adequacy of systemic oxygen transport is characterized by SaO_2. The severity of EIAH is defined by the reduction in SaO_2 with mild EIAH as 93 % to 95 %, moderate EIAH as 88 % to 93 %, and severe EIAH as <88 % [23]. The widening of the A-aDO_2 (due ventilation–perfusion mismatch, shunts, and diffusion limitation), VO_{2max}, and inadequate hyperventilation contribute to EIAH. It is currently thought that the widening of the A-aDO_2 contributes 35 %, VO_{2max} 25 %, and inadequate hyperventilation 60 % to EIAH [23]. EIAH is rarely seen in healthy untrained men exercising at sea level. In 1984, Dempsey and colleagues measured arterial blood gases during an incremental exercise test in endurance-trained men. Twelve of 16 men experienced EIAH during submaximal and maximal exercise [25]. The prevalence of EIAH is ~50 % in endurance-trained men during maximal exercise [29]. On the other hand, the prevalence of EIAH in women during maximal exercise is considerably higher (~65–75 %) compared to men [30–32]. Both untrained and endurance-trained women experience EIAH during submaximal and maximal exercise [30, 31]. What are possible mechanisms that explain this increased prevalence of EIAH in women? Although intrapulmonary shunts contribute to the widening of the A-aDO_2 during exercise, there are no sex differences in the opening of the intrapulmonary shunts during exercise [33]. Additionally, sex differences do not exist in V/Q mismatch during exercise [34]. However, the higher prevalence of ventilatory constraints (i.e., expiratory flow limitation) [35] and lower lung diffusion surface [16, 17] of women compared to men likely contribute to their higher prevalence of EIAH.

Ventilation–Perfusion Mismatch

Due to the gravitational effects on both air and blood, the matching of ventilation and perfusion (blood flow) in the different regions of the lung is heterogeneous (i.e., V/Q mismatch). From rest to maximal exercise, there is a drastic increase in alveolar ventilation (15–20x), while cardiac output increases a modest 5–7x, which will lead to a larger V/Q mismatch. However, because both ventilation and cardiac output increase during exercise, the lung has a higher V/Q leading to higher P_AO_2 and P_aO_2. Thus, the contribution of V/Q to A-aDO_2 is similar during exercise to rest; however, in some subjects it can contribute to the majority of the A-aDO_2 during maximal exercise [36]. The degree of V/Q mismatch is not different across VO_{2max} [37]. A sex differences does not exist in the degree of V/Q mismatch during exercise [37].

Shunts

Pulmonary shunts are pathways in which blood bypasses the gas exchange portions of the lung. Extrapulmonary (e.g., Thebesian vein and bronchial circulation), intra-cardiac (patent foramen ovale), and/or intrapulmonary shunts occur at rest and during exercise. The prevalence of intracardiac shunts specifically patent foramen ovale is ~30 % [38] and the prevalence of intrapulmonary shunts is ~90 % [33] in healthy humans. Shunts can lead to impairment of pulmonary gas exchange because the deoxygenated blood is mixed with the oxygenated blood from the lungs returning to the arterial circulation. Approximately 1 % of the total cardiac output flows through shunts [23] and therefore bypasses pulmonary gas exchange. At rest, a portion of cardiac output flows through extrapulmonary and intracardiac shunts [39], which contributes to the resting A-aDO$_2$. During exercise, a portion of cardiac output flows through intrapulmonary shunts [33, 40] and to a lesser degree intracardiac shunts [39]. The increased cardiac output flowing through shunts during exercise contributes to the widening of the A-aDO$_2$. Therefore, shunts can impair resting and exercising pulmonary gas exchange, but there is no sex difference in the opening of the shunts during exercise [33].

Diffusion Limitation

Diffusion limitations can also lead to widening of the A-aDO$_2$ during exercise. The contribution of diffusion limitation to the widening of A-aDO$_2$ is similar to *V/Q* mismatch [23]. A diffusion limitation is any impairment in diffusion of oxygen from the atmosphere to the hemoglobin in the pulmonary capillaries. Diffusion of oxygen is reliant on the rate of equilibrium of the mixed venous blood with the P$_A$O$_2$ (lung diffusion capacity) and the mean transit time of red blood cells through the lung.

Lung diffusion capacity (D_{LCO}) is the capability for the atmospheric oxygen to diffuse across the alveolar-capillary membrane, diffuse across the blood, and bind with the hemoglobin in the pulmonary capillary. Historically, diffusion capacity has been characterized as resistances and simplified in the following equation:

$$\frac{1}{D_{LCO}} = \frac{1}{D_M} + \frac{1}{\theta \cdot V_C}$$

where $1/D_M$ is the resistance to diffusion by the alveolar-capillary membrane and $1/\theta^*V_C$ is the resistance of uptake of oxygen to the hemoglobin (θ) in the pulmonary blood volume (V_C) [41]. Women have smaller lungs, less alveoli (and therefore lung surface area), and lower resting D_{LCO} compared to height-matched men [16, 17]. The lower lung diffusion capacity results from a lower pulmonary blood volume. During incremental exercise, there is a proportional increase in D_{LCO} due to increases in pulmonary blood volume. At rest, pulmonary blood volume is ~70 mL and during exercise it can increase to 150–200 mL because of pulmonary capillary recruitment and distention. These sex differences in lung diffusion capacity and pulmonary blood volume at rest likely exist during exercise. In fact, the D_{LCO} in men at maximal exercise is almost doubled compared to women (64.7 vs. 37.7 mL/mmHg/min) due to their 40 % higher pulmonary blood volume compared to women [125]. A smaller lung diffusion capacity can decrease the rate of diffusion of oxygen from the atmosphere to the pulmonary capillaries impairing pulmonary gas exchange.

The pulmonary blood volume associated with D_{LCO} is also very important for transit time of the pulmonary red blood cells. Mean red blood cell transit times are calculated by dividing pulmonary blood volume by cardiac output. At rest, the mean transit time is ~0.8 s which is usually adequate time for equilibration. If pulmonary blood volume did not increase during heavy and maximal exercise, pulmonary red blood cell transit times would fall below 0.25 s leading to diffusion limitation and widening of the A-aDO$_2$. The 2–3x increase in pulmonary blood volume is extremely important to allow adequate time for the red blood cell to become oxygenated in the pulmonary capillary during exercise. Mean red blood cell transit time decreases during exercise, but remains above ~0.25 s to allow for complete equilibration. However, in endurance-trained men, cardiac output may increase up to ~30 L/min, while pulmonary blood volume is similar to an untrained individual (~150–200 mL), which can lead to insufficient time for diffusion equilibration and widening of the A-aDO$_2$. The smaller pulmonary blood volume of women during maximal exercise will lead to a lower mean pulmonary red blood cell transit time compared to men. It is quite possible, especially in endurance-trained women, the mean pulmonary red blood cell transit time may fall <0.25 s, which would not allow for complete diffusion equilibrium. The incomplete diffusion equilibrium will lead to pulmonary gas impairments and contribute to the higher prevalence of EIAH in women.

Inadequate Hyperventilation

Inadequate hyperventilation during exercise does not increase the widening of the A-aDO$_2$, but still contributes to the onset of EIAH. Inadequate hyperventilation is present when the P$_a$CO$_2$ is >~38 mmHg during heavy exercise [23]. Inadequate ventilation is due to altered chemosensitivity [43] and mechanical constraints [7]. Specifically, resting hypercapnic and hypoxic chemosensitivity is lower in men who experience EIAH at maximal exercise compared to men without EIAH [43]. Chemosensitivity is not different between men and women [44]. This suggests that the development of EIAH is at least partially due to decreased chemosensitivity in men and women leading to an inadequate hyperventilatory response.

Mechanical constraints of the airways also can limit the hyperventilatory response during exercise. Expiratory flow limitation (EFL) (explained below) can limit ventilation during heavy exercise. This was demonstrated by using a heliox inspirate (increases the maximum flow-volume loop by ~20–35 %) to reduce EFL during exercise. Without EFL (via the heliox inspirate), alveolar ventilation, tidal volume, and breathing frequency were all higher compared to exercising with EFL [7, 45]. However, breathing the heliox inspirate during heavy to maximal exercise only prevented 30–40 % of EIAH, suggesting that mechanical constraints do not fully explain the development of EIAH [23]. In fact, endurance-trained men who inadequately ventilate during maximal exercise would need to further increase their ventilation ~50 L/min to fully prevent the development of EIAH. However, endurance-trained men use ~85 % of their maximum ventilatory capacity so increasing ventilation ~50 L/min is not possible [23]. Due to morphological differences, women have a higher prevalence of expiratory flow limitation and higher severity of EFL at similar ventilations compared to men [35]. With more of their tidal volume expiratory flow limited, ventilation during exercise is likely to be limited to a greater extent in women compared to men. Additionally, endurance-trained women exhibit more EFL during exercise compared to non-endurance-trained women, suggesting that endurance-trained women are more likely to develop EIAH [7]. The higher prevalence and severity of EFL in women contributes to the inadequate hyperventilation and the increased development of EIAH.

Ventilation

The normal ventilatory response to exercise includes increasing minute ventilation (V_E), which is accomplished by increases in both tidal volume (V_T) and breathing frequency (f_b). At exercise less than 50 % of vital capacity (VC), V_T increases with minimal increases in f_b. The greater tidal-volume loop causes decreases in both inspiratory and expiratory reserve volumes (IRV, ERV, respectively), but still is capable of maintaining pulmonary gas exchange and adequate ventilation within the maximum flow-volume loop (MFVL) [46]. Figure 1.3 shows an MFVL as well as end-expiratory lung volume (EELV), end-inspiratory lung volume (EILV), inspiratory reserve volume, and expiratory reserve volume [47]. Increases in V_T occur to maintain the greatest compliance with the least resistive work of breathing (WOB) in the pressure–volume relationship [48] (see section "Work of Breathing").

The greater V_T is accomplished by decreasing EELV below functional residual capacity (FRC) by recruitment of the expiratory muscles. The activity of the expiratory

Fig. 1.3 Maximal flow-volume loop and lung volumes. *MFVL* maximal flow-volume loop, *TLC* total lung capacity, *EILV* end-inspiratory lung volume, *IRV* inspiratory reserve volume, *IC* inspiratory capacity, V_T tidal volume, *EELV* end-expiratory lung volume, *ERV* expiratory reserve volume, *RV* residual volume, *ext FVL* exercise flow-volume loop, V_{FL} volume expiratory flow limited

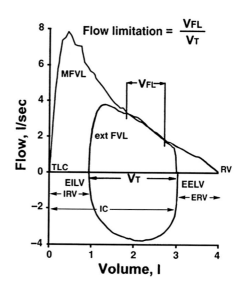

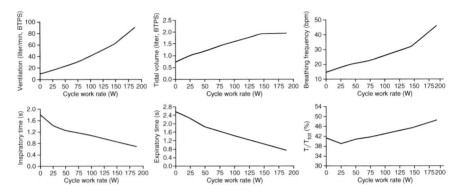

Fig. 1.4 The ventilatory response to incremental exercise during cycling in one healthy subject. There is an initial rise in tidal volume (V_T), followed by an increase in breathing frequency when V_T plateaus

muscles in the reduction of EELV enables greater expiratory flow rates, lowers intra-abdominal pressure, and enables the diaphragm to function at optimal length for generating force [49]. Lastly, the expiratory muscles that allow lung volume to decrease below FRC will cause subsequent decreases in inspiratory muscle work by allowing for the storage of elastic energy in the chest and abdominal walls during expiration. This energy can be used for the following inspiration and reduce the total WOB [50, 51]. Additional increases in EILV also maximize the V_T.

During exercise where V_E exceeds 50–60 % of VC, further increases in V_E are met solely by increases in f_b [46]. This is accomplished by decreasing inspiratory and expiratory time (T_I and T_E, respectively) [52]. There is a greater T_E relative to T_I relative to total breath time (T_{TOT}), with a T_I/T_{TOT} as high as 0.55 during maximal exercise [53]. Regulation of airway caliber also helps achieve high ventilatory rates by decreasing airway resistance during heavy exercise. As inspiratory and expiratory flow increase, dilation and stiffening of intrathoracic and extrathoracic airways occur to reduce turbulent airflow [54, 55]. The pulmonary system is extraordinarily built for maintaining V_E, and the increases in V_T and f_B throughout exercise maximize alveolar gas exchange and minimize WOB. The ventilatory response to increasing exercise is displayed in Fig. 1.4, adapted from Sheel and Romer [52].

The literature investigating the breathing mechanics and control of ventilation in men and women at rest and during exercise is contradictory and inconclusive. Current research suggests that exercise values for V_E, V_T, and f_b are similar between men and women, and the plateau in V_T is the same in men and women when controlling for FVC [7]. Habedank et al. [56] and Blackie et al. [57] each reported no difference between breathing reserves in men and women, although their reported absolute values were about 20 % different (~61 % reserve and ~41 % reserve, respectively). This discrepancy is more likely due to the mode of exercise utilized in the study design (cycling versus treadmill running) rather than differences in breathing pattern during exercise [58].

The control of V_E during exercise is multifaceted. Exercise ventilation during submaximal or steady-state exercise increases in three distinct phases. The first phase is an immediate increase in ventilation upon the onset of exercise, while the second is a further slow, gradual increase between 5 s and 2–3 min. The third is a stable phase where ventilation is sustained for several minutes, but can drift during prolonged time of exercise. Control of ventilation has primarily been attributed to the mechanisms that contribute and regulate exercise hyperpnea to prevent hypercapnia and hypoxemia [46]. These include (1) feedforward influences including central command and CO_2 flow, (2) feedback from the exercising limbs, and (3) contribution from carotid chemoreceptors. Feedforward deals with a sensor (e.g., respiratory sensors: chemoreceptors and sensory receptors) transmitting information to the central nervous system, where it integrates the information and further increases or reinitiates signals to the effectors (e.g., the respiratory muscles). Feedback occurs when the sensor transmits information, and when the information is received, there will be a subsequent decrease or increase in drive back to the effectors that will attempt to return the body back to homeostasis. Due to the complexity of control of breathing during exercise, we partitioned the control of breathing into two categories (feedforward and feedback) as has been previously done by Sheel and Romer [52].

Central command (neural signals that originate from the hypothalamus) has a recognized and definite contribution to regulation of exercise hyperpnea, although the magnitude of the input is uncertain. Eldridge and colleagues [59, 60] conducted several studies to understand the role of central command in the control of breathing using an anaesthetized brain model and anaesthetized decorticate cats. This animal model allowed their research team to investigate locomotor, respiratory, and cardiovascular responses when feedback mechanisms were eliminated. The findings concluded respiratory responses began before peripheral feedback mechanisms, indicating feedforward systems contribute to control of breathing that originates in the central nervous system. Carbon dioxide increases at the onset of exercise, and V_E closely tracks VCO_2 to prevent CO_2 and H+ accumulation in arterial blood. Although this is not a causal relationship between VCO_2 and ventilation [61], there has been strong evidence from research investigating ventilatory–metabolic coupling via this feedforward mechanism [62–64]. Conflicting research exists, particularly in animal studies that show CO_2 flow is minimally altered with exercise hyperpnea [65–67]. Still no known CO_2 receptors have been identified so the feedforward mechanism for CO_2 flow is based primarily on strong correlative data.

Feedback mechanisms come from (1) the limb locomotor muscles and (2) the carotid chemoreceptors. In skeletal muscles, thinly myelinated muscle afferents (group III and group IV) are present that sense mechanical and chemical changes. During exercise, these afferents are stimulated and send feedback to the medulla to increase V_E. Both human and animal studies have used electrical stimulation of these muscle afferents and reported an increase in V_E. Still, it remains unclear to what extent these afferents contribute to the exercise hyperpnea. The carotid bodies also provide feedback because they are sensitive to hypercapnia, hypoxemia, hyperkalemia, and acidosis. Studies support the ventilatory response to hypoxia and hypercapnia is greater during exercise than at rest ([68, 69], respectively). However, the carotid bodies may play a larger role during hyperventilation during heavy exercise [70, 71]. For a comprehensive reviw on the control of breathing, refer to Forster and colleagues [123]

Published literature investigating sex differences in the control of breathing yields conflicting and inconclusive results, although the literature is scarce. These existing studies report either an increased V_E during exercise while subjects are in the luteal phase compared to the follicular phase [5, 72, 126] or no change between phases [6, 73–75]. Additional studies have reported minimal improvements in VO_{2max} [9] depending on menstrual phase, while others have shown no difference [2, 76, 77]. Jurkowski and colleagues [72] reported a significant improvement in cycling time to exhaustion at 90 % peak power during the luteal phase and conclude the increased time to exhaustion was due to 30 % lower lactate accumulation at end-exercise. Most studies show dissimilar results and show no performance improvements across the menstrual cycle [78, 79].

Expiratory Flow Limitation

Expiratory flow limitation (EFL) is defined as the point when the tidal-volume loop intersects with the MFVL, as displayed in Fig. 1.5. Regulation of EELV and EILV, as described earlier, contributes to the ventilatory constraint experienced during exercise [48]. As EELV decreases below FRC, expiratory reserve volume (ERV) is reduced. As the exercising tidal-volume loop encroaches upon the maximal expiratory flow portion of the flow-volume loop, EELV will begin to rise to prevent EFL [80]. This causes EILV to increase and can approach total lung capacity (TLC) [45]. Johnson et al. [47] termed this dynamic hyperinflation, which can cause decreases in elastic muscle strength and inspiratory muscle endurance, and increased work of breathing and oxygen cost of breathing. Dynamic hyperinflation, due to EFL or impending EFL, reduces inspiratory muscle length and compromises force generation [81]. The decreased force generation of the inspiratory muscles places a greater pressure generation on them to operate at higher lung volumes, increasing the WOB.

Smaller airway diameters in women compared to men make women more prone to show EFL during exercise. Women have greater mechanical constraints than men due to a smaller pulmonary envelope compared to that of men [35]. The increased ventilatory drive coupled with the decreased pulmonary envelope contributes to EFL during exercise [7], and women may therefore experience EFL at a lower minute ventilation and oxygen consumption (VO_2) than men. Indeed, women experience more EFL at a lower V_E and VO_2 as well as exhibit more dynamic hyperinflation compared to their male counterparts [35]. As a consequence of the EFL for a given VO_2, a woman is more vulnerable to higher levels of WOB that occurs at high exercise intensities and ultimately to other adverse outcomes including increased perception of labored breathing (dyspnea), respiratory muscle fatigue, and gas exchange impairments.

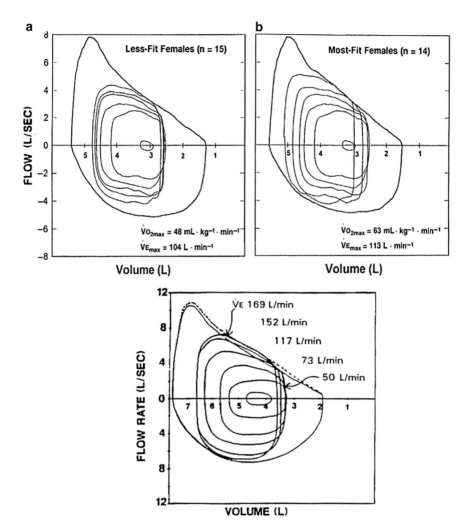

Fig. 1.5 *Top* represents mean flow-volume loops in young adult women while *figure on the bottom* represents young adult men: (**a**) is less-fit women while (**b**) is highly fit women at rest, then during light (55% VO_{2max}), moderate (74% VO_{2max}), and heavy (90% VO_{2max}), all the way to near maximal (96% VO_{2max}), plotted relative to the group mean maximal flow-volume loop; V_{Emax}, maximal ventilation. Flow limitation occurs when the tidal-volume flow loop intersects with the maximal expiratory flow-volume loop

Dyspnea (i.e., the perceived exertion of breathing) increases with exercise, and often limits exercise tolerance via labored breathing and discomfort from both the respiratory system and locomotor muscles. EFL has been reported to be a strong predictor of dyspnea during exercise [82], and imposed EFL in healthy adults causes substantial dyspnea [83]. The perception of discomfort in breathing is associated with increases in inspiratory muscle work from EFL and may limit exercise tolerance.

Respiratory Work/Muscles

Work of Breathing

The respiratory work or work of breathing performed by the respiratory muscles is divided into the elastic and resistive work components. The elastic components include the work needed to overcome lung elastic recoil, chest recoil, and surface tension. The resistive components include the work needed to overcome airway resistance. Figure 1.6 shows how work of breathing changes across a range of exercising ventilation from rest to maximal exercise. It is evident from Fig. 1.6 that with increasing ventilation there is an increase in the work of breathing. However, the work of breathing will increase out of proportion to ventilation at higher ventilations due to expiratory flow limitation (EFL), dynamic hyperinflation, and increased turbulent flow. At the onset of EFL, dynamical hyperinflation (increase EELV) will occur allowing for higher expiratory flow rates [84]. Breathing at a higher EELV lies on the less compliant portion of the lung compliance curve and will consequently lead to increased work of breathing. Additionally, dynamic hyperinflation will lead to increased EILV to ~90–95 % lung capacity at which the inspiratory muscles are no longer at their optimal length for pressure generation [81] and there is an increased VO_2 requirement by the respiratory muscles [85]. Women have disproportionally smaller airways (dysanapsis) for a given lung volume compared to men [15]. Additionally, smaller lungs and dysanapsis lead to the onset and increased severity of expiratory flow limitation [42, 45]. In agreement, women have a higher prevalence of EFL during exercise compared to men. Figure 1.7 shows the operating lung volumes of endurance-trained men (A) and women (B) during an incremental exercise test to exhaustion [35]. Both men and women demonstrate a decreased EELV and increased EILV compared to rest during incremental exercise. However, at ~80 % VO_{2max},

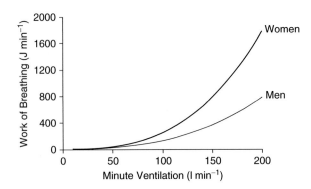

Fig. 1.6 Work of breathing in men and women over exercising ventilations. With increasing ventilation, there is an increase in work of breathing. At ~50 L/min, the work of breathing is higher in women compared to men

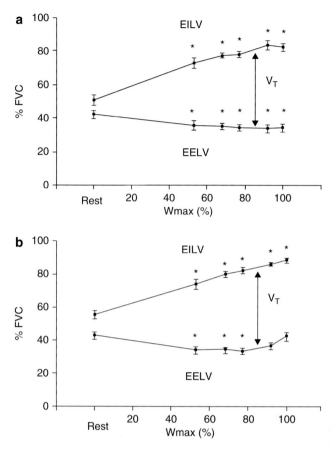

Fig. 1.7 Operating lung volumes during incremental exercise in men and women. End-expiratory and end-inspiratory lung volumes (EELV, EILV) from rest to maximal exercise. From rest to exercise, men (**a**) and women (**b**) decrease EELV and increase EILV. At higher intensities, women dynamically hyperinflate (increase EELV), while men maintain EELV near resting values

women increase their EELV near resting values indicating dynamically hyperinflation, while men maintain their EELV below resting values. Figure 1.6 shows the work of breathing in both endurance men and women during incremental exercise [35]. The work of breathing is similar between men and women at rest until a ventilation of ~50 L/min at which the work of breathing in women disproportionally increases. At a ventilation of ~90 L/min, the work of breathing is twice as high in women compared to men. Smaller lungs and airways as well as dynamic hyperinflation contribute to the higher work of breathing in women compared to men during exercise. The Campbell diagram (Fig. 1.8) is used to determine the contribution of the elastic (inspiratory and expiratory) and resistive (inspiratory and expiratory) components to the total work of breathing. With increasing intensity, there is an increase in inspiratory elastic,

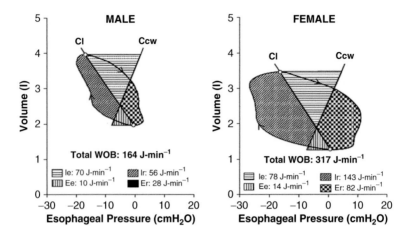

Fig. 1.8 Sex differences in elastic and resistive work of breathing. The Campbell diagram shows inspiratory and expiratory elastic as well as resistive components of work of breathing. The endurance-trained male and female were matched for ventilation, tidal volume, breathing frequency, and body mass exercising during exercise. The female had higher inspiratory and expiratory resistive work of breathing compared to the male, but similar elastic components

expiratory elastic, inspiratory resistive, and expiratory resistive. During submaximal workloads, women have higher inspiratory resistive work [86] due to their smaller airways. At maximal exercise, men have higher inspiratory elastic work due to their large tidal volumes and higher maximal ventilation compared to women [86]. To illustrate this, Fig. 1.8 shows the Campbell diagram for an endurance-trained men and women matched for ventilation, tidal volume, breathing frequency, and body mass exercising during exercise [86]. The inspiratory and expiratory resistive work is higher in the women compared to the men with similar inspiratory and expiratory elastic work for the same ventilation. This figure illustrates how the smaller airways in women largely contribute to the higher work of breathing compared to men.

Metabolic Cost of Breathing

The respiratory muscles, like other skeletal muscles, require an increase in oxygen uptake and a portion of cardiac output during exercise. The oxygen cost of breathing (VO_2 required by the respiratory muscles) is investigated by having subjects perform voluntary hyperpnea at similar exercising ventilations and measuring the oxygen cost of the respiratory muscles. The oxygen cost of breathing at rest is ~3–5 % of VO_{2total} and increases up to 10 % VO_{2max} in untrained men and 12–15 % VO_{2max} in endurance-trained men at maximal exercise [87]. In endurance-trained men, respiratory muscle blood flow increases in proportion to the work of breathing and cost of breathing [88]. In addition, 14–16 % of the total cardiac output is distributed to the diaphragm and respiratory muscles during maximal exercise [30, 31]. Due to the higher work of breathing, it is likely that the cost of breathing is higher in women compared to men; however, this is not yet known.

Exercise-Induced Respiratory Muscle Fatigue

The diaphragm of humans is composed of primarily oxidative fibers, approximately 55 % Type I and 21 % Type IIa [89]. The diaphragm exhibits different morphological characteristics compared to other skeletal muscles including higher oxidative capacity, capillary density, maximum blood flow, and resistance to fatigue [90]. Despite these morphological differences between the diaphragm and other skeletal muscles, the diaphragm can fatigue during high-intensity exercise [91]. Fatigue is defined as a reduction in the maximal capacity for force or pressure generation of a muscle compared to resting conditions, which is reversible by rest [92]. Respiratory muscle and/or diaphragmatic fatigue had been linked to respiratory muscle work, respiratory muscle blood flow, glycogen depletion, hypoxia, and reactive oxygen species [93–96]. Although each of these can contribute to exercise-induced respiratory muscle fatigue, respiratory muscle work and respiratory muscle blood flow are largely responsible [93, 94]. When the respiratory muscles are experimentally unloaded via a proportional assist ventilator during heavy exercise, diaphragmatic fatigue does not occur because the work of breathing is reduced by ~50 % [93]. Additionally, diaphragmatic fatigue does not occur at similar exercising ventilations performed at rest during voluntary hyperpnea because there is an adequate reserve of cardiac output that can supply the respiratory muscles [94]. In fact, ventilations 50 % higher than these exercising ventilations are needed to induce diaphragmatic fatigue at rest [94]. Therefore, high work of breathing and whole-body heavy exercise are both required for the development of respiratory muscle fatigue.

Diaphragmatic fatigue occurs following continuous exercise at >85 % VO_{2max} to exhaustion in men and women [91, 97]. As stated in the above section, women have a higher work of breathing during exercise above a ventilation of ~50 L/min compared to men due to their smaller lungs and airways as well as their higher prevalence of expiratory flow limitation and consequently dynamic hyperinflation [35]. Therefore, logically women should also exhibit increased diaphragmatic fatigue following heavy exercise compared to men. However, it should be noted that women exhibit attenuated skeletal muscle fatigue compared to men when exercising at the same relative intensity [98]. Although the mechanisms are yet to be elucidated, muscle mass, skeletal muscle morphology, and substrate utilization are thought to contribute to this skeletal fatigue resistance in women [99]. In agreement with the findings in other skeletal muscle, women have attenuated diaphragmatic fatigue following heavy exercise compared to men [100].

Despite the fatigue of the respiratory muscles, the ventilatory response is not altered during heavy exercise in men and women. Even though exercise hyperpnea is not affected by respiratory muscle fatigue, respiratory muscle fatigue has cardiovascular consequences during exercise. This has been investigated by altering the work of breathing (both unloading and loading) and measuring exercising leg blood flow during maximal cycling exercise. With an increase in the work of breathing (~150 % of control) during maximal exercise, leg blood flow decreased ~7 %, and with a reduction in work of breathing (~50 % of control), leg blood flow increased ~4 % [101]. However, while exercising at submaximal intensity exercise (50 % and 75 % VO_{2max}), leg blood flow and leg vascular conductance was not altered with increases in work of breathing [102]. The fatiguing respiratory muscles lead to a metaboreflex originating from the respiratory muscles leading to a systemic increase in muscle sympathetic nerve activity [103, 104] leading to an increase in blood pressure and reduction in blood flow [105]. Although never measured, it is likely women will exhibit an attenuated inspiratory metaboreflex due to their greater fatigue-resistant inspiratory muscles [100]. Increasing both the work of breathing and respiratory muscle fatigue during heavy exercise also increases exercise-induced peripheral fatigue [106, 107]. Altering the work of breathing and prior inducing respiratory muscle fatigue has also been shown to negatively impact exercise performance. Pre-fatiguing of the inspiratory muscles leads to a 23 % reduction in time to exhaustion [108]. Similarly by increasing the work of breathing time to exhaustion decreases by ~15 % and decreasing the work of breathing increases time to exhaustion by ~14 % [26, 27]. At this time, it is not known how respiratory muscle fatigue affects peripheral fatigue or exercise performance in women. However, it is likely that women will be affected less due to their greater skeletal muscle fatigue resistance compared to men.

Across the Life span (Children to Aging)

Children

During childhood, lung capacity increases proportionally to the growth of the thoracic capacity [109]. Additionally, lung elastic recoil increases during childhood [110], which is evident by histology studies showing increases in elastic fibers during this time [111]. Children also have smaller airways in proportion to lung size compared to adults [15]. In prepubescent children, boys have larger resting lung capacities, expiratory flow rates, and lung diffusion capacity compared to age-matched girls [112]. During puberty, the increase in expiratory flow rates and lung capacity begins and peaks (~12 years) earlier in girls compared to boys (~15 years) [113]. Additionally, pulmonary function increases curvilinearly in boys and linear in girls during puberty [113]. During exercise, prepubescent children have a higher ventilatory equivalent for carbon dioxide (V_E/VCO_2) leading to higher ventilations during exercise for a given VCO_2 compared to adults. Prepubescent girls have lower ventilation, tidal volume, and VO_{2max} compared to prepubescent boys during exercise [114].

Can these differences in pulmonary function between children and adults lead to ventilatory limitations (e.g., expiratory flow limitation)? Indeed, the smaller airways for a given lung volume and the increased drive to breathe lead to the occurrence of EFL. The prevalence of EFL in children is ~95 % and is considerably higher compared to adults [112]. In addition, the prevalence of EFL is similar between boys and girls [112]. Despite having a larger maximum flow-volume loop, boys also had EFL during maximal exercise due to their larger exercise ventilation. The girls had lower ventilation rates during maximal exercise, but also a smaller maximal flow-volume loop leading to EFL. Dynamic hyperinflation occurred similarly in boys and girls during exercise most likely leading to higher work of breathing. Although never directly measured, it is likely that children would exhibit more respiratory muscle fatigue compared to adults following heavy exercise due to their higher incidence of EFL and small airways. Despite the high prevalence of EFL in prepubescent children, EIAH is not present during maximal exercise in neither boys nor girls [112]. In spite of the high prevalence of EFL in children, imperfections in pulmonary gas exchange (EIAH) are rarely experienced [112].

Aging

Healthy aging leads to changes in pulmonary function at rest and during exercise. During aging, there is a decrease in elastic recoil [115] most likely due to alterations in the cross-linking of the elastin and collagen matrix in the lung. Interestingly, women have an augmented reduction in elastic recoil compared to men [116]. The loss in elastic recoil leads to a reduced vital capacity, expiratory flow rates, and increased functional residual capacity and residual volume leading to a smaller maximum flow-volume loop [117]. In addition, lung diffusion capacity and respiratory muscle strength decrease with aging [118]. Dead space ventilation also increases with aging [118]. These aging-induced anatomical and functional changes at rest affect ventilation and pulmonary gas exchange during exercise.

Due to the aging-induced alterations to pulmonary structure and function, the ventilatory response is negatively affected. Because of the increased dead space ventilation, ventilation will be higher during exercise and the increased ventilation will be accomplished by an increased breathing frequency due to the mechanical constraints. Indeed with aging, there is an increased prevalence of EFL during exercise [118]. The perception of breathing or dyspnea is higher with aging compared to younger subjects during incremental exercise [119]. Although never measured, it is likely that older women will also have a higher prevalence of EFL compared to older men. Additionally, older women experience more dyspnea during incremental exercise compared to age-matched men [120]. Compared to younger women, older women are more likely to have EFL as well as more dyspnea and leg discomfort during exercise for a given absolute workload [119].

The reduced pulmonary function due to the loss of elastic recoil leads to pulmonary consequences during exercise. During exercise, the more severe EFL and hyperinflation leads to a considerably higher work of breathing and cost of breathing in older individuals [121]. It is likely that older women will have a higher work of breathing at similar absolute workloads during exercise compared to older men. This higher work of breathing with aging will lead to an earlier onset of respiratory muscle fatigue and consequently the earlier onset of the respiratory metaboreflex. EFL, the increased dead space ventilation, and decreased cardiac output and lung diffusion capacity also lead to increased ventilation–perfusion mismatch during exercise [122]. This will lead to widening of the A-aDO2 during exercise compared to younger adults. Despite the increased expiratory flow limitation, ventilation–perfusion mismatch, and decreased lung diffusion capacity, pulmonary gas exchange during exercise is rarely impaired in the aging population [118]. At this time, research has not been performed investigating sex differences in pulmonary gas exchange during exercise in aging. However, it would be speculated based on the sex differences seen in the adult population and the augmented decline in elastic recoil that elderly women would be more susceptible to pulmonary gas exchange impairments during exercise.

Summary

Traditionally, the lung is not believed to limit exercise tolerance. However, increasing evidence suggests that the pulmonary system may not always exceed the metabolic demand of exercise. Pulmonary limitations to exercise are found in individuals of varying fitness levels and both sexes. However, women may be more prone to pulmonary limitations during heavy exercise (and perhaps submaximal intensities) than men due to the influence of the reproductive hormones (estrogen and progesterone) combined with a reduced pulmonary capacity. In particular, a greater ventilatory work associated with increased expiratory flow limitation during exercise and gas exchange impairments seem to be of primary concern. It should be emphasized, however, that the amount of literature investigating these issues is limited. Certainly, much more research is needed to substantiate these ideas.

References

1. Lebrun CM. Effect of different phases of the menstrual cycle and oral contraceptives on athletic performance. Sports Med. 1993;16(6):400–30.
2. Lebrun CM, McKenzie DC, Prior JC, Taunton JE. Effects of menstrual cycle phase on athletic performance. Med Sci Sports Exerc. 1995;27(3):437–44.
3. Moore LG, McCullough RE, Weil JV. Increased HVR in pregnancy: relationship to hormonal and metabolic changes. J Appl Physiol. 1987;62:158–63.
4. England SJ, Farhi LE. Fluctuations in alveolar CO_2 and in base excess during the menstrual cycle. Respir Physiol. 1976;26:157–61.
5. Schoene RB, Robertson HT, Pierson DJ. Respiratory drives and exercise in menstrual cycles of athletic and nonathletic women. J Appl Physiol. 1981;50:1300–5.

6. Dombovy ML, Bonekat HW, Williams TJ, Staats BA. Exercise performance and ventilatory response in the menstrual cycle. Med Sci Sports Exerc. 1987;19(2):111–7.

7. McClaran SR, Harms CA, Pegelow DF, Dempsey JA. Smaller lungs in women affect exercise hyperpnea. J Appl Physiol. 1998;84:1872–81.

8. Zhao XJ, McKerr G, Dong Z, Higgins CA, Carson J, Yang ZQ, Hannigan BM. Expression of oestrogen and progesterone receptors by mast cells alone, but not lymphocytes, macrophages, or other immune cells in human upper airways. Thorax. 2001;56:205–11.

9. Beidleman BA, Rock PB, Muza SR, et al. Exercise VE and physical performance at altitude are not affected by menstrual cycle phase. J Appl Physiol. 1999;86:1519–26.

10. White DP, Douglas NJ, Pickett CK, et al. Sexual influence on control of breathing. J Appl Physiol. 1983;54:874–9.

11. Aitken ML, Franklin JL, Pierson DJ, et al. Influence of body size and gender on control of ventilation. J Appl Physiol. 1986;60:1894–9.

12. Carlberg KA, Fregly MJ, Fahey M. Effects of chronic estrogen treatment on water exchange in rats. Am J Physiol. 1984;247(1):E101–10.

13. Sansores RH, Abboud RT, Kennell C, Haynes N. The effect of menstruation on the pulmonary carbon monoxide diffusing capacity. Am J Respir Crit Care Med. 1995;152:381–4.

14. Dempsey JA. Is the lung built for exercise? Med Sci Sports Exerc. 1986;18:161–75.

15. Mead J. Dysanapsis in normal lungs assessed by the relationship between maximal flow, static recoil, and vital capacity. Am Rev Respir Dis. 1980;121:339–42.

16. Thurlbeck WM. Postnatal human lung growth. Thorax. 1982;37:564–71.

17. Schwartz J, Katz SA, Fegley RW, Tockman MS. Sex and race differences in the development of lung function. Am Rev Respir Dis. 1988;138:1415–21.

18. Rohrbach MC, Perret C, Kayser B, Boutellier U, Spengler CM. Task failure from inspiratory resistive loaded breathing: a role from inspiratory muscle fatigue? Eur J Appl Physiol. 2003;90:405–10.

19. Johnson BD, Saupe KW, Dempsey JA. Mechanical constraints on exercise hyperpnea in endurance athletes. J Appl Physiol. 1992;73:874–86.

20. Brooks LJ, Byard PJ, Helms RC, Foulke JM, Strohl KP. Relationship between lung volume and trachea size assessed by acoustic reflection. J Appl Physiol. 1988;64(3):1050–4.

21. Green M, Mead J, Turner JM. Variability of maximum expiratory flow-volume curves. J Appl Physiol. 1974;37(1):67–74.

22. Sheel AW, Guenette JA, Yuan R, Holy L, Mayo JR, McWilliams Lam S, Coxson HO. Evidence for dysanapsis using computed tomographic imaging of the airways in older ex-smokers. J Appl Physiol. 2009;107(5):1622–8.

23. Dempsey JA, Wagner PD. Exercise-induced arterial hypoxemia. J Appl Physiol. 1999;87:1997–2006.

24. Amann M, Eldridge MW, Lovering AT, Stickland MK, Pegelow DF, Dempsey JA. Arterial oxygenation influences central motor output and exercise performance via effects on peripheral locomotor muscle fatigue in humans. J Physiol. 2006;575:937–52.

25. Dempsey JA, Hanson PG, Henderson KS. Exercise-induced arterial hypoxaemia in healthy subjects at sea level. J Physiol. 1984;355:161–75.

26. Harms CA, McClaran SR, Nickele GA, Pegelow DF, Nelson WB, Dempsey JA. Effect of exercise-induced arterial O2 desaturation on VO_{2max} in women. Med Sci Sports Exerc. 2000;32:1101–8.

27. Harms CA, Wetter TJ, St. Croix CM, Pegelow DF, Dempsey JA. Effects of respiratory muscle work on exercise performance. J Appl Physiol. 2000;89:131–8.

28. Romer LM, Haverkamp HC, Lovering AT, Pegelow DF, Dempsey JA. Effect of exercise-induced arterial hypoxemia on quadriceps muscle fatigue in healthy humans. Am J Physiol Regul Integr Comp Physiol. 2006;290:R365–75.

29. Powers SK, Dodd S, Lawler J, Landry G, Kirtley M, McKnight T, Grinton S. Incidence of exercise induced hypoxemia in elite endurance athletes at sea level. Eur J Appl Physiol Occup Physiol. 1988;58:298–302.

30. Harms CA, McClaran SR, Nickele GA, Pegelow DF, Nelson WB, Dempsey JA. Exercise-induced arterial hypoxaemia in healthy young women. J Physiol. 1998;507:619–28.
31. Harms CA, Wetter TJ, McClaran SR, Pegelow DF, Nickele GA, Nelson WB, et al. Effects of respiratory muscle work on cardiac output and its distribution during maximal exercise. J Appl Physiol. 1998;85:609–18.
32. Richards JC, McKenzie DC, Warburton DER, Road JD, Sheel AW. Prevalence of exercise-induced arterial hypoxemia in healthy women. Med Sci Sports Exerc. 2004;36:1514–21.
33. Eldridge MW, Dempsey JA, Haverkamp HC, Lovering AT, Hokanson JS. Exercise-induced intrapulmonary arteriovenous shunting in healthy humans. J Appl Physiol. 2004;97:797–805.
34. Hopkins SR, Barker RC, Brutsaert TD, Gavin TP, Entin P, Olfert IM, Wagner PD. Pulmonary gas exchange during exercise in women: effects of exercise type and work increment. J Appl Physiol. 2000;89:721–30.
35. Guenette JA, Witt JD, McKenzie DC, Road JD, Sheel AW. Respiratory mechanics during exercise in endurance-trained men and women. J Physiol. 2007;581:1309–22.
36. Hopkins SR, McKenzie DC, Schoene RB, Glenny RW, Robertson HT. Pulmonary gas exchange during exercise in athletes. I. Ventilation-perfusion mismatch and diffusion limitation. J Appl Physiol. 1994;77:912–7.
37. Hopkins SR, Harms CA. Gender and pulmonary gas exchange during exercise. Exerc Sport Sci Rev. 2004;32:50–6.
38. Hagen PT, Scholz DG, Edwards WD. Incidence and size of patent foramen ovale during the first 10 decades of life: an autopsy study of 965 normal hearts. Mayo Clin Proc. 1984;59:17–20.
39. Lovering AT, Stickland MK, Amann M, O'Brien MJ, Hokanson JS, Eldridge MW. Effect of a patent foramen ovale on pulmonary gas exchange efficiency at rest and during exercise. J Appl Physiol. 2011;110:1354–61.
40. Stickland MK, Welsh RC, Haykowsky MJ, Petersen SR, Anderson WD, Taylor DA, et al. Intra-pulmonary shunt and pulmonary gas exchange during exercise in humans. J Physiol. 2004;561:321–9.
41. Roughton FJW, Forster RE. Relative importance of diffusion and chemical reaction rates in determining rate of exchange of gases in the human lung with special reference to true diffusing capacity of pulmonary membrane and volume of blood in the lung capillaries. J Appl Physiol. 1957;11:290–302.
42. Smith JR, Rosenkranz SK, Harms CA. Dysanapsis ratio as a predictor for expiratory flow limitation. Respir Phys Neurobiol. 2014;198:25–31.
43. Harms CA, Stager JM. Low chemoresponsiveness and inadequate hyperventilation contribute to exercise-induced hypoxemia. J Appl Physiol. 1995;79:575–80.
44. MacNutt MJ, De Souza MJ, Tomczak SE, Homer JL, Sheel AW. Resting and exercise ventilatory chemosensitivity across the menstrual cycle. J Appl Physiol. 2012;112(5):737–47.
45. McClaran SR, Wetter TJ, Pegelow DF, Dempsey JA. Role of expiratory flow limitation in determining lung volumes and ventilation during exercise. J Appl Physiol. 1999;86:1357–66.
46. Dempsey JA, Forster HV, Ainsworth DM. Regulation of hyperpnea, hyperventilation, and respiratory muscle recruitment during exercise. Regulation of breathing. New York: Marcel Dekker; 1995. p. 1064–134.
47. Johnson BD, Weisman IM, Zeballos RJ, Beck KC. Emerging concepts in the evaluation of ventilatory flow limitation during exercise: the exercise tidal-volume loop. Chest. 1999;116(2):488–503.
48. Henke KG, Sharrat M, Pegelow D, Dempsey JA. Regulation of end-expiratory lung volume during exercise. J Appl Physiol. 1988;64:135–46.
49. DeTroyer A, Wilson TA. Effects of acute inflation on the mechanics of the inspiratory muscles. J Appl Physiol. 2009;107:315–23.
50. Ainsworth DM, Smith CA, Eicker SW, Henderson KS, Dempsey JA. The effects of locomotion of respiratory muscle activity in the awake dog. Respir Physiol. 1989;78:145–62.

51. Grassino AE, Derenne JP, Almirall J, Milic-Emili J, Whitelaw W. Configuration of the chest wall and occlusion pressures in the awake humans. J Appl Physiol. 1981;50:134–42.

52. Sheel AW, Romer LM. Ventilation and respiratory mechanics. Comp Physiol. 2012;2: 1093–142.

53. McParland C, Krishnan B, Lobo J, Gallagher CG. Effect of physical training on breathing pattern during progressive exercise. Respir Physiol. 1992;90:311–23.

54. Cole P, Forsyth R, Haight JS. Respiratory resistance of the oral airway. Am Rev Respir Dis. 1982;125:363–5.

55. England SJ, Bartlett DJ. Changes in respiratory movements of the human vocal cords during hyperpnea. J Appl Physiol. 1982;52:780–5.

56. Habedank D, Reindl I, Vietzke G, et al. Ventilatory efficiency and exercise tolerance in 101 healthy volunteers. Eur J Appl Physiol Occup Physiol. 1998;77:421–6.

57. Blackie SP, Fairbarn MS, McElvaney NG, et al. Normal values and ranges for ventilation and breathing pattern at maximal exercise. Chest. 1991;100:136–42.

58. Sheel AW, Richards JC, Foster GE, Guenette JA. Sex difference in respiratory exercise physiology. Sports Med. 2004;34(9):567–79.

59. Elridge FL, Millhorn DE, Kiley JP, Waldrop TG. Stimulation by central command of locomotion, respiration and circulation during exercise. Respir Physiol. 1985;59:313–37.

60. Elridge FL, Willhorn DE, Waldrop TG. Exercise hyperpnea and locomotion: parallel activation from the hypothalamus. Science. 1981;211:844–6.

61. Haouzi P. Theories on the nature of the coupling between ventilation and gas exchange during exercise. Respir Physiol Neurobiol. 2006;151:267–79.

62. Phillipson EA, Duffin J, Cooper JD. Critical dependence on respiratory rhythmicity on metabolic CO_2 load. J Appl Physiol. 1981;50:45–54.

63. Tallman RDJ, Marcolin R, Howie M, McDonald JS, Stafford T. Cardiopulmonary response to extracorporeal venous CO_2 removal in awake spontaneously breathing dogs. J Appl Physiol. 1986;61:516–22.

64. Yamamoto WS, Edwards MWJ. Homeostasis of carbon dioxide during intravenous infusion of carbon dioxide. J Appl Physiol. 1960;15:807–18.

65. Bennett FM, Tallman RDJ, Grodin FS. Role of VCO_2 in control of breathing of awake exercising dogs. J Appl Physiol. 1984;56:1335–9.

66. Bisgard GE, Forster HV, Mesina J, Sarazin RG. Role of carotid body in hyperpnea of moderate exercise in goats. J Appl Physiol. 1982;52:1216–22.

67. Pan JG, Forster HV, Bisgard GE, Kaminski RP, Dorsey SM, Busch MA. Hyperventilation in ponies at the onset of and during steady-state exercise. J Appl Physiol. 1983;54: 1394–402.

68. Asmussen E, Nielson M. Ventilatory response to CO2 during work at normal and at low oxygen tensions. Acta Physiol Scand. 1957;39:27–35.

69. Weil JV, Bryne-Quinn E, Sodal IE, Kline JS, McCullough RE, Filley GF. Augmentation of chemosensitivity during mild exercise in normal man. J Appl Physiol. 1972;33:813–9.

70. Heigenhauser GL, Sutton JR, Jones NL. Effect of glycogen depletion on the ventilatory response to exercise. J Appl Physiol. 1983;54:470–4.

71. Wasserman K, Whipp BJ, Koyal SN, Cleary MG. Effect of carotid body resection on ventilatory and acid-base control during exercise. J Appl Physiol. 1975;39:354–8.

72. Jurkowski JE, Jones NL, Toews CJ, et al. Effects of menstrual cycle on blood lactate, O_2 delivery, and performance during exercise. J Appl Physiol. 1981;51:1493–9.

73. Bemben DA, Salm PC, Salm AJ. Ventilatory and blood lactate responses to maximal treadmill exercise during the menstrual cycle. J Sports Med Phys Fit. 1995;35:257–62.

74. Cassaza GA, Suh SH, Miller BF, et al. Effects of oral contraceptives on peak exercise capacity. J Appl Physiol. 2002;93:1698–702.

75. De Souza MJ, Maguire MS, Rubin KR, et al. Effects of menstrual phase and amenorrhea on exercise performance in runners. Med Sci Sports Exerc. 1990;22:575–80.

76. Bryner RW, Toffle RCUIH, et al. Effect of low dose oral contraceptives on exercise performance. Br J Sports Med. 1996;30:36–40.

77. Hackney AC, Curley CS, Nicklas BJ. Physiological responses to submaximal exercise at the mid-follicular, ovulatory, and mid-luteal phases of the menstrual cycle. Scand J Med Sci Sport. 1991;1:94–8.
78. Hessemer V, Bruck K. Influence of menstrual cycle on thermoregulatory, metabolic, and heart rate responses to exercise at night. J Appl Physiol. 1991;59:1911–7.
79. Miskec CM, Potteiger JA, Nau KL, et al. Do varying environmental and menstrual cycle conditions affect anaerobic power output in female athletes? J Strength Cond Res. 1997;11:219–23.
80. Babb TG, Viggiano R, Hurley B, Staats B, Rodarte JR. Effect of mild to moderate airflow limitation on exercise capacity. J Appl Physiol. 1991;70(1):223–30.
81. Roussos C, Fixley M, Gross D, Macklem PT. Fatigue of inspiratory muscles and their synergic behavior. J Appl Physiol. 1979;46:897–904.
82. Eltayara L, Becklake MR, Volta CA, Milic-Emili J. Relationship between chronic dyspnea and expiratory flow limitation in patients with chronic obstructive pulmonary disease. Am J Respir Crit Care Med. 1996;154(6):1726–34.
83. Iandelli I, Aliverti A, Kayser B, et al. Determinants of exercise performance in normal men with externally imposed expiratory flow limitation. J Appl Physiol. 2002;92(5):1943–52.
84. Pellegrino R, Brusasco V, Rodarte JR, Babb TG. Expiratory flow limitation and regulation of end-expiratory lung volume during exercise. J Appl Physiol. 1993;74:2552–8.
85. Collett PW, Engel LA. Influence of lung volume on oxygen cost of resistive breathing. J Appl Physiol. 1986;61:16–24.
86. Guenette JA, Querido JS, Eves ND, Chua R, Sheel AW. Sex differences in the resistive and elastic work of breathing during exercise in endurance-trained athletes. Am J Physiol Regul Integr Comp Physiol. 2009;297:R166–75.
87. Aaron EA, Seow KC, Johnson BD, Dempsey JA. Oxygen cost of exercise hyperpnea: implications for performance. J Appl Physiol. 1992;72:1818–25.
88. Guenette JA, Vogiatzis I, Zakynthinos S, Athanasopoulos D, Koskolou M, Golemati S, Bouscel R. Human respiratory muscle blood flow measured by near-infrared spectroscopy and indocyanine green. J Appl Physiol. 2008;104:1202–10.
89. Lieberman DA, Faulkner JA, Craig AB, Maxwell LC. Performance and histochemical composition of guinea pig and human diaphragm. J Appl Physiol. 1973;34:233–7.
90. Edwards RHT, Faulkner JA. Structure and function of the respiratory muscles. In: Roussos C, editor. The thorax. Part A: Physiology. New York: Marcel Dekker; 1995. p. 185–217.
91. Johnson BD, Babcock MA, Suman OE, Dempsey JA. Exercise-induced diaphragmatic fatigue in healthy humans. J Physiol (London). 1993;460:385–405.
92. NHLBI Workshop Respiratory Muscle Fatigue. Report of the respiratory muscle fatigue workshop group. Am Rev Respir Dis. 1990;142:474–80.
93. Babcock MA, Pegelow DF, Harms CA, Dempsey JA. Effects of respiratory unloading on exercise-induced diaphragm fatigue. J Appl Physiol. 2002;93:201–6.
94. Babcock MA, Pegelow DF, McClaran SR, Suman OE, Dempsey JA. Contribution of diaphragmatic power output to exercise-induced diaphragm fatigue. J Appl Physiol. 1995; 78:1710–9.
95. Fregosi RF, Dempsey JA. Effects of exercise on normoxia and acute hypoxia on respiratory muscle metabolites. J Appl Physiol. 1986;60:1274–83.
96. Shindoh C, DiMarco A, Thomas A, Manubay P, Supinski G. Effect of N-acetylcysteine on diaphragm fatigue. J Appl Physiol. 1990;68:2107–13.
97. Mador MJ, Magalang UJ, Rodis A, Kufel TJ. Diaphragmatic fatigue after exercise in healthy human subjects. Am Rev Respir Dis. 1993;148:1571–5.
98. Fulco CS, Rock PB, Muza SR, Lammi E, Cymerman A, Butterfield G, Lewis SF. Slower fatigue and faster recovery of the adductor pollicis muscle in women matched for strength with men. Acta Physiol Scand. 1999;167:233–9.
99. Hicks AL, Kent-Braun J, Ditor DS. Sex differences in human skeletal muscle fatigue. Exerc Sport Sci Rev. 2001;29:109–12.

100. Guenette JA, Romer LM, Querido JS, Chua R, Eves ND, Road JD, et al. Sex differences in exercise-induced diaphragmatic fatigue in endurance-trained men. J Appl Physiol. 2010;109:35–46.
101. Harms CA, Babcock MA, McClaran SR, Pegelow DF, Nickele GA, Nelson WB, Dempsey JA. Respiratory muscle work compromises leg blood flow during maximal exercise. J Appl Physiol. 1997;82:1573–83.
102. Wetter TJ, Harms CA, Nelson WB, Pegelow DF, Dempsey JA. Influence of respiratory muscle work on VO_2 and leg blood flow during submaximal exercise. J Appl Physiol. 1999;87:643–51.
103. Derchak PA, Sheel AW, Morgan BJ, Dempsey JA. Effect of expiratory muscle work on muscle sympathetic nerve activity. J Appl Physiol. 2002;92:1539–52.
104. St. Croix CM, Morgan BJ, Wetter TJ, Dempsey JA. Fatiguing inspiratory muscle work causes reflex sympathetic activation in humans. J Physiol. 2000;529:493–504.
105. Sheel AW, Derchak PA, Morgan BJ, Pegelow DF, Jacques AJ, Dempsey JA. Fatiguing inspiratory muscle work causes reflex reduction in resting leg blood flow in humans. J Physiol. 2001;537:227–89.
106. Romer LM, Lovering AT, Haverkamp HC, Pegelow DF, Dempsey JA. Effect of inspiratory muscle work on peripheral fatigue of locomotor muscles in healthy humans. J Physiol. 2006;571:425–39.
107. Wuthrich TU, Notter DA, Spengler CM. Effect of inspiratory muscle fatigue on exercise performance taking into account the fatigue-induced excess respiratory drive. Exp Physiol. 2013;98:1705–17.
108. Mador MJ, Acevedo FA. Effect of respiratory muscle fatigue on subsequent exercise performance. J Appl Physiol. 1991;70:2059–65.
109. Kivastik J, Kingisepp P. Differences in lung function and chest dimensions in school-age girls and boys. Clin Physiol. 1997;17:149–57.
110. DeTroyer A, Yernault JC, Englert M, Baran D, Paiva M. Evolution of intrathoracic airway mechanics during lung growth. J Appl Physiol. 1978;44:521–7.
111. Loosli CG, Potter EL. Pre and postnatal development of the respiratory portion of the human lung with special reference to the elastic fibers. Am Rev Respir Dis. 1959;80:5–23.
112. Swain KE, Rosenkranz SK, Beckman B, Harms CA. Expiratory flow limitation during exercise in prepubescent boys and girls: prevalence and implications. J Appl Physiol. 2010;108:1267–74.
113. Wang X, Dockery DW, Wypij D, Gold DR, Speizer FE, Ware JH, Ferris BG. Pulmonary function growth velocity in children 6 to 18 years of age. Am Rev Respir Dis. 1993;148:1502–8.
114. Armstrong N, Kirby BJ, McManus AM, Welsman JR. Prepubescents' ventilatory responses to exercise with reference to sex and body size. Chest. 1997;112:1554–60.
115. Knudson RJ, Clark DF, Kennedy TC, Knudson DE. Effect of aging alone on mechanical properties of the normal adult human lung. J Appl Physiol. 1977;43:1054–62.
116. Bode FR, Dosman J, Martin RR, Ghezzo H, Macklem PT. Age and sex differences in lung elasticity, and in closing capacity in nonsmokers. J Appl Physiol. 1976;41:129–35.
117. Johnson BD, Reddan WG, Pegelow DF, Seow KC, Dempsey JA. Flow limitation and regulation of functional residual capacity during exercise in a physically active aging population. Am Rev Respir Dis. 1991;143:960–7.
118. Taylor BJ, Johnson BD. The pulmonary circulation and exercise responses in the elderly. Semin Respir Crit Care Med. 2010;31:528–38.
119. Wilkie SS, Guenette JA, Dominelli PB, Sheel AW. Effects of an aging pulmonary system on expiratory flow limitation and dyspnea during exercise in healthy women. Eur J Appl Physiol. 2012;112:2195–204.
120. Ofir D, Laveneziana P, Webb KA, Lam YM, O'Donnell DE. Sex differences in the perceived intensity of breathlessness during exercise with advancing age. J Appl Physiol. 2008;104:1583–93.
121. Johnson BD, Reddan WG, Seow KC, Dempsey JA. Mechanical constraints on exercise hyperpnea in a fit aging population. Am Rev Respir Dis. 1991;143:968–77.

122. Cardius J, Burgos F, Diaz O, Roca J, Barbera JA, Marrades RM, Rodriguez-Roisin R, Wagner PD. Increase in pulmonary ventilation-perfusion inequality with age in healthy individuals. Am J Respir Crit Care Med. 1997;156:648–53.
123. Forster HV, Haozi P, Dempsey JA. Control of breathing during exercise. Comp Physiol. 2012;2:743–77.
124. Harms CA, Rosenkranz SR. Sex differences in pulmonary function during exercise. Med Sci Sports Exerc. 2008;40:664–8.
125. Smith JR, Brown KR, Murphy JD, Harms CA. Does menstrual cycle phase affect lung diffusion capacity during exercise? Respir Phys Neurobiol. 2015;205:99–104.
126. Williams, TJ, Krahenbuhl, GS. Menstrual cycle phase and running economy. Medicine and Science in Sport and Exercise. 1997;29:1609–1618.

Chapter 2
Sex Hormone Signaling in the Lung in Health and Disease: Airways, Parenchyma, and Pulmonary Vasculature

Andrea L. Frump and Tim Lahm

Abstract Gender and sex differences have been implicated in many major lung diseases, such as asthma, chronic obstructive pulmonary disease, cystic fibrosis, pulmonary arterial hypertension, and lung cancer. Sex differences and sex hormone-mediated effects emerge in the lung as early as during prenatal development and persist well into adulthood. In addition, significant sex hormone-mediated differences may occur even within the same individual, resulting from fluctuations in sex hormone levels as a function of age and/or menstrual cycle. While the exact role of sex hormones in many lung diseases has not been fully characterized, it is now evident that all major cell types in the lung appear to be targets of sex hormones. Many of these effects, however, are heterogenous and often not fully understood. This chapter will review the effects of the most relevant sex hormones on lung parenchyma, airways, and vasculature in health, thus providing a segue for the individual disease states reviewed in later chapters of this textbook. The biogenesis, signaling mechanisms, and regulation of the three main classes of sex hormones (estrogens, progestogens, and androgens) will be reviewed, followed by an examination of the role of sex hormones in healthy lung development and homeostasis. Finally, the current understanding of the role of steroid signaling in the healthy lung will be reviewed via a compartment-based approach, highlighting current knowledge gaps and identifying research opportunities. Where appropriate, the impact of sex hormones on pulmonary disease and their clinical implications will be discussed.

A.L. Frump, PhD
Department of Medicine, Division of Pulmonary, Critical Care, Occupational and Sleep Medicine, Indiana University School of Medicine, Indianapolis, IN, USA

T. Lahm, MD (✉)
Department of Medicine, Division of Pulmonary, Critical Care, Occupational and Sleep Medicine, Indiana University School of Medicine, Indianapolis, IN, USA

Richard L. Roudebush VA Medical Center, Indianapolis, IN, USA

980 W. Walnut Street, Room C-410, Indianapolis, IN 46202, USA
e-mail: tlahm@iu.edu

© Springer International Publishing Switzerland 2016
A.R. Hemnes (ed.), *Gender, Sex Hormones and Respiratory Disease*,
Respiratory Medicine, DOI 10.1007/978-3-319-23998-9_2

Introduction

Chronic lung diseases are a major public health problem. Nearly 400,000 mortalities each year are due to chronic pulmonary diseases, which have become the third leading cause of death in America [1]. Over 35 million Americans are diagnosed with a chronic lung disease and the number of annual mortalities is predicted to increase [1]. The spectrum of chronic pulmonary diseases encompasses several highly prevalent disorders such as asthma, chronic obstructive pulmonary disease (COPD), pulmonary hypertension (PH), interstitial lung disease, and lung cancers. While each of these disease states affects different compartments and structures of the lung and while their etiologies and pathophysiological processes are complex and multifactorial, epidemiological evidence increasingly demonstrates that one commonality between many of these pulmonary diseases is the influence of sex and gender on disease prevalence, susceptibility, and severity [1–7]. The observed sex differences and gender disparities in pulmonary disease have been linked, at least in part, to physiologically and pathophysiologically relevant effects of sex hormones, resulting in developmental and physiological differences between the sexes [5, 6]. Sex differences and differences in sex hormone signaling in the lung emerge as early as during prenatal development and persist well into adulthood [8]. Furthermore, significant differences may occur even within individuals of the same sex, resulting from fluctuations in sex hormone levels as a function of age and/or menstrual cycle [9–12].

As evidence for sex as not only an epidemiological characteristic but also as a biological variable in pulmonary disease mounts, the importance of sex-specific development, disease pathogenesis, outcome, and therapeutic interventions in both clinical and basic science researches has taken on increased significance. This is evidenced by recent statements by the Institute of Medicine [13] and the National Institutes of Health calling for a greater focus on the investigation of sex and sex differences in preclinical studies [14].

While sex hormones are best characterized as being responsible for the development of secondary sex characteristics and reproductive processes in females and males, they have increasingly been shown to play important roles in the development, homeostasis, and disease pathogenesis of many other biological systems including the brain, cardiovascular, immune, and respiratory systems [15–17]. Consequentially, research has begun to examine the impact of sex differences on the structure and function of the healthy and diseased lung.

In order to understand these sex differences in chronic lung disease, it is imperative to understand the physiologic effects of sex hormones on pulmonary homeostasis. This chapter will review the effects of the most relevant sex hormones on lung parenchyma, airways, and vasculature in health, thus providing a segue for the individual disease states reviewed in later chapters of this textbook. In particular, we will review the biogenesis, signaling mechanisms, and regulation of the three main classes of sex hormones (estrogens, progestogens, and androgens). We will then examine the role of sex hormones in healthy lung development and homeostasis.

Where appropriate, we will briefly review the impact of sex hormones on pulmonary disease and their clinical implications. Finally, we will discuss our current understanding of the role of steroid signaling in the lung with an emphasis on current gaps in knowledge and likely future directions of sex hormone research in the pulmonary field. According to scientific guidelines, we will use the term "gender" when discussing a cultural or behavioral concept and use the term "sex" when referring to biological concepts [18, 19].

Overview of Sex Hormone Synthesis, Signaling, and Regulation

Sex Hormone Synthesis and Metabolism

The following section is a brief overview of sex hormone synthesis and metabolism. For a more comprehensive review of sex hormone steroidogenesis and metabolism, the reader is referred to detailed reviews of the topic [20, 21]. Sex hormone steroidogenesis occurs primarily in the ovaries of women of reproductive age and, to a lesser extent, in the breast, uterus, and placenta of pregnant women [17, 22]. In men of reproductive age, steroidogenesis primarily occurs in the adrenal cortex and testes [15]. Another site of sex hormone steroidogenesis that is particularly important in men and women of post-reproductive age is the adipose tissue [16, 17]. The three major estrogen metabolites and five androgen metabolites are synthesized from cholesterol through a series of monooxygenase reactions facilitated primarily by the cytochrome P450 (CYP) superfamily of enzymes (summarized in Fig. 2.1) [23]. Briefly, the biosynthesis of steroid hormones begins by oxidative cleavage of the side chain of cholesterol by CYP11A [24], resulting in the removal of six methyl groups converting cholesterol to pregnenolone, a progestogen [25]. Progestogens are precursors to all other steroids, and this conversion is the rate-limiting step of steroidogenesis [21, 26]. Pregnenolone can be converted to progesterone by 3-beta-hydroxysteroid dehydrogenase (3β-HSD) [26] or to dehydroepiandrosterone (DHEA), an androgen, by CYP17A1 (through its 17,20-lyase activity), resulting in the loss of two methyl groups [27]. DHEA can be ester-sulfated via the enzyme sulfotransferase to DHEA sulfate (DHEA-S) [28]. DHEA and DHEA-S are produced at the highest quantities of all the circulating sex hormones, typically as the less potent DHEA-S [29]. While less potent than DHEA, DHEA-S is more abundant and more easily measurable as it is more stable. DHEA-S can be converted back to the slightly more bioactive DHEA by steroid sulfatase [30]. DHEA then is hydroxylated to androstenedione via 3β-HSD. Of note, androstenedione can also be generated from progesterone. Androstenedione is then oxidized to testosterone by 17β-hydroxysteroid dehydrogenase (17β-HSD). In a next step, testosterone is converted to the more active androgen metabolite, dihydrotestosterone (DHT) by the enzyme 5α-reductase [31]. Additionally, testosterone, through hydroxylation and

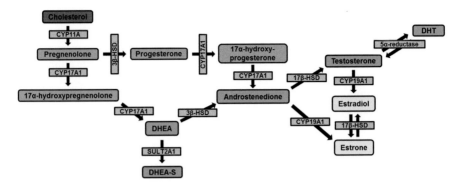

Fig. 2.1 Simplified overview of sex hormone steroidogenesis. Synthesis of progestogens (*blue*), androgens (*green*), and estrogens (*yellow*) from cholesterol (*red*). Enzymes are shown in *orange boxes*. Abbreviations: *3β-HSD* 3-beta-hydroxysteroid dehydrogenase, *17β-HSD* 17-beta-hydroxysteroid dehydrogenase, *CYP19A1* aromatase, *CYP* cytochrome, *DHEA* dehydroepiandrosterone, *DHEA-S* dehydroepiandrosterone-sulfate, *DHT* dihydrotestosterone, *SULT2A1* sulfotransferase 2A1

removal of a single methyl group, can be converted by aromatase (CYP19A1) to 17β-estradiol (E2) [32]. Aromatase also facilitates the conversion of androstenedione to estrone (E1). Finally, E1 can be converted to E2 and vice versa through 17β-HSD [33]. Once synthesized, sex hormones can act by an autocrine, paracrine, or juxtacrine mechanism on target cells and organs [34–38]. The concentrations of the three main circulating sex hormones in healthy adults are listed in Table 2.1. Briefly, women of reproductive age have lower levels of testosterone but higher levels of estrogen and progesterone compared to men [39]. Pregnant women have the highest levels of circulating progesterone, estrogen, and testosterone. Men have the highest amounts of circulating testosterone and DHEA/DHEA-S and lowest levels of estrogen and progesterone. Menopausal women have similar levels of progesterone and testosterone to their reproductive-aged counterparts, but have estrogen levels similar to those detected in men. Finally, as men and women age, circulating hormone levels decrease steeply [6, 40, 41]. However, in older individuals, biologically relevant amounts of estrogens can be generated in adipocytes (especially in obese individuals) and possibly also in fibroblasts of the skin [42]. Uterine bleeding, endometrial hyperplasia, and cancer development have been linked to this extraglandular estrogen production in older women [42].

While circulating sex hormones have been implicated in the development and homeostasis of the normal lung [8], recent evidence has shown that sex hormones can also be synthesized in peripheral tissues such as the brain, skin, adipose tissue, bone, heart, and blood vessels [17, 43, 44]. In case of the latter, this occurs in both vascular endothelial cells (ECs) and smooth muscle cells (SMCs) [44, 45]. Important for the focus of this textbook, enzymes involved in sex hormone synthesis have been detected in the lung. Examples include aromatase (CYP19A1), 17β-HSD, CYP1B1, and CYP1A1 [8, 46–48]. This provides compelling evidence that not only does sex hormone-mediated modulation of the lung occur through the *passive* exposure to sex hormones in the systemic circulation but also that the lung has the capability to *actively* modulate sex hormone synthesis at the cellular level.

Table 2.1 Circulating sex hormone levels in the human adult

	Men <70 years	Men >70 years	Follicular	Preovulatory	Luteal	Pregnant women	Postmenopausal women
Estradiol	15–50 pg/ml	n/a	20–100 pg/ml	150–400 pg/ml	60–200 pg/ml	10,000–40,000 pg/ml	10–30 pg/ml
Progesterone	0.25–0.9 ng/ml	n/a	0.3–1.2 ng/ml	0.7–2.5 ng/ml	1–18 ng/ml	9–300 ng/ml	<0.2–1.1 ng/ml
Testosterone	2–15 ng/ml	1.8–7.5 ng/ml	0.2–0.8[a] ng/ml	0.2–0.8[a] ng/ml	0.2–0.8[a] ng/ml	1–1.4 ng/ml	0.2–0.8[a] ng/ml
DHEA-S	3470[b] ng/ml	670 ng/ml	2470[a] ng/ml	2470[a] ng/ml	2470[a] ng/ml	2470[a] ng/ml	450 ng/ml

Approximate physiological levels of sex hormones in the adult circulation [6, 39, 249–251]

[a]Hormone concentrations have not been dissected according to stage of menstrual cycle

[b]Concentration in men under 30 years of age; levels decrease with older age. n/a = no data available

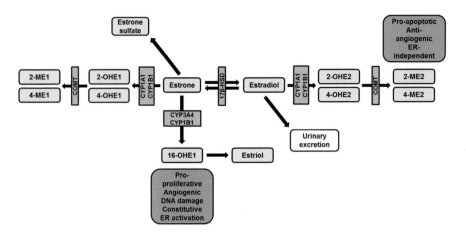

Fig. 2.2 Simplified overview of estrogen metabolism. Enzymes are shown in *orange boxes.* Abbreviations: *2-ME1* 2-methoxyestrone, *2-ME2* 2-methoxyestradiol, *2-OHE1* 2-hydroxyestrone, 2-hydroxyestradiol (2-OHE2), *4-ME1* 4-methoxyestrone, *4-ME2* 4-methoxyestradiol, *4-OHE1* 4-hydroxyestrone, *4-OHE2* 4-hydroxyestradiol, *16-OHE1* 16-alpha-hydroxyestrone, *17β-HSD* 17-beta-hydroxysteroid dehydrogenase, *COMT* catechol-O-methyltransferase, *CYP* cytochrome P450

The Role of Biologically Active Estrogen Metabolites (Fig. 2.2)

Three major estrogens are produced during steroidogenesis: estrone (E1), estradiol (E2), and estriol (E3). E2 is the primary circulating estrogen during reproductive years, whereas E1 is the primary circulating estrogen during and after menopause. E3 is primarily expressed during pregnancy and is the dominant circulating estrogen at that time [40]. Subsequent metabolism of estrogens is mediated by members of the cytochrome P450 superfamily: CYP1A1, CYP1B1, CYP3A4, and catechol-O-methyltransferase (COMT) [49]. Several of the CYPs are highly expressed in the lung, in particular CYP1B1 and CYP1A1 [46–48]. CYP1A1 and CYP1B1 facilitate the oxidation of estrogen into 2-hydroxy- (2-OHE), 4-hydroxy- (4-OHE), and 16α-hydroxy-estrogens [50, 51]. 2-OHE and 4-OHE metabolites have a short half-life and are rapidly converted to the more stable and biologically active 2-methoxy-estradiol (2-ME2) and 4-methoxy-estradiol (4-ME2). Of these, 2-ME2 has been shown to have antiproliferative, anti-angiogenic, anti-inflammatory, and pro-apoptotic effects on target organs that are independent of estrogen receptors [49, 50, 52]. Conversely, studies have demonstrated 4-ME2 and 16α-OHE1 to have pro-proliferative and pro-inflammatory effects on target tissues. In contrast to 2-ME-2, 16α-hydroxy-estrone (16α-OHE1)-mediated effects appear to be due, at least in part, to the constitutive activation of estrogen receptors, particularly estrogen receptor (ER)β [53]. 16α-OHE1 has also been shown to induce DNA damage [54, 55], leading to an association between individuals producing more 16α-OHE1 and an increased risk for diseases characterized by DNA damage, inflammation, or hyperproliferation such as cancer and pulmonary arterial hypertension [2, 56–60], whereas individuals producing more 2-ME2 may be protected from these diseases [61, 62].

Mechanisms of Estrogen-Mediated Signaling

There are three known estrogen receptors: two classical steroid hormone receptors, ERα and ERβ [63–65], as well as a third less well-characterized G-protein-coupled receptor, GPR30 [66]. These receptors are widely, but differentially, expressed throughout the body including the cardiovascular, respiratory, immune, central nervous, and skeletal systems. ER expression and activity in these compartments are regulated by sex, age, diet, and sex steroid concentration (reviewed below).

ERα and ERβ are coded by different genes located on chromosomes 6 and 14, respectively. Despite these differences in chromosomal location, ERα and ERβ exhibit strong homology in their DNA-binding domain sequences (97 %). Both ERs also contain structural similarities in their ligand-binding domain and in their AF1 domain, through which different protein binding partners interact. However, these domains are less homologous than the DNA-binding regions; the ligand-binding domains of ERα and ERβ are 60 % homologous, whereas the AF1 domains are only 18 % homologous. ERα and ERβ are localized to the cell surface membrane, cytoplasm, and nucleus, whereas GPR30 is localized primarily to the cell surface [67]. ER localization is dependent at least in part on which signaling mechanism pathway is activated [63, 66]. In general, there are four major signaling mechanisms through which ERs exert their effects [2, 63–65, 68, 69]. The *classical or genomicpathway* is a common mechanism shared by the steroid receptor superfamily, including progesterone and androgen receptors. Briefly, estrogen binds to cytoplasmic ERα or ERβ which leads to a conformation change of the receptor, the dissociation of regulatory proteins, dimerization with another estrogen–ER complex (either as homodimer with the same ER subtype [e.g., ERα–ERα] or as heterodimer with the other subtype [e.g., ERα–ERβ]), and translocation to the nucleus. Once localized to the nucleus, the estrogen–ER dimer binds to estrogen responsive elements (EREs) on target genes where it then regulates transcriptional activity as a classical transcription factor. In a second pathway, the estrogen–ER dimer *indirectly modulates transcriptional activity* by interacting with other transcription factors. The third mechanism of ER activation occurs through an *estrogen-independent mechanism*. In this scenario, the ER is activated through phosphorylation by a non-estrogen growth factor (i.e., epidermal growth factor [71]). The ER then dimerizes, translocates to the nucleus, and regulates the transcription of target genes. The fourth mechanism is known as the *non-genomic signaling pathway*. In this pathway, estrogen binds to ER localized at the cell membrane. This ligand–receptor complex then trans-activates cytoplasmic protein kinases such as PI3K or MAPK [72]. Examples for non-genomic estrogen signaling include rapid effects on endothelial nitric oxide synthase (eNOS) or calcium channel activity in the vasculature [73, 79]. This mechanism of estrogen-mediated effects was initially described for GPR30, but recently ERα and ERβ have also been shown to mediate estrogen signaling through this pathway [72, 74]. The non-genomic pathway occurs rapidly (within seconds or minutes after the receptor is activated by estrogen) and is likely an important pathway in tissues where a rapid cellular response to injury is required, i.e., the cardiovascular system [75–79]. This is in contrast to signaling via genomic pathways, which occurs over several hours or even days [2, 69].

Regulation of Estrogen Signaling

Estrogen-mediated signaling is a highly complex process that is regulated in several ways [68]. Globally, estrogens are regulated through the differential cell-type and tissue-specific expression pattern of ERs [6, 8]. Sex, age, and the presence of health versus disease are major mediators of estrogen signaling [9, 43, 80]. ER expression is also temporally regulated based on the phase of menstrual cycle and by abundance of circulating estrogen levels [81–83]. Nutritional influences may also interfere with ER expression and/or activity. For example, indole-3-carbinol, a key ingredient of cruciferous vegetables, is a negative regulator of estrogen signaling [61]. On the other hand, xenoestrogens introduced into the environment through industrial, agricultural, and chemical processes exert pro-estrogenic effects [84, 85]. On a molecular level, estrogen signaling is modulated through heat shock protein chaperone interactions with ERs and through post translational modification of the receptors [86]. For example, ERs can be S-nitrosylated or acetylated, with the first modification inhibiting and the latter process enhancing the transcriptional activity of ERs [87]. Additionally, ER gene promoters themselves can be methylated, thus reducing ER mRNA levels [88]. Conversely, estrogen has been shown to upregulate ER transcription, while other sex hormones (e.g., progesterone) can negatively regulate the expression of ER mRNA [89, 90]. Other transcription factors, such as MEF2 and HDAC2, may inhibit ER signaling, and ubiquitination and proteasomal degradation decrease ER abundance. Lastly, several splice variants of ERα and ERβ are able to interact and positively or negatively modulate the activity of ERs, thus adding another layer of complexity to regulation of estrogen-mediated signaling [63, 91].

Progesterone and Androgen-Mediated Signaling

Progestogens are a class of steroid hormones characterized by their ability to bind to and activate progesterone receptors (PR). Progesterone is the most abundant and biologically active progestogen. Other endogenous progestogens include 17-hydroxyprogesterone, 5α-dihydroprogesterone, and 11-deoxycorticosterone, all of which are converted to other intermediates in the steroidogenesis pathway [15, 22, 92]. As multiple cell and tissue types have the capacity to convert cholesterol to steroid hormones, progestogens are found in many cell types [93, 94].

There are several major *androgens*. These include testosterone and dihydrotestosterone (DHT), DHEA/DHEA-S, androstenediol, androstenedione, and androsterone. DHEA/DHEA-S and androstenediol are considered weak steroids and precursors for testosterone and estrogen synthesis [28]. However, there is increasing interest in the effects of DHEA/DHEA-S on the cardiopulmonary system [2], and androstenediol plays a role as a major regulator of gonadotropin secretion [95]. While testosterone and DHT exert multiple biologically relevant effects, they (together with androstenedione) also function as important estrogen precursors. Consequentially, androgen pathways and their receptors are expressed in a wide range of tissues throughout the body, including the cardiopulmonary system [96–98].

Progestogens and androgens mediate their effects on lung function in health and disease through two progesterone receptors (PR-A and PR-B) and an androgen receptor (AR), respectively. ARs, used by testosterone and DHT, and PRs are found widely throughout the body, and both receptors are present in the human lung [93, 98], vascular ECs [99, 100], SMCs [101, 102], and the heart [97, 103], suggesting relevant physiologic effects in these organs. In general, AR and PR signaling occurs in a similar manner to ER signaling, via genomic or non-genomic pathways. Vasodilatory effects of testosterone, however, appear to be independent of the AR [104]. Little is known about receptor signaling pathways employed by DHEA in the cardiopulmonary system, and no specific DHEA receptor has been identified. While DHEA actions appear to be independent of ERs or ARs [105], DHEA has been reported to bind to a specific EC membrane receptor coupled to G-alpha i2,3 with subsequent activation of eNOS [106]. In addition, DHEA stimulates Akt/eNOS signaling through activation and/or upregulation of sigma-1 receptor. Non-genomic DHEA signaling has been described as well [69].

Regulation of Progesterone and Androgen Signaling

Similar to ERs, PRs and AR regulate steroid hormone effects through cell- and tissue-type-specific expression patterns, which are modulated by sex, age, sex hormone concentrations, and menstrual cycle [107, 108]. Like ERs, PRs and ARs are regulated by chaperone proteins and by degradation via the proteasome. Both receptor types can also be posttranslationally modified to enhance or repress transcriptional activity of target genes. Progesterone plays a major role in regulating expression of the PRs. PR-B is the primary activator of progesterone-mediated gene transcription, whereas PR-A exerts inhibitory effects and can act as a repressor of PR-B signaling. In addition to progesterone, estrogen regulates PR expression, indicating significant cross-talk between ER and PR pathways. For example, the presence of estrogen may enhance the effects of PR-B, whereas the presence of androgens or PR-A can inhibit estrogen and progesterone pathways, again demonstrating the importance of sex hormone balance to maintain tissue homeostasis [92, 109–111].

Sex Hormones and Lung Development

Sex Hormones and the Prenatal and Early Postnatal Lung

Sex hormones have been shown to modulate lung development as early 16–24 weeks of gestation [8, 112]. The lung itself continues to develop after birth until 2–4 years of age and continues to change in complexity until early adolescence [8,

113–116]. During neonatal lung development, androgens inhibit surfactant production in the developing neonates, causing delayed surfactant production and delayed alveolar maturation in male neonates compared to female neonates [114, 117]. Additionally, androgens enhance lung airway branching leading to the development of larger lungs in male neonates [8, 117, 118]. These two roles of androgens in the developing lung are clinically relevant, as male neonates exhibit an increased incidence and mortality of infant respiratory distress syndrome, a condition that mainly results from surfactant deficiency and incomplete fetal lung maturation [112, 114, 117]. Mechanisms of androgen-mediated enhancement of airway branching and inhibition of surfactant production appear to involve upregulation of epidermal growth factor (EGF) and transforming growth factor (TGF)-β pathways. However, while this has been demonstrated in vitro and in animal models, it remains unclear if these mechanisms are also responsible for surfactant inhibition in humans [119–121].

The fetal lung also contains ERs, which have been implicated in alveolar development [112, 118, 121]. For example, genetic deletion of ERα or ERβ in mice decreases the number and increases the size of alveoli; these changes are more pronounced in female mice [120]. These ER-mediated effects on alveoli size are likely mediated through effects on platelet-derived growth factor (PDGF) signaling [122]. Morphologically and structurally, compared to male lungs, female lungs are smaller and have fewer respiratory bronchioles. The larger lung size of males at any given age results in an increase in the number of alveoli and alveolar surface area as compared to females; however when normalized for unit area and lung volume, the number of alveoli, at least at birth, is not different between sexes [6, 112, 118].

Additional evidence that steroid hormones regulate fetal lung development comes from studies of the expression of steroidogenesis enzymes such as 17β-HSD, 3β-HSD, 5α-reductase, and aromatase in human fetal lung tissue [8, 122]. Although these studies strongly suggest active modulation of sex hormone pathways in the human fetal lung, it is unlikely that de novo synthesis of sex hormones from cholesterol occurs during this time because CYP17A1 (the enzyme responsible for converting progestogens to androgens) is not detectable [123]. Thus, the presence of several steroidogenesis enzymes suggests that the conversion of precursors into biologically active sex hormones occurs locally in the prenatal and early postnatal lung and that these hormones play a role in mediating lung development.

Taken together, the data reviewed in this section suggest a significant role for estrogens and androgens in lung development, implying them in alveolarization and surfactant production.

Sex Differences in the Pubescent Lung

Female airways and lung parenchyma grow proportionally during childhood and puberty; in males, however, airway growth lags behind the development and growth of other lung structures, resulting in fewer alveoli for the number of airways as well as narrower airways, a phenomenon called dysanapsis [115, 116, 124, 125]. This disproportional growth of lungs and airways results in higher airway resistance in males [112]. On the other hand, males have larger conducting airways than females throughout adolescence and into adulthood. During adolescence, males have higher respiratory pressures compared to females. This difference is attributed to the role of testosterone in changing the shape of the thorax and respiratory muscles during puberty [126]. Other sex differences observed in neonates and children are maintained through puberty, with the dysanaptic growth of the airways in males maintained into adulthood.

Sex Differences in the Aging Lung

Sex differences also occur in the aging lung. During the aging process, there is a decrease in elastic recoil of the lung and large airways as well as of alveolar air volume, whereas abundance of connective tissue increases [127, 128]. However, these changes appear to be less pronounced in females compared to males and occur at a later age [129]. Menopause has significant effects on lung function. For example, during menopause, which is associated with low levels of progesterone and estrogen, women are less likely to develop asthma compared to men [3]. Furthermore, the aging-mediated associated decrease in sex hormone production negatively affects alveolar fluid clearance [130]. Finally, loss of anabolic effects of sex steroids on muscle structure and function during aging is associated with a generalized loss of muscle mass; this results in changes in chest wall architecture and a general loss of respiratory muscle strength [131].

Taken together, the reviewed sex differences during lung development and throughout aging illustrates how minor changes in lung structure and development can have a major impact on health in later life. Despite emerging evidence of the role of sex hormones in regulating lung development, architecture, and function, further understanding of these processes is required to determine their role in aging.

Effects of Sex Hormones on the Healthy Lung

Nearly every major cell type of the lung is affected by sex hormones. This section will review these effects using a compartment-based approach that focuses on bronchial and alveolar epithelium, airway smooth muscle cells, lung parenchyma, the pulmonary vasculature, as well as lung immune cells, concluding with a brief review of sex hormone effects on respiratory mechanics and respiratory drive. Table 2.2 provides a synopsis of the reviewed data.

Table 2.2 Sex hormone effects on major cell types of the lung

Pulmonary cell type	Estrogen	Progesterone	Androgen
Bronchial epithelium	↑ Nitric oxide generation	↑ Nitric oxide generation	Unknown
	↑ Cell proliferation	↓ Cell proliferation	↑ Cell proliferation
Alveolar epithelium	↑ Alveolar regeneration and development	Unknown	↓ Alveolar maturation
	↑ Alveolar fluid clearance	↑ Alveolar fluid clearance	↓ Surfactant production
	↑ ENaC expression	↑ ENaC expression	Unknown
Airway smooth muscle	↓ Intracellular calcium relaxation	↓ Intracellular calcium relaxation	↓ Intracellular calcium relaxation
	↑ Cell proliferation	↓ Cell proliferation	Unknown
Parenchyma (ECM/ fibroblasts)	↓ Fibroblast proliferation	Fibroblast apoptosis	Unknown
	↑ Laminin/fibronectin	Unknown	↓ Laminin/fibronectin
	↓ MMPs	↓ MMPs	↑ MMPs
Pulmonary artery smooth muscle	↓ Intracellular calcium relaxation	↓ Intracellular calcium relaxation	↓ Intracellular calcium relaxation
	↑ Cell proliferation	Unknown	Unknown
	↓ Proliferation at supraphysiological concentrations	Unknown	Unknown
Pulmonary artery endothelium	↑ Nitric oxide generation	↑ Nitric oxide generation	Unknown
	↑ Cell proliferation	Unknown	Unknown
	↓ Proliferation at supraphysiological concentrations and during hypoxia	Unknown	Unknown
Immune cells	Th2 profile	Th2 profile	Th1 profile
	↑ Mast cell degranulation	↓ Mast cell degranulation	↑ Mast cell degranulation
	↑ Eosinophil degranulation	Unknown	Unknown

↑ = increase; ↓ = decrease. *ECM* extracellular matrix; *ENaC* epithelial sodium channel; *MMP* matrix metalloproteinase

Bronchial Epithelium

The bronchial epithelium functions as a barrier between the body and external pathogens, allergens, and pollutants as well as a modulator of airway tone [132]. Inflammation of the bronchial epithelium is a key step in the pathogenesis of a number of diseases including asthma and chronic bronchitis [133]. Likewise, the bronchial epithelium is the starting point for several lung cancers [134]. Despite the importance of the bronchial epithelium, little is known about the role of sex hormones in this tissue.

Both ERs are expressed in bronchial epithelial cells (BECs). Whereas in immortalized airway epithelial cell lines ERβ is expressed more abundantly, in primary BECs both ERs are expressed at similar levels [135, 136]. These data emphasize that results derived from studies of ER expression in immortalized cells cannot be extrapolated to primary cells or the in vivo scenario. Expression of PR or AR in the bronchial epithelium has not been studied.

Nitric Oxide (NO) Signaling One mechanism by which estrogens modulate BECs is through the regulation of NO signaling. The main source of NO production in the airways in response to inflammation is through inducible NO synthase (iNOS) [137, 138]. However, endothelial NOS (eNOS) also plays a major role in the bronchial epithelium through the regulation of airway blood flow [139]. NO generated as a result of BEC iNOS and eNOS can be quantified as exhaled NO (eNO) and is used clinically as an indicator of airway inflammation [140]. iNOS and eNOS facilitate the conversion of L-arginine to L-citrulline and thus the release of NO, a by-product of this reaction and a potent bronchodilator [137]. Studies in the vascular endothelium have shown that estrogens facilitate the dissociation of inactive eNOS from caveolae, leading to eNOS activation and a subsequent increase in NO production and vasodilation [141, 142]. Whether the same phenomenon also occurs in BECs is unknown. However, what is known is that in immortalized BEC lines, E2 acutely increases eNOS activity [135]. This is inhibited by the ER antagonist, fulvestrant, suggesting an ER dependence of effects. Similarly, activation of ERα or ERβ with selective receptor agonists in primary BECs results in eNOS phosphorylation and increased NO production [143]. This effect occurs within minutes, strongly implicating a role of non-genomic estrogen signaling in NO production in the bronchial epithelium. Additional evidence from isolated human female bronchial rings shows that physiological concentrations of estrogens are sufficient to produce a robust bronchodilator response. Denuding the epithelium blunts this effect, suggesting that estrogens non-genomically induce NO production in the bronchial epithelium and thus modulate bronchodilation [143]. This mechanism is remarkably similar to what has been described in the vascular endothelium, where estrogen-mediated non-genomic stimulation of eNOS in endothelial cells results in vasodilation [78].

Exhaled NO production in humans may fluctuate with menstrual cycle status; however there are several studies with conflicting results. For example, one study showed that eNO levels decreased when estrogen levels were high and increased when progesterone levels were high [140]. Women taking an oral contraceptive did not have such fluctuations in eNO production [144, 145]. On the other hand, data also exists indicating that the menstrual cycle does not significantly affect NO levels [81, 146].

BEC Proliferation In addition to mediating bronchodilator responses in BECs, estrogens may affect BEC proliferation. While sex hormones are known to regulate cell proliferation pathways in other tissues and cell types [147, 148], data on estrogen-mediated proliferative responses in BECs are sparse. While in some lung adenocarcinoma cell lines pro-proliferative responses were mediated through ER activation, this did not occur in all cell lines studied [136]. In particular, lung adenocarcinoma cell lines from female, but not male, patients appear to be responsive to pro-proliferative effects of E2, an effect that was linked to differences in nuclear localization of ERα. Effects of other sex hormones on BECs remain uncharacterized.

Mucus Clearance Lastly, E2 has been shown to regulate chloride secretion, implicating estrogens in a role for susceptibility to infection and impaired mucus clearance in the bronchiolar epithelium [82]. This role has particular significance for female cystic fibrosis patients, who have cyclical decreases in lung function correlating with menstrual cycle [82]. Taken together, these data suggest estrogens as modulators of BEC NO production, proliferation, and chloride secretion. Effects of other sex hormones and expression patterns and roles of AR and PR remain poorly characterized.

Alveolar Epithelium

The alveolar epithelium consists of type I cells which are squamous epithelial cells comprising the structure of the alveolar wall and type II cells which are cuboidal epithelial cells responsible for producing and secreting surfactant. ERs, PRs, and AR have been detected in alveolar epithelial cells (AECs) of normal lung tissue and in cell lines [98, 149]. Several steroidogenesis enzymes, including 17β-HSD and aromatase, are found in AECs, indicating that sex hormone precursors may be modified to biologically active sex hormones locally [150]. However, as with the bronchial epithelium, most studies in AECs have focused on the role of sex hormones in the context of disease. It is thus difficult to extrapolate a role for sex hormone signaling and function in the healthy alveolar epithelium.

Surfactant Production, Alveolar Development, and Regeneration One area where the role of sex hormones in the healthy lung is relatively well defined is the role of androgens in delaying maturation of type II AECs and surfactant production in the prenatal lung [151]. Here, androgens inhibit surfactant production through modulation of EGF and TGF-β pathways (which are positive and negative regulators of lung maturation, respectively [119–121]). In fact, an androgen-induced delay in EGF receptor binding during lung development has been described in rabbits [152]. Alternatively, exposure of female fibroblasts to DHT results in a dose-dependent increase of TGF-β1 activity [119].

Estrogens modulate AECs through multiple mechanisms. For example, E2 regulates type I AEC development and regeneration [153, 154]. In mouse studies, ovariectomy (OVX) of sexually immature wild-type female mice results in a decrease in the number of alveoli during development and lung maturation. Treatment with E2, on the other hand, restores alveolar numbers in OVX mice [154]. Furthermore, ERα or ERβ knockout mice exhibit similar alveolar developmental defects, demonstrating that both ERα and ERβ are required for the normal development of pulmonary alveoli in female mice [154]. OVX of wild-type adult female mice results in the loss of 40 % of alveoli. E2 treatment induces alveolar regeneration through a distinct ERα-dependent mechanism and restores alveoli number and lung volume [153]. These data thus demonstrate a role for estrogen-mediated signaling in alveolar development and regeneration and provide a mechanism for increases in FVC and FEV1 observed in postmenopausal women undergoing hormone replacement therapy [155].

Alveolar Fluid Homeostasis Sex hormones also regulate alveolar fluid homeostasis in healthy AECs. Estrogens and progestogens (specifically E2 and progesterone) have been identified as key mediators of alveolar fluid clearance, a process that occurs through regulation of epithelial sodium channel (ENaC) expression, abundance, and activity [130, 156, 157]. ENaCs are essential for sodium transport and fluid balance in the alveolar space. In particular, fluid is absorbed into AECs through ENaCs and extruded from the cell through Na/K+ ATPases [158]. These channels are often dysregulated in pulmonary diseases such as cystic fibrosis and acute respiratory distress syndrome (ARDS), leading to abnormal fluid clearance of the alveolar space [159]. Interestingly, aging and the associated decrease in sex hormone production can lead to deficiencies in alveolar fluid clearance [130]. On the other hand, E2 treatment of adult type II AECs causes, through a GPR30-dependent mechanism, an increase in ENaC abundance and localization to the apical membrane [130]. Similarly, treatment of fetal type II AECs with progesterone leads to an increase in ENaC expression and activity [156].

Airway Smooth Muscle

The airway smooth muscle (ASM) is responsible for modulating the tone of the bronchial airways by constricting or dilating the airway. The role sex hormones in the regulation of ASM function is better understood than their role in other lung compartments, in part due to increasing interest in the investigation of sex differences in asthma and COPD.

Regulation of Airway Tone In general, estrogens exert bronchodilatory effects, but time- and dose-dependent differences seem to exist. These effects are mediated through both epithelium-dependent and epithelium-independent mechanisms leading to decreased intracellular Ca^{2+} levels. Chronic administration of low doses of E2 (10 μg/kg) increases the concentration of inhaled acetylcholine (ACh) necessary to double airway resistance in OVX rats [160, 161]. On the other hand, OVX rats treated with high doses of E2 (100 μg/kg) exhibited increased responsiveness to ACh-induced vasoconstriction [161]. Together, these data suggest a dose-specific effect of E2 on ASM responses to ACh. Studies in rabbit tracheal strips pre-constricted with ACh showed that treatment with 100 µM E2 was able to relax the airway smooth muscle layer in an epithelium-independent manner [162, 163]. E2-mediated effects were found to be due in part to increased prostaglandin synthesis with downstream increases in cAMP levels, as well as through increases in cGMP signaling, both leading to attenuation of muscle tone through inhibition of Ca^{2+} influx [163].

In addition to indirectly regulating Ca^{2+} concentrations via cAMP and cGMP, estrogen is also able to directly modulate Ca^{2+}-mediated responses via effects on Ca^{2+} channels [164]. For example, in human ASM cells, physiologically relevant concentrations of E2 (100 pM–10 nM) substantially decrease Ca^{2+} responses to histamine through an ERα-mediated mechanism [165]. E2 effects on ASM are regulated, in part, through decreased Ca^{2+} influx through regulation of L-type channels and store-operated entry [165]. Taken together, these studies indicate that estrogen-mediated bronchodilation in ASM occurs via reduction of intracellular Ca^{2+} concentrations through ER-dependent mechanisms.

The effects of progesterone on ASM tone are less well defined. Progesterone potentiates the dilatory effect of isoprenaline in constricted pig bronchial rings [166]. In these studies, progesterone, although administered at a high dose (40 µM), had a more robust dilatory effect than testosterone, but was less effective than estradiol. Progesterone also prevents histamine- or carbachol-induced contraction in guinea pig trachea [167]. Progesterone-mediated regulation is proposed to occur through direct inhibition of Ca^{2+} influx [168]. Combined, these studies provide evidence for a bronchodilator effect of progesterone on ASM similar to, but not as robust as, that of estrogen.

Similar to estrogen and progesterone treatment, testosterone treatment causes a dose-dependent bronchodilator effect on ASM, as shown in pre-constricted rabbit tracheal strips [162]. However, unlike estrogen and progesterone treatment, whose bronchodilatory effects are both epithelial dependent and independent, removal of the epithelium in testosterone-treated tracheal strips completely attenuates the dilatory response, suggesting testosterone-mediated relaxation is epithelial dependent. Interestingly, inhibition of AR with flutamide does not alter the dilatory effects of testosterone, suggesting an AR-independent mechanism of action. Furthermore, dilatory effects were maintained after administration of bovine serum albumin (BSA)-conjugated (and thus cell membrane-impermeable) testosterone, a phenomenon consistent with non-genomic signaling [162]. Similar to the previous study, removal of the epithelium attenuated the testosterone response. Taken together, these studies suggest that testosterone is mediating bronchodilator effects through non-genomic interaction at the cell surface with the AR receptor. These bronchodilator effects are mediated through voltage-gated Ca^{2+} channel antagonism.

Of clinical relevance, in asthma, a disease characterized by both inflammation and hyperresponsiveness of the airway, there is greater prevalence and morbidity in adult women compared to men [169, 170]. Women also have more severe and more frequent asthma exacerbations than men [113], with 40–50 % of women having cyclic variations and exacerbations during the premenstrual/late luteal phase of their menstrual cycle [171]. At this point in the menstrual cycle, estrogen levels are at their lowest, and progesterone levels are increased [39, 172]. Studies in healthy volunteers and asthma patients demonstrate that the luteal phase of the menstrual cycle is characterized by the lowest FVC and FEV1, suggesting a direct effect between sex hormone levels and lung function [81]. Along these lines, postmenopausal women exhibit decreased airway function [173], and postmenopausal asthma patients are characterized by more severe disease compared to men and reproductive-aged women [173]. Together, while the exact mechanism is unclear, these studies suggest that sex hormones modulate airway tone and asthma prevalence and severity [3, 81]. However, these relationships are complex, as there is also evidence that administration of estrogen to menopausal women is associated with increased rates of newly diagnosed asthma [174]. Disparate effects on airway tone vs. airway inflammatory responses and ASM proliferation may contribute to these complex relationships. Environmental effects on ERs and estrogen metabolism may also play a role (e.g., hyperoxia) [48].

ASM Proliferation Evidence also exists that sex steroids, in addition to affecting ASM tone, exert physiologically relevant effects on ASM proliferation. For example, E2 has been shown to enhance proliferation of ASM cells [175]. Such effects have been linked to worsening effects of estrogens on airway remodeling in asthma [176]. DHEA, on the other hand, inhibits rat tracheal smooth muscle cell proliferation after stimulation by fetal bovine serum or PDGF through inhibition of activator protein-1 [177]. However, more detailed exploration of the role of sex hormones on ASM proliferation is required; such studies would help to further decipher the role of these hormones in airway diseases such as asthma.

Parenchyma

For the purpose of this chapter, the lung parenchyma refers specifically to the alveolar tissue with respiratory bronchioles, alveolar ducts, and terminal bronchioles. The parenchyma provides structural support, participates in gas exchange, and is the site of extracellular signaling and regulation. The role of sex hormones on extracellular matrix deposition and modulation of enzyme regulators of the extracellular matrix is of clinical interest since men are more likely to develop and die from idiopathic pulmonary fibrosis than women [112]. Studies in the bleomycin model of pulmonary fibrosis, however, suggest female sex hormones as being pro-fibrotic [178]. Along those lines, female rats treated with bleomycin developed more severe fibrosis than males. OVX female rats, on the other hand, had less severe fibrosis compared to intact females, and E2 replenishment restored fibrosis levels to those of intact females [178]. In vitro studies suggest that the pro-fibrotic effect of E2 is likely mediated through upregulation of procollagen 1 and TGF-β1 gene expression in fibroblasts [178]. Studies in the mouse bleomycin model of pulmonary fibrosis, however, suggest a greater degree of fibrosis in male animals [179]. Here, castration of male mice is protective against the development of pulmonary fibrosis, while DHT replenishment attenuates this protective effect [179]. Taken together, even though discrepant with regard to protection versus harm, the reported in vivo and human data suggest sex hormones as potential modulators of fibrotic processes. Effects on proliferation may also play a role in this process. For example, high concentrations (5 μg/ml) of E2, testosterone, or progesterone decrease proliferation of human fetal lung fibroblasts [180, 181]. Furthermore, decreased proliferation was noted in lung myofibroblasts treated with E2, mediated through non-genomic signaling via activation of the Raf1–ERK–MAPK pathway [181]. However, the relevance of these in vitro studies to the in vivo scenario remains unknown.

Collagen, fibronectin, laminin, and other components of the extracellular matrix of the parenchyma are important for the structural integrity and regulation of lung homeostasis, and their dysregulation can result in various pathologies. However, effects of sex hormones on extracellular matrix components have only recently been explored and have yet to be studied in the lung. Studies using mouse skin biopsies have shown that adult male mice have 25 % more lung hydroxyproline (representative of collagen deposition) present than age-matched females [182]. AR knockout mice did not have such an increase in hydroxyproline, implicating male sex hormones as potential modulators of collagen deposition in the parenchyma of the lung [182]. Despite these studies, the exact mechanisms of sex hormone regulation of the lung parenchyma are mostly unknown.

Pulmonary Vasculature

Due to the well-described gender differences in pulmonary arterial hypertension (PAH) [2, 70, 73, 183–185], there has been increasing interest in the study of sex hormone effects on the pulmonary vasculature. While a significant body of knowledge has been derived from specific study of the pulmonary vasculature, other data have been extrapolated from studies of systemic vascular cells. Studies from our laboratory demonstrate that both ERα and ERβ are expressed in pulmonary artery endothelial cells (PAECs) as well as smooth muscle cells (PASMCs) [186, 187] (Fig. 2.3). In addition, enzymes critical for estrogen synthesis and metabolism have been detected in lung blood vessels; these include aromatase and CYP1B1 [46, 47], suggesting that local estrogen production and metabolism occur in the pulmonary vasculature. This is of importance, as alterations in estrogen synthesis have recently been linked to PAH pathogenesis [2, 188]. GPR30, while present in the lung (Lahm, Frump; unpublished), has not yet been described in the pulmonary vasculature, but has been found in systemic vascular cells [189]. Similarly, AR and PR have been detected in vascular ECs [99, 100] and SMCs [101, 102].

Estradiol Effects on Vasomotor Tone In general, sex hormones serve as vasodilators of the vasculature, with most data being available for E2. Multiple pathways have been implicated in E2's vasodilator effects. Non-genomic stimulation of eNOS appears to be the most prominent mechanism. In particular, in PAECs, estrogen acutely activates eNOS with subsequent production of NO, and both ERs have been implicated in these effects via two different non-genomic signaling mechanisms

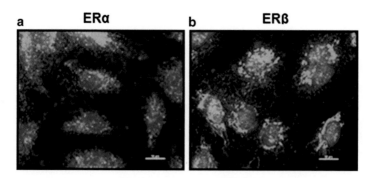

Fig. 2.3 ERα and ERβ are expressed in human pulmonary artery endothelial cells (HPAECs). Representative immunocytochemistry images of cultured HPAECs. Expressions of ERα (*green*, **a**) and ERβ (*green*, **b**) are shown. Note that localization of both ERs correlates with expression in cytoplasm and nucleus. Cell nuclei are stained with DAPI (*blue*). Images are 40x; scale bar indicates 10 μm

[190, 191]. While such effects have been demonstrated in various cell types as well as in isolated pulmonary artery (PA) rings, various downstream mediators have been implicated in these findings. For example, in transformed rat lung vascular ECs, eNOS activation was mediated through an ERα- and Akt-dependent mechanism [192, 193]. In PAECs, on the other hand, estrogen-mediated eNOS activation occurred through ERβ localized to caveolae [76]. In isolated PA rings from healthy rats, both ERs have been implicated in E2's non-genomic vasodilator effects, with ERα attenuating potassium-induced vasocontraction and ERβ attenuating hypoxic vasoconstriction (HPV) [194]. These effects are mediated in an endothelial cell- and NO-dependent manner. Such effects are physiologically relevant, as PA rings from proestrus rats exhibit less HPV than arteries from animals with lower circulating E2 levels, such as estrus or diestrus rats as well as male rats [83].

E2 also targets other vasoactive mediators. For example, in PAECs, E2 attenuates hypoxia-induced upregulation of the vasoconstrictor endothelin-1, an effect mediated by interfering with activity of hypoxia-inducible factor (HIF)-1α [195]. Lastly, E2 enhances prostacyclin synthase activity and prostacyclin production through an ERβ- and calcium-dependent mechanism and also regulates the upstream mediators, cyclooxygenase-1 and cyclooxygenase-2 [73].

While many of E2's PAEC effects ultimately affect PASMC tone, direct effects on PASMCs may also contribute to E2's pulmonary vasodilator effects. However, such data mostly stem from the systemic circulation, where E2 has a vasodilatory effect on SMCs. For example, E2 hyperpolarizes calcium-dependent potassium channels (BK_{Ca}) in a cGMP-mediated manner, thus leading to SMC relaxation [196]. Estrogens are also purported to promote SMC relaxation through inhibition of the Rho kinase pathway [197]. Despite robust evidence for the role of estrogen on systemic vascular SMCs, there is little direct evidence for the role of estrogens on PASMCs, although such effects are hypothesized [198]; consequentially, this still represents a knowledge gap in the field.

While the described effects of estrogens on PAECs and PASMCs are relevant for maintaining vascular homeostasis in healthy individuals under baseline conditions, they also play a major role in attenuating HPV [2, 73, 199, 200] and in inducing pulmonary vasodilation during pregnancy [73].

Estradiol Effects on PA Cell Proliferation In contrast to the small number of studies evaluating vasorelaxor effects of estrogens on PASMCs, multiple studies have evaluated E2 effects on PASMC proliferation. The observation that ERs, aromatase, and CYP1B1 are expressed in PASMCs indicates that conversion of sex hormone precursors into biologically active estrogens and metabolites may be regulated locally in PASMCs [186–188]. Many of the currently published investigations identified estrogens as inducers of PASMC proliferation [201, 202]. However, in hypoxic PASMCs, the opposite seems to be the case, and E2 has been identified in this context as an inhibitor of PASMC proliferation [203, 204]. Interestingly, PASMCs isolated from proestrus rats exhibited less proliferation under hypoxia conditions than cells from estrus or male rats [204]. Mitogenic effects of E2 also seem to be dose dependent, as at least one study suggests a shift toward anti-mitogenic effects on PASMCs at higher concentrations [205]. Similar dose-dependent effects on proliferation have also been described for PAECs, with physiological concentrations promoting, but supraphysiological concentrations inhibiting, proliferation [205]. Our laboratory found that proliferative E2 effects on rat PAECs are context dependent, with pro-proliferative effects being detected in room air conditions, but antiproliferative effects being observed during hypoxia (1 % O_2) [206]. Similar hypoxia-specific effects were seen when evaluating ERK1/2 activation and VEGF secretion, both of which were attenuated in hypoxia, but not normoxia. Along these lines, expression of the cell cycle inhibitor p27^{kip1} was decreased by E2 at room air, but enhanced during hypoxia. These effects appear to be mediated in an ER-dependent manner, with effects on ERK1/2 activation being attenuated by both ERα and ERβ blockades, thus implicating both ERs in these effects. Hypoxia-induced upregulation of ERβ PAEC expression may mediate such hypoxia-specific effects (Fig. 2.2) [186, 187]. Biologically active effects of estrogen metabolites also seem to regulate PASMC and PAEC proliferation, with 2-ME acting as a mitogen [205], while 16α-OHE1 appears to mediate pro-proliferative signaling [46].

Taken together, the current body of literature suggests context-dependent E2 effects on PAEC and PASMC proliferation, with antiproliferative effects predominantly being seen during hypoxia and/or at supraphysiological concentrations. Genetic alterations (e.g., BMPR2 mutations) and environmental exposures (e.g., drugs interfering with serotonin signaling, such as appetite inhibitors) may affect such responses.

E2 Effects on Angiogenesis Cyclic angiogenic changes occur in the lung parallel with cyclic gas exchange changes that occur during the menstrual cycle [207]. Specifically, over the course of their menstrual cycle, healthy women exhibit variable lung diffusion capacity, with the nadir occurring during the follicular phase. This decrease in lung diffusion capacity was accompanied by a 25 % decrease in vascular capillary blood volume and a 24 % decrease in CD34+ CD133+ circulating endothelial progenitor cells [207]. Expression of the pro-angiogenic cytokine stem cell factor (SCF) correlated with these changes; however vascular endothelial growth factor (VEGF) did not. Interestingly, OVX mice with estrogen replenishment exhibited an increased number of microvessels compared to OVX mice without estrogen replacement [207]. This suggests that pulmonary vascular angiogenesis is regulated by estrogen and that lung microvascular density and diffusion capacity vary throughout the menstrual cycle, thus paralleling a pattern that has been described previously in uterine endometrium [208, 209].

Effects of Progesterone, Testosterone, and DHEA The effects of progesterone on the pulmonary vasculature are less well characterized. In a study of isolated PAs, progesterone had the strongest vasodilatory effect compared to estrogen and testosterone [210]. This vasodilatory effect of progesterone treatment was due in part to endothelial-dependent NO mechanisms. Treatment with an NOS inhibitor reduced progesterone-mediated vasodilation. Additional study demonstrated that the vasodilatory effects of progesterone were also mediated through inhibition of voltage-gated and receptor-mediated Ca^{2+} channels [211]. Further mechanisms of pulmonary vasomotor tone regulation by progesterone are largely unknown.

Testosterone-mediated effects in the pulmonary vasculature are not well studied. Two studies identified testosterone as a more potent vasodilator of isolated PAs than E2, with PAs from male rats being more sensitive to the effects of testosterone than those from female rats [104, 210]. Testosterone's vasodilator effect is mediated at least in part through inhibition of voltage-gated and receptor-mediated Ca^{2+} channels, while AR, NO, or prostaglandins do not appear to be involved [104]. Such vasodilator effects were recapitulated in human PAs and isolated perfused human lungs, but no sex differences were noted in this context [212]. Further studies demonstrated that most robust vasodilator effects of testosterone were observed at physiological concentrations and only in the presence of an intact endothelium [213].

DHEA effects in the pulmonary vasculature are slightly better understood. Several studies identified DHEA acts as a pulmonary vasodilator. In isolated ferret lungs preconstricted with the K+ inhibitor tetraethylammonium, DHEA treatment, through a cAMP- and cGMP-independent mechanism, stimulated the opening of K^+ channels and decreased pulmonary artery pressure [214]. In another study using isolated rat lungs and PAs, DHEA treatment, through a prostaglandin-, endothelial-, NO-, and cGMP-independent mechanism, opened voltage-gated K+ channels leading to the relaxation of PAs. The mechanism is believed to be through reduced NADPH expression and a change in PASMC redox status [215]. One specific mechanism by which DHEA is thought to regulate vasodilation is through its role as a noncompetitive inhibitor of glucose-6-phosphate dehydrogenase [216]. This, in turn, inhibits the pentose phosphate pathway and NADPH production, changing the redox state of the cell. This mechanism was also linked to potential antiproliferative effects of DHEA in the pulmonary vasculature [217]. Lastly, DHEA has also been shown to exert antiproliferative effects via eNOS activation in ECs [218]. DHEA's role in these pathways makes it an interesting target for PH, and in fact several studies have investigated DHEA effects in PH with promising results [219–222].

Immune Cells

The following section will briefly focus on the interplay between sex steroids and immune cells with regard to their implications for pulmonary disease. As in other cell types, the effects of sex hormone function on the immune system are dependent on hormone levels, ER expression, concentration, and duration of sex hormone exposure, as well as context.

Sex Steroid Effects on Lymphocytes and Th1/Th2 Balance Lymphocytes are an important target cell of sex steroids. For example, T-cell regulation by sex hormones has been described previously [223, 224]. E2 binds to peripheral blood mononuclear cells (PBMCs) and thymic cells, while androgens only bind to thymic cells. ERα-46, a splice variant of ERα, and ERβ are strongly expressed in lymphocytes, suggesting a role in modulating the function of these cells [225]. Specifically, estrogen-mediated T-cell activation has been described, but the exact mechanism of sex hormone modulation of these cells is unknown. In the context of disease, such as asthma, high estrogen levels at the luteal phase of the menstrual cycle and during pregnancy shift the immune system to a Th2 response, leading to increased IL-4 and IL-10 secretion [223]. Along those lines, secretion of TNF-α, a Th1-specific cytokine, is attenuated at higher physiological concentrations of estrogen [226]. These effects are regulated primarily through ERα [223, 227]. On the other hand, in natural killer (NK) cells, estrogen promotes secretion of the Th1 cytokine interferon (IFN)-γ, which can then, via iNOS and cyclooxygenase-2, contribute to inflammatory processes via this pathway [223].

Progesterone's effects on T cells are similar to those of estrogen; however the expression of PR in immune cells has not been confirmed [228, 229]. Furthermore, progesterone inhibits Th1-type cell signaling in humans, induces Th2-type cytokines, and inhibits NF-κB and TNF-α [230, 231]. In women, progesterone and estrogen may have synergistic effects on Th1/Th2 balance, a phenomenon that has been linked to exacerbations of asthma [168].

Androgens, on the other hand, are purported to cause a T-cell switch toward a Th1 immune response. For example, testosterone increases IFN-γ and IL-2 secretion in mice [232, 233]. Similarly, DHEA may regulate the Th1/Th2 balance; this has been linked to DHEA-mediated attenuation of allergic airway inflammation in mice [234].

Taken together, these data suggest that sex hormones modulate immune responses and Th1/Th2 balance, with a shift toward a Th2 phenotype in women and a shift toward a Th1 phenotype in males [233, 235].

Sex Steroid Effects on Eosinophils and Mast Cells Eosinophils have been shown to bind E2, leading to degranulation and increased adhesiveness [224, 236, 237]. Progesterone has been shown to increase airway hyperresponsiveness [168], but since PR has not been detected on eosinophils, underlying mechanisms of this response are not clear; progesterone conversion to estrogen may play a role. There is currently no known role for androgens in modulating eosinophil responses.

Mast cells express both ERs and PRs, but do not express AR [224, 238]. Estrogen is a known stimulator of mast cell degranulation and histamine secretion [239, 240]. Conversely, progesterone inhibits mast cell migration and histamine release [238, 241]. Finally, testosterone is able to indirectly stimulate mast cell degranulation [241]. While some of these effects may be context dependent, sex steroids are recognized as physiologically relevant modulators of allergic responses. This has clinically relevant implications for allergic airway diseases such as asthma, a phenomenon that will be reviewed later in this textbook.

Sex Hormone Effects on Respiratory Mechanics and Respiratory Control

Sex hormones have relevant effects on chest wall architecture and respiratory drive that are relevant for changes in respiratory mechanics associated with pregnancy or aging. For example, estrogen- and progesterone-mediated effects on architecture of the thoracic ligament apparatus cause the subcostal angle to increase from 68° up to more than 100° in the first trimester of pregnancy. Similarly, the chest diameter increases resulting in a "barrel chest" appearance of the thorax [242–244]. These changes in the connective tissue compartment result at least in part from a general loosening of the underlying structures, likely mediated through sex hormone effects on matrix metalloproteinases as well as other components of the extracellular matrix. On the other hand, loss of anabolic effects of sex steroids on muscle function and structure during aging is associated with a generalized loss of muscle mass, a phenomenon that leads to changes in chest wall architecture and a loss of strength of respiratory muscles [131]. Lastly, progesterone exerts significant effects on regulation of respiratory drive in the medulla oblongata; this is exemplified by a significant increase in tidal volume that is mediated by progesterone during pregnancy [245, 246].

Table 2.2 summarizes sex hormone signaling effects in each pulmonary cell type discussed.

Clinical Implications

Even though much work needs to be done to further define the effects of sex hormones on lung function in health and disease, the currently available data suggest sex hormones as potent modifiers of pulmonary processes. While sex hormones play an important role in the healthy lung, alterations in their levels, release patterns, receptor expression, and signaling, as well as their metabolism, caused by genetic or environmental factors, have emerged as significant disease modifiers. A detailed understanding of sex hormone effects in health and disease may allow for identification of novel therapeutic targets for both male and female patients with lung disease. The availability of potent and specific modifiers of sex hormone synthesis and signaling already in clinical use for hormone-dependent cancers or endocrine diseases represents a major advantage for the development of novel therapeutic targets. Examples include the use of ER antagonists (e.g., fulvestrant), aromatase inhibitors (e.g., anastrozole), 5α-reductase inhibitors (e.g., finasteride, used to block conversion of testosterone to DHT), and selective ER modulators (SERMs). In addition, preclinical studies have used specific ERα and ERβ agonists and antagonists. Similarly, GPR30 signaling can be enhanced or inhibited with specific agonists and antagonists (G1 and G15, respectively). Finally, conversion of sex hormones to their biologically active metabolites is modifiable with CYP or COMT inhibitors (e.g., 2,3′,4,5′-tetramethoxystilbene [TMS], 1-ABT or OR-486). Interestingly, literature exists that sex hormones can also be modified non-pharmacologically through nutritional interventions. For example, a reduction of dietary fats is purported to decrease production of 16α-OH-E1 [247], whereas a diet rich in indole-3-carbanole (through ingestion of cruciferous vegetables) promotes E2 conversion to 2-ME2 [61]. 2-ME2 is currently in clinical trials for breast and ovarian cancer [248].

Feasibility of modifying sex hormone signaling in lung disease has been demonstrated preclinically in the context of asthma, ARDS, PAH, and HPV (reviewed in [6, 191]). In particular, estrogen signaling in PAH has recently gained interest (reviewed in [2, 73]), and a clinical trial of aromatase inhibition in patients with PAH (clinicaltrials.gov identifier NCT01545336) is currently underway. An already established example of successful modification of sex hormone signaling for a chronic lung disease is the use of anti-estrogen strategies for patients with lymphangioleiomyomatosis.

Conclusions and Future Directions

Gender and sex differences, as well as biologically relevant effects of sex hormones, have been implicated in many major lung diseases, such as asthma, COPD, cystic fibrosis, PAH, and lung cancer. Sex differences and sex hormone-mediated effects emerge in the lung as early as during prenatal development and persist well into adulthood. Furthermore, significant differences may occur even within individuals of the same sex, resulting from fluctuations in sex hormone levels as a function of age and/or menstrual cycle. While the exact role of sex hormones in many of these diseases has not been fully characterized, it is now evident that all major cell types in the lung appear to be targets of sex hormones. The effects of these hormones on many of the cell types reviewed in this chapter are heterogenous and often not fully understood. What is known, however, is that many of the effects of sex hormones appear to be context, time, and/or dose dependent. While playing a critical role for lung homeostasis, alterations in sex hormone abundance and/or signaling may contribute to or worsen a variety of lung diseases (e.g., asthma or PAH). Further studies should focus on better defining the effects of estrogens, progestogens, androgens, and their receptors and metabolites on normal lung function. Novel pathways employed by sex hormones to influence the structure and function of the major cell types in the normal lung need to be identified. A better understanding of genetic, epigenetic, and environmental modifiers of sex hormone synthesis and signaling may allow for identifying the basis of sex differences in lung disease and may provide novel targets to be harnessed therapeutically.

References

1. CDC. National vital statistics reports, Deaths: Final data for 2004. Volume 55. DeKalb County: Centers for Disease Control and Prevention; 2007.
2. Austin ED, Lahm T, West J, Tofovic SP, Johansen AK, et al. Gender, sex hormones and pulmonary hypertension. Pulm Circ. 2013;3:294–314.
3. Balzano G, Fuschillo S, Melillo G, Bonini S. Asthma and sex hormones. Allergy. 2001;56:13–20.
4. Belani CP, Marts S, Schiller J, Socinski MA. Women and lung cancer: epidemiology, tumor biology, and emerging trends in clinical research. Lung Cancer. 2007;55:15–23.
5. Caracta CF. Gender differences in pulmonary disease. Mt Sinai J Med. 2003;70:215–24.
6. Townsend EA, Miller VM, Prakash YS. Sex differences and sex steroids in lung health and disease. Endocr Rev. 2012;33:1–47.
7. Bonds RS, Midoro-Horiuti T. Estrogen effects in allergy and asthma. Curr Opin Allergy Clin Immunol. 2013;13:92–9. doi:10.1097/ACI.1090b1013e32835a32836dd32836.
8. Seaborn T, Simard M, Provost PR, Piedboeuf B, Tremblay Y. Sex hormone metabolism in lung development and maturation. Trends Endocrinol Metab. 2010;21:729–38.
9. Tam A, Morrish D, Wadsworth S, Dorscheid D, Man SF, et al. The role of female hormones on lung function in chronic lung diseases. BMC Womens Health. 2011;11:24.
10. Barr RG, Camargo Jr CA. Hormone replacement therapy and obstructive airway diseases. Treat Respir Med. 2004;3:1–7.
11. Koledova VV, Khalil RA. Sex hormone replacement therapy and modulation of vascular function in cardiovascular disease. Expert Rev Cardiovasc Ther. 2007;5:777–89.
12. Barr RG, Wentowski CC, Grodstein F, Somers SC, Stampfer MJ, et al. Prospective study of postmenopausal hormone use and newly diagnosed asthma and chronic obstructive pulmonary disease. Arch Intern Med. 2004;164:379–86.
13. Institute of Medicine. Sex-specific reporting of scientific research - Workshop summary. Washington, DC: Institute of Medicine; 2012.
14. U.S. Department of Health and Human Services, NIoH, Office of Research on Women's Health, editors. Strategic Plan: Moving into the future with new dimensions and strategies: a vision for 2020 for women's health research; 2010.
15. Luu-The V, Labrie F. The intracrine sex steroid biosynthesis pathways. Prog Brain Res. 2010;181:177–92.
16. Labrie F, Simard J, Luu-The V, Trudel C, Martel C, et al. Expression of 3 beta-hydroxysteroid dehydrogenase/delta 5-delta 4 isomerase (3 beta-HSD) and 17 beta-hydroxysteroid dehydrogenase (17 beta-HSD) in adipose tissue. Int J Obes. 1991;15 Suppl 2:91–9.
17. Labrie F. Extragonadal synthesis of sex steroids: intracrinology. Ann Endocrinol (Paris). 2003;64:95–107.
18. Wizeman TM, Pardue ML. Exploring the Biological Contributions to Human Health: Does Sex Matter? Washington, DC: National Academy Press, 2001, p. 288.
19. Committee AMAMoS. American Medical Association manual of style: a guide for editors, Correct and Preferred Usage. 10th ed. Oxford: Oxford University Press; 2007.

20. Ghayee HK, Auchus RJ. Basic concepts and recent developments in human steroid hormone biosynthesis. Rev Endocr Metab Disord. 2007;8:289–300.
21. Payne AH, Hales DB. Overview of steroidogenic enzymes in the pathway from cholesterol to active steroid hormones. Endocr Rev. 2004;25:947–70.
22. Tuckey RC. Progesterone synthesis by the human placenta. Placenta. 2005;26:273–81.
23. Hanukoglu I. Steroidogenic enzymes: structure, function, and role in regulation of steroid hormone biosynthesis. J Steroid Biochem Mol Biol. 1992;43:779–804.
24. Guo IC, Shih MC, Lan HC, Hsu NC, Hu MC, et al. Transcriptional regulation of human CYP11A1 in gonads and adrenals. J Biomed Sci. 2007;14:509–15.
25. Shih MC, Chiu YN, Hu MC, Guo IC, Chung BC. Regulation of steroid production: analysis of Cyp11a1 promoter. Mol Cell Endocrinol. 2011;336:80–4.
26. Chapman JC, Polanco JR, Min S, Michael SD. Mitochondrial 3 beta-hydroxysteroid dehydrogenase (HSD) is essential for the synthesis of progesterone by corpora lutea: an hypothesis. Reprod Biol Endocrinol. 2005;3:11.
27. Soucy P, Luu-The V. Conversion of pregnenolone to DHEA by human 17alpha-hydroxylase/17, 20-lyase (P450c17). Evidence that DHEA is produced from the released intermediate, 17alpha-hydroxypregnenolone. Eur J Biochem. 2000;267:3243–7.
28. Labrie F, Luu-The V, Labrie C, Simard J. DHEA and its transformation into androgens and estrogens in peripheral target tissues: intracrinology. Front Neuroendocrinol. 2001;22:185–212.
29. Labrie F, Luu-The V, Labrie C, Belanger A, Simard J, et al. Endocrine and intracrine sources of androgens in women: inhibition of breast cancer and other roles of androgens and their precursor dehydroepiandrosterone. Endocr Rev. 2003;24:152–82.
30. Reed MJ, Purohit A, Woo LW, Newman SP, Potter BV. Steroid sulfatase: molecular biology, regulation, and inhibition. Endocr Rev. 2005;26:171–202.
31. Zhu YS, Imperato-McGinley JL. 5alpha-reductase isozymes and androgen actions in the prostate. Ann NY Acad Sci. 2009;1155:43–56.
32. Miller WL. Androgen biosynthesis from cholesterol to DHEA. Mol Cell Endocrinol. 2002;198:7–14.
33. Labrie F, Luu-The V, Lin SX, Labrie C, Simard J, et al. The key role of 17 beta-hydroxysteroid dehydrogenases in sex steroid biology. Steroids. 1997;62:148–58.
34. Babiker FA, De Windt LJ, van Eickels M, Thijssen V, Bronsaer RJP, et al. 17β-estradiol antagonizes cardiomyocyte hypertrophy by autocrine/paracrine stimulation of a guanylyl cyclase A receptor-cyclic guanosine monophosphate-dependent protein kinase pathway. Circulation. 2004;109:269–76.
35. Risbridger GP, Ellem SJ, McPherson SJ. Estrogen action on the prostate gland: a critical mix of endocrine and paracrine signaling. J Mol Endocrinol. 2007;39:183–8.
36. Hatthachote P, Gillespie JI. Complex interactions between sex steroids and cytokines in the human pregnant myometrium: evidence for an autocrine signaling system at term. Endocrinology. 1999;140:2533–40.
37. Richards JA, Petrel TA, Brueggemeier RW. Signaling pathways regulating aromatase and cyclooxygenases in normal and malignant breast cells. J Steroid Biochem Mol Biol. 2002;80:203–12.
38. Dontu G, El-Ashry D, Wicha MS. Breast cancer, stem/progenitor cells and the estrogen receptor. Trends Endocrinol Metab. 2004;15:193–7.
39. Elmlinger MW, Kuhnel W, Ranke MB. Reference ranges for serum concentrations of lutropin (LH), follitropin (FSH), estradiol (E2), prolactin, progesterone, sex hormone-binding globulin (SHBG), dehydroepiandrosterone sulfate (DHEAS), cortisol and ferritin in neonates, children and young adults. Clin Chem Lab Med. 2002;40:1151–60.
40. Tulchinsky D, Hobel CJ, Yeager E, Marshall JR. Plasma estrone, estradiol, estriol, progesterone, and 17-hydroxyprogesterone in human pregnancy. I. Normal pregnancy. Am J Obstet Gynecol. 1972;112:1095–100.
41. Labrie F, Belanger A, Luu-The V, Labrie C, Simard J, et al. DHEA and the intracrine formation of androgens and estrogens in peripheral target tissues: its role during aging. Steroids. 1998;63:322–8.

42. Bulun SE, Zeitoun K, Sasano H, Simpson ER. Aromatase in aging women. Semin Reprod Endocrinol. 1999;17:349–58.
43. Thakur MK, Paramanik V. Role of steroid hormone coregulators in health and disease. Horm Res. 2009;71:194–200.
44. Simpson ER. Sources of estrogen and their importance. J Steroid Biochem Mol Biol. 2003;86:225–30.
45. Harada N, Sasano H, Murakami H, Ohkuma T, Nagura H, et al. Localized expression of aromatase in human vascular tissues. Circ Res. 1999;84:1285–91.
46. White K, Johansen AK, Nilsen M, Ciuclan L, Wallace E, et al. Activity of the estrogen-metabolizing enzyme cytochrome P450 1B1 influences the development of pulmonary arterial hypertension. Circulation. 2012;126:1087–98.
47. Dempsie Y, MacRitchie NA, White K, Morecroft I, Wright AF, et al. Dexfenfluramine and the oestrogen-metabolizing enzyme CYP1B1 in the development of pulmonary arterial hypertension. Cardiovasc Res. 2013;99:24–34.
48. Martin YN, Manlove L, Dong J, Carey WA, Thompson MA, et al. Hyperoxia-induced changes in estradiol metabolism in postnatal airway smooth muscle. Am J Physiol Lung Cell Mol Physiol. 2015;308:L141–6.
49. Parl FF, Dawling S, Roodi N, Crooke PS. Estrogen metabolism and breast cancer: a risk model. Ann NY Acad Sci. 2009;1155:68–75.
50. Nebert DW. Elevated estrogen 16 alpha-hydroxylase activity: is this a genotoxic or nongenotoxic biomarker in human breast cancer risk? J Natl Cancer Inst. 1993;85:1888–91.
51. Tsuchiya Y, Nakajima M, Yokoi T. Cytochrome P450-mediated metabolism of estrogens and its regulation in human. Cancer Lett. 2005;227:115–24.
52. Yager JD, Davidson NE. Estrogen carcinogenesis in breast cancer. N Engl J Med. 2006;354:270–82.
53. Zhu BT, Han GZ, Shim JY, Wen Y, Jiang XR. Quantitative structure-activity relationship of various endogenous estrogen metabolites for human estrogen receptor alpha and beta subtypes: insights into the structural determinants favoring a differential subtype binding. Endocrinology. 2006;147:4132–50.
54. Bolton JL, Thatcher GR. Potential mechanisms of estrogen quinone carcinogenesis. Chem Res Toxicol. 2008;21:93–101.
55. Roy D, Cai Q, Felty Q, Narayan S. Estrogen-induced generation of reactive oxygen and nitrogen species, gene damage, and estrogen-dependent cancers. J Toxicol Environ Health B Crit Rev. 2007;10:235–57.
56. Eliassen AH, Missmer SA, Tworoger SS, Hankinson SE. Circulating 2-hydroxy- and 16alpha-hydroxy estrone levels and risk of breast cancer among postmenopausal women. Cancer Epidemiol Biomarkers Prev. 2008;17:2029–35.
57. Kaaks R, Rinaldi S, Key TJ, Berrino F, Peeters PH, et al. Postmenopausal serum androgens, oestrogens and breast cancer risk: the European prospective investigation into cancer and nutrition. Endocr Relat Cancer. 2005;12:1071–82.
58. Missmer SA, Eliassen AH, Barbieri RL, Hankinson SE. Endogenous estrogen, androgen, and progesterone concentrations and breast cancer risk among postmenopausal women. J Natl Cancer Inst. 2004;96:1856–65.
59. Muti P, Bradlow HL, Micheli A, Krogh V, Freudenheim JL, et al. Estrogen metabolism and risk of breast cancer: a prospective study of the 2:16alpha-hydroxyestrone ratio in premenopausal and postmenopausal women. Epidemiology. 2000;11:635–40.
60. Muti P, Westerlind K, Wu T, Grimaldi T, De Berry 3rd J, et al. Urinary estrogen metabolites and prostate cancer: a case-control study in the United States. Cancer Causes Control. 2002;13:947–55.
61. Michnovicz JJ, Bradlow HL. Altered estrogen metabolism and excretion in humans following consumption of indole-3-carbinol. Nutr Cancer. 1991;16:59–66.
62. Kanasaki K, Palmsten K, Sugimoto H, Ahmad S, Hamano Y, et al. Deficiency in catechol-O-methyltransferase and 2-methoxyoestradiol is associated with pre-eclampsia. Nature. 2008;453:1117–21.

63. Heldring N, Pike A, Andersson S, Matthews J, Cheng G, et al. Estrogen receptors: how do they signal and what are their targets. Physiol Rev. 2007;87:905–31.
64. Mendelsohn ME, Karas RH. The protective effects of estrogen on the cardiovascular system. N Engl J Med. 1999;340:1801–11.
65. Mendelsohn ME, Karas RH. Molecular and cellular basis of cardiovascular gender differences. Science. 2005;308:1583–7.
66. Hsieh YC, Yu HP, Frink M, Suzuki T, Choudhry MA, et al. G protein-coupled receptor 30-dependent protein kinase A pathway is critical in nongenomic effects of estrogen in attenuating liver injury after trauma-hemorrhage. Am J Pathol. 2007;170:1210–8.
67. Thomas P, Pang Y, Filardo EJ, Dong J. Identity of an estrogen membrane receptor coupled to a G protein in human breast cancer cells. Endocrinology. 2005;146:624–32.
68. Murphy E. Estrogen signaling and cardiovascular disease. Circ Res. 2011;109:687–96.
69. Simoncini T, Mannella P, Fornari L, Caruso A, Varone G, et al. Genomic and non-genomic effects of estrogens on endothelial cells. Steroids. 2004;69:537–42.
70. Rich S, Dantzker DR, Ayres SM, Bergofsky EH, Brundage BH, et al. Primary pulmonary hypertension. A national prospective study. Ann Intern Med. 1987;107:216–23.
71. Curtis SW, Washburn T, Sewall C, DiAugustine R, Lindzey J, et al. Physiological coupling of growth factor and steroid receptor signaling pathways: estrogen receptor knockout mice lack estrogen-like response to epidermal growth factor. Proc Natl Acad Sci USA. 1996;93:12626–30.
72. Simoncini T, Hafezi-Moghadam A, Brazil DP, Ley K, Chin WW, et al. Interaction of oestrogen receptor with the regulatory subunit of phosphatidylinositol-3-OH kinase. Nature. 2000;407:538–41.
73. Lahm T, Tuder RM, Petrache I. Progress in solving the sex hormone paradox in pulmonary hypertension. Am J Physiol Lung Cell Mol Physiol. 2014;307:L7–26.
74. Simoncini T, Genazzani AR, Liao JK. Nongenomic mechanisms of endothelial nitric oxide synthase activation by the selective estrogen receptor modulator raloxifene. Circulation. 2002;105:1368–73.
75. Hisamoto K, Ohmichi M, Kurachi H, Hayakawa J, Kanda Y, et al. Estrogen induces the Akt-dependent activation of endothelial nitric-oxide synthase in vascular endothelial cells. J Biol Chem. 2001;276:3459–67.
76. Chambliss KL, Yuhanna IS, Anderson RG, Mendelsohn ME, Shaul PW. ERbeta has nongenomic action in caveolae. Mol Endocrinol. 2002;16:938–46.
77. Sherman TS, Chambliss KL, Gibson LL, Pace MC, Mendelsohn ME, et al. Estrogen acutely activates prostacyclin synthesis in ovine fetal pulmonary artery endothelium. Am J Respir Cell Mol Biol. 2002;26:610–6.
78. Chen Z, Yuhanna IS, Galcheva-Gargova Z, Karas RH, Mendelsohn ME, et al. Estrogen receptor alpha mediates the nongenomic activation of endothelial nitric oxide synthase by estrogen. J Clin Invest. 1999;103:401–6.
79. Shaul PW. Rapid activation of endothelial nitric oxide synthase by estrogen. Steroids. 1999;64:28–34.
80. Taraseviciute A, Voelkel NF. Severe pulmonary hypertension in postmenopausal obese women. Eur J Med Res. 2006;11:198–202.
81. Farha S, Asosingh K, Laskowski D, Hammel J, Dweik RA, et al. Effects of the menstrual cycle on lung function variables in women with asthma. Am J Respir Crit Care Med. 2009;180:304–10.
82. Johannesson M, Ludviksdottir D, Janson C. Lung function changes in relation to menstrual cycle in females with cystic fibrosis. Respir Med. 2000;94:1043–6.
83. Lahm T, Patel KM, Crisostomo PR, Markel TA, Wang M, et al. Endogenous estrogen attenuates pulmonary artery vasoreactivity and acute hypoxic pulmonary vasoconstriction: the effects of sex and menstrual cycle. Am J Physiol Endocrinol Metab. 2007;293:E865–71.
84. Card JW, Zeldin DC. Hormonal influences on lung function and response to environmental agents: lessons from animal models of respiratory disease. Proc Am Thorac Soc. 2009;6:588–95.

85. Melgert BN, Ray A, Hylkema MN, Timens W, Postma DS. Are there reasons why adult asthma is more common in females? Curr Allergy Asthma Rep. 2007;7:143–50.
86. Gougelet A, Bouclier C, Marsaud V, Maillard S, Mueller SO, et al. Estrogen receptor alpha and beta subtype expression and transactivation capacity are differentially affected by receptor-, hsp90- and immunophilin-ligands in human breast cancer cells. J Steroid Biochem Mol Biol. 2005;94:71–81.
87. Garban HJ, Marquez-Garban DC, Pietras RJ, Ignarro LJ. Rapid nitric oxide-mediated S-nitrosylation of estrogen receptor: regulation of estrogen-dependent gene transcription. Proc Natl Acad Sci USA. 2005;102:2632–6.
88. Martinez-Galan J, Torres-Torres B, Nunez MI, Lopez-Penalver J, Del Moral R, et al. ESR1 gene promoter region methylation in free circulating DNA and its correlation with estrogen receptor protein expression in tumor tissue in breast cancer patients. BMC Cancer. 2014;14:59.
89. Katzenellenbogen BS. Mechanisms of action and cross-talk between estrogen receptor and progesterone receptor pathways. J Soc Gynecol Investig. 2000;7:S33–7.
90. Kraus WL, Weis KE, Katzenellenbogen BS. Inhibitory cross-talk between steroid hormone receptors: differential targeting of estrogen receptor in the repression of its transcriptional activity by agonist- and antagonist-occupied progestin receptors. Mol Cell Biol. 1995;15:1847–57.
91. Levin ER. Cell localization, physiology, and nongenomic actions of estrogen receptors. J Appl Physiol. 1985;91:1860–7.
92. Giangrande PH, McDonnell DP. The A and B isoforms of the human progesterone receptor: two functionally different transcription factors encoded by a single gene. Recent Prog Horm Res. 1999;54:291–313. discussion 313–4.
93. Barberis MC, Veronese S, Bauer D, De Juli E, Harari S. Immunocytochemical detection of progesterone receptors. A study in a patient with primary pulmonary hypertension. Chest. 1995;107:869–72.
94. Cahill MA. Progesterone receptor membrane component 1: an integrative review. J Steroid Biochem Mol Biol. 2007;105:16–36.
95. Swerdloff RS, Walsh PC, Odell WD. Control of LH and FSH secretion in the male: evidence that aromatization of androgens to estradiol is not required for inhibition of gonadotropin secretion. Steroids. 1972;20:13–22.
96. Lamont KR, Tindall DJ. Androgen regulation of gene expression. Adv Cancer Res. 2010;107:137–62.
97. Marsh JD, Lehmann MH, Ritchie RH, Gwathmey JK, Green GE, et al. Androgen receptors mediate hypertrophy in cardiac myocytes. Circulation. 1998;98:256–61.
98. Mikkonen L, Pihlajamaa P, Sahu B, Zhang FP, Janne OA. Androgen receptor and androgen-dependent gene expression in lung. Mol Cell Endocrinol. 2010;317:14–24.
99. Welter BH, Hansen EL, Saner KJ, Wei Y, Price TM. Membrane-bound progesterone receptor expression in human aortic endothelial cells. J Histochem Cytochem. 2003;51:1049–55.
100. Bonnet S, Dumas-de-La-Roque E, Begueret H, Marthan R, Fayon M, et al. Dehydroepiandrosterone (DHEA) prevents and reverses chronic hypoxic pulmonary hypertension. Proc Natl Acad Sci USA. 2003;100:9488–93.
101. Fujimoto R, Morimoto I, Morita E, Sugimoto H, Ito Y, et al. Androgen receptors, 5 alpha-reductase activity and androgen-dependent proliferation of vascular smooth muscle cells. J Steroid Biochem Mol Biol. 1994;50:169–74.
102. Nakamura Y, Suzuki T, Inoue T, Tazawa C, Ono K, et al. Progesterone receptor subtypes in vascular smooth muscle cells of human aorta. Endocr J. 2005;52:245–52.
103. Ingegno MD, Money SR, Thelmo W, Greene GL, Davidian M, et al. Progesterone receptors in the human heart and great vessels. Lab Invest. 1988;59:353–6.
104. Jones RD, English KM, Pugh PJ, Morice AH, Jones TH, et al. Pulmonary vasodilatory action of testosterone: evidence of a calcium antagonistic action. J Cardiovasc Pharmacol. 2002;39:814–23.
105. Williams MR, Ling S, Dawood T, Hashimura K, Dai A, et al. Dehydroepiandrosterone inhibits human vascular smooth muscle cell proliferation independent of ARs and ERs. J Clin Endocrinol Metab. 2002;87:176–81.

106. Liu D, Dillon JS. Dehydroepiandrosterone activates endothelial cell nitric-oxide synthase by a specific plasma membrane receptor coupled to Galpha(i2,3). J Biol Chem. 2002;277:21379–88.
107. Beato M, Klug J. Steroid hormone receptors: an update. Hum Reprod Update. 2000;6:225–36.
108. McKenna NJ, O'Malley BW. Minireview: nuclear receptor coactivators–an update. Endocrinology. 2002;143:2461–5.
109. Edwards DP. Regulation of signal transduction pathways by estrogen and progesterone. Annu Rev Physiol. 2005;67:335–76.
110. Lee YF, Shyr CR, Thin TH, Lin WJ, Chang C. Convergence of two repressors through heterodimer formation of androgen receptor and testicular orphan receptor-4: a unique signaling pathway in the steroid receptor superfamily. Proc Natl Acad Sci USA. 1999;96:14724–9.
111. Zhou ZX, Wong CI, Sar M, Wilson EM. The androgen receptor: an overview. Recent Prog Horm Res. 1994;49:249–74.
112. Carey MA, Card JW, Voltz JW, Arbes Jr SJ, Germolec DR, et al. It's all about sex: gender, lung development and lung disease. Trends Endocrinol Metab. 2007;18:308–13.
113. Becklake MR, Kauffmann F. Gender differences in airway behaviour over the human life span. Thorax. 1999;54:1119–38.
114. Dezateux C, Stocks J. Lung development and early origins of childhood respiratory illness. Br Med Bull. 1997;53:40–57.
115. Thurlbeck WM. Postnatal growth and development of the lung. Am Rev Respir Dis. 1975;111:803–44.
116. Thurlbeck WM, Angus GE. Growth and aging of the normal human lung. Chest. 1975;67:3s–6.
117. Torday JS, Nielsen HC. The sex difference in fetal lung surfactant production. Exp Lung Res. 1987;12:1–19.
118. Fleisher B, Kulovich MV, Hallman M, Gluck L. Lung profile: sex differences in normal pregnancy. Obstet Gynecol. 1985;66:327–30.
119. Dammann CE, Ramadurai SM, McCants DD, Pham LD, Nielsen HC. Androgen regulation of signaling pathways in late fetal mouse lung development. Endocrinology. 2000;141:2923–9.
120. Nielsen HC, Martin A, Volpe MV, Hatzis D, Vosatka RJ. Growth factor control of growth and epithelial differentiation in embryonic lungs. Biochem Mol Med. 1997;60:38–48.
121. Caniggia I, Tseu I, Han RN, Smith BT, Tanswell K, et al. Spatial and temporal differences in fibroblast behavior in fetal rat lung. Am J Physiol. 1991;261:L424–33.
122. Pezzi V, Mathis JM, Rainey WE, Carr BR. Profiling transcript levels for steroidogenic enzymes in fetal tissues. J Steroid Biochem Mol Biol. 2003;87:181–9.
123. Provost PR, Tremblay Y. Genes involved in the adrenal pathway of glucocorticoid synthesis are transiently expressed in the developing lung. Endocrinology. 2005;146:2239–45.
124. Mead J. Dysanapsis in normal lungs assessed by the relationship between maximal flow, static recoil, and vital capacity. Am Rev Respir Dis. 1980;121:339–42.
125. Taussig LM, Cota K, Kaltenborn W. Different mechanical properties of the lung in boys and girls. Am Rev Respir Dis. 1981;123:640–3.
126. Schrader PC, Quanjer PH, Olievier IC. Respiratory muscle force and ventilatory function in adolescents. Eur Respir J. 1988;1:368–75.
127. Turner JM, Mead J, Wohl ME. Elasticity of human lungs in relation to age. J Appl Physiol. 1968;25:664–71.
128. Gibson GJ, Pride NB, O'Cain C, Quagliato R. Sex and age differences in pulmonary mechanics in normal nonsmoking subjects. J Appl Physiol. 1976;41:20–5.
129. Pride NB. Ageing and changes in lung mechanics. Eur Respir J. 2005;26:563–5.
130. Greenlee MM, Mitzelfelt JD, Yu L, Yue Q, Duke BJ, et al. Estradiol activates epithelial sodium channels in rat alveolar cells through the G protein-coupled estrogen receptor. Am J Physiol Lung Cell Mol Physiol. 2013;305(11):L878–89.

131. Tolep K, Kelsen SG. Effect of aging on respiratory skeletal muscles. Clin Chest Med. 1993;14:363–78.
132. Velden VH, Versnel HF. Bronchial epithelium: morphology, function and pathophysiology in asthma. Eur Cytokine Netw. 1998;9:585–97.
133. Levine SJ. Bronchial epithelial cell-cytokine interactions in airway inflammation. J Investig Med. 1995;43:241–9.
134. Stavrides JC. Lung carcinogenesis: pivotal role of metals in tobacco smoke. Free Radic Biol Med. 2006;41:1017–30.
135. Kirsch EA, Yuhanna IS, Chen Z, German Z, Sherman TS, et al. Estrogen acutely stimulates endothelial nitric oxide synthase in H441 human airway epithelial cells. Am J Respir Cell Mol Biol. 1999;20:658–66.
136. Ivanova MM, Mazhawidza W, Dougherty SM, Klinge CM. Sex differences in estrogen receptor subcellular location and activity in lung adenocarcinoma cells. Am J Respir Cell Mol Biol. 2010;42:320–30.
137. Barnes PJ. Nitric oxide and airway disease. Ann Med. 1995;27:389–93.
138. Watkins DN, Garlepp MJ, Thompson PJ. Regulation of the inducible cyclo-oxygenase pathway in human cultured airway epithelial (A549) cells by nitric oxide. Br J Pharmacol. 1997;121:1482–8.
139. Krasteva G, Pfeil U, Filip AM, Lips KS, Kummer W, et al. Caveolin-3 and eNOS colocalize and interact in ciliated airway epithelial cells in the rat. Int J Biochem Cell Biol. 2007;39:615–25.
140. Mandhane PJ, Hanna SE, Inman MD, Duncan JM, Greene JM, et al. Changes in exhaled nitric oxide related to estrogen and progesterone during the menstrual cycle. Chest. 2009;136:1301–7.
141. Sud N, Wiseman DA, Black SM. Caveolin 1 is required for the activation of endothelial nitric oxide synthase in response to 17beta-estradiol. Mol Endocrinol. 2010;24:1637–49.
142. Hamad AM, Clayton A, Islam B, Knox AJ. Guanylyl cyclases, nitric oxide, natriuretic peptides, and airway smooth muscle function. Am J Physiol Lung Cell Mol Physiol. 2003;285:L973–83.
143. Townsend EA, Meuchel LW, Thompson MA, Pabelick CM, Prakash YS. Estrogen increases nitric-oxide production in human bronchial epithelium. J Pharmacol Exp Ther. 2011;339:815–24.
144. Kharitonov SA, Logan-Sinclair RB, Busset CM, Shinebourne EA. Peak expiratory nitric oxide differences in men and women: relation to the menstrual cycle. Br Heart J. 1994;72:243–5.
145. Oguzulgen IK, Turktas H, Erbas D. Airway inflammation in premenstrual asthma. J Asthma. 2002;39:517–22.
146. Morris NH, Sooranna SR, Steer PJ, Warren JB. The effect of the menstrual cycle on exhaled nitric oxide and urinary nitrate concentration. Eur J Clin Invest. 1996;26:481–4.
147. Vihko P, Herrala A, Harkonen P, Isomaa V, Kaija H, et al. Control of cell proliferation by steroids: the role of 17HSDs. Mol Cell Endocrinol. 2006;248:141–8.
148. Folkerd EJ, Dowsett M. Influence of sex hormones on cancer progression. J Clin Oncol. 2010;28:4038–44.
149. Marquez-Garban DC, Chen HW, Fishbein MC, Goodglick L, Pietras RJ. Estrogen receptor signaling pathways in human non-small cell lung cancer. Steroids. 2007;72:135–43.
150. Plante J, Simard M, Rantakari P, Cote M, Provost PR, et al. Epithelial cells are the major site of hydroxysteroid (17beta) dehydrogenase 2 and androgen receptor expression in fetal mouse lungs during the period overlapping the surge of surfactant. J Steroid Biochem Mol Biol. 2009;117:139–45.
151. Provost PR, Simard M, Tremblay Y. A link between lung androgen metabolism and the emergence of mature epithelial type II cells. Am J Respir Crit Care Med. 2004;170:296–305.
152. Marquez DC, Lee J, Lin T, Pietras RJ. Epidermal growth factor receptor and tyrosine phosphorylation of estrogen receptor. Endocrine. 2001;16:73–81.

153. Massaro D, Clerch LB, Massaro GD. Estrogen receptor-alpha regulates pulmonary alveolar loss and regeneration in female mice: morphometric and gene expression studies. Am J Physiol Lung Cell Mol Physiol. 2007;293:L222–8.
154. Massaro D, Massaro GD. Estrogen regulates pulmonary alveolar formation, loss, and regeneration in mice. Am J Physiol Lung Cell Mol Physiol. 2004;287:L1154–9.
155. Pata Ö, Atiş S, Utku Öz A, Yazici G, Tok E, et al. The effects of hormone replacement therapy type on pulmonary functions in postmenopausal women. Maturitas. 2003;46:213–8.
156. Schmidt C, Klammt J, Thome UH, Laube M. The interaction of glucocorticoids and progesterone distinctively affects epithelial sodium transport. Lung. 2014;192:935–46.
157. Laube M, Kuppers E, Thome UH. Modulation of sodium transport in alveolar epithelial cells by estradiol and progesterone. Pediatr Res. 2011;69:200–5.
158. Fronius M. Treatment of pulmonary edema by ENaC activators/stimulators. Curr Mol Pharmacol. 2013;6:13–27.
159. Collawn JF, Lazrak A, Bebok Z, Matalon S. The CFTR and ENaC debate: how important is ENaC in CF lung disease? Am J Physiol Lung Cell Mol Physiol. 2012;302(11):L1141–6.
160. Degano B, Prevost MC, Berger P, Molimard M, Pontier S, et al. Estradiol decreases the acetylcholine-elicited airway reactivity in ovariectomized rats through an increase in epithelial acetylcholinesterase activity. Am J Respir Crit Care Med. 2001;164:1849–54.
161. Degano B, Mourlanette P, Valmary S, Pontier S, Prevost MC, et al. Differential effects of low and high-dose estradiol on airway reactivity in ovariectomized rats. Respir Physiol Neurobiol. 2003;138:265–74.
162. Kouloumenta V, Hatziefthimiou A, Paraskeva E, Gourgoulianis K, Molyvdas PA. Non-genomic effect of testosterone on airway smooth muscle. Br J Pharmacol. 2006;149:1083–91.
163. Pang JJ, Xu XB, Li HF, Zhang XY, Zheng TZ, et al. Inhibition of beta-estradiol on trachea smooth muscle contraction in vitro and in vivo. Acta Pharmacol Sin. 2002;23:273–7.
164. Dimitropoulou C, White RE, Ownby DR, Catravas JD. Estrogen reduces carbachol-induced constriction of asthmatic airways by stimulating large-conductance voltage and calcium-dependent potassium channels. Am J Respir Cell Mol Biol. 2005;32:239–47.
165. Townsend EA, Thompson MA, Pabelick CM, Prakash YS. Rapid effects of estrogen on intracellular Ca^{2+} regulation in human airway smooth muscle. Am J Physiol Lung Cell Mol Physiol. 2010;298:L521–30.
166. Foster PS, Goldie RG, Paterson JW. Effect of steroids on beta-adrenoceptor-mediated relaxation of pig bronchus. Br J Pharmacol. 1983;78:441–5.
167. Perusquia M, Hernandez R, Montano LM, Villalon CM, Campos MG. Inhibitory effect of sex steroids on guinea-pig airway smooth muscle contractions. Comp Biochem Physiol C Pharmacol Toxicol Endocrinol. 1997;118:5–10.
168. Hellings PW, Vandekerckhove P, Claeys R, Billen J, Kasran A, et al. Progesterone increases airway eosinophilia and hyper-responsiveness in a murine model of allergic asthma. Clin Exp Allergy. 2003;33:1457–63.
169. de Marco R, Locatelli F, Sunyer J, Burney P. Differences in incidence of reported asthma related to age in men and women. A retrospective analysis of the data of the European Respiratory Health Survey. Am J Respir Crit Care Med. 2000;162:68–74.
170. Postma DS. Gender differences in asthma development and progression. Gend Med. 2007;4(Suppl B):S133–46.
171. Murphy VE, Gibson PG. Premenstrual asthma: prevalence, cycle-to-cycle variability and relationship to oral contraceptive use and menstrual symptoms. J Asthma. 2008;45:696–704.
172. Hanley SP. Asthma variation with menstruation. Br J Dis Chest. 1981;75:306–8.
173. Bellia V, Augugliaro G. Asthma and menopause. Monaldi Arch Chest Dis. 2007;67:125–7.
174. Ticconi C, Pietropolli A, Piccione E. Estrogen replacement therapy and asthma. Pulm Pharmacol Ther. 2013;26:617–23.
175. Stamatiou R, Paraskeva E, Papagianni M, Molyvdas PA, Hatziefthimiou A. The mitogenic effect of testosterone and 17beta-estradiol on airway smooth muscle cells. Steroids. 2011;76:400–8.

176. Lazaar AL, Panettieri Jr RA. Airway smooth muscle: a modulator of airway remodeling in asthma. J Allergy Clin Immunol. 2005;116:488–95. quiz 496.
177. Dashtaki R, Whorton AR, Murphy TM, Chitano P, Reed W, et al. Dehydroepiandrosterone and analogs inhibit DNA binding of AP-1 and airway smooth muscle proliferation. J Pharmacol Exp Ther. 1998;285:876–83.
178. Gharaee-Kermani M, Hatano K, Nozaki Y, Phan SH. Gender-based differences in bleomycin-induced pulmonary fibrosis. Am J Pathol. 2005;166:1593–606.
179. Voltz JW, Card JW, Carey MA, Degraff LM, Ferguson CD, et al. Male sex hormones exacerbate lung function impairment after bleomycin-induced pulmonary fibrosis. Am J Respir Cell Mol Biol. 2008;39:45–52.
180. Kondo H, Kasuga H, Noumura T. Effects of various steroids on in vitro lifespan and cell growth of human fetal lung fibroblasts (WI-38). Mech Ageing Dev. 1983;21:335–44.
181. Flores-Delgado G, Bringas P, Buckley S, Anderson KD, Warburton D. Nongenomic estrogen action in human lung myofibroblasts. Biochem Biophys Res Commun. 2001;283:661–7.
182. Markova MS, Zeskand J, McEntee B, Rothstein J, Jimenez SA, et al. A role for the androgen receptor in collagen content of the skin. J Investig Dermatol. 2004;123:1052–6.
183. Badesch DB, Raskob GE, Elliott CG, Krichman AM, Farber HW, et al. Pulmonary arterial hypertension: baseline characteristics from the REVEAL Registry. Chest. 2010;137:376–87.
184. Benza RL, Miller DP, Gomberg-Maitland M, Frantz RP, Foreman AJ, et al. Predicting survival in pulmonary arterial hypertension: insights from the Registry to Evaluate Early and Long-Term Pulmonary Arterial Hypertension Disease Management (REVEAL). Circulation. 2010;122:164–72.
185. Humbert M, Sitbon O, Chaouat A, Bertocchi M, Habib G, et al. Pulmonary arterial hypertension in France: results from a national registry. Am J Respir Crit Care Med. 2006;173:1023–30.
186. Selej M, Brown J, Lockett A, Albrecht M, Schweitzer K, et al. Hypoxia increases expression of estrogen receptor (ER)-beta in vivo and in vitro. Am J Respir Crit Care Med. 2013;187:A2257.
187. Selej M, Lockett A, Albrecht M, Petrache I, Lahm T. Hypoxia increases estrogen receptor beta expression in cultured rat pulmonary artery endothelial cells. Am J Respir Crit Care Med. 2012;185:A4817.
188. Mair KM, Wright AF, Duggan N, Rowlands DJ, Hussey MJ, et al. Sex-dependent influence of endogenous estrogen in pulmonary hypertension. Am J Respir Crit Care Med. 2014;190:456–67.
189. Filardo EJ, Quinn JA, Frackelton Jr AR, Bland KI. Estrogen action via the G protein-coupled receptor, GPR30: stimulation of adenylyl cyclase and cAMP-mediated attenuation of the epidermal growth factor receptor-to-MAPK signaling axis. Mol Endocrinol. 2002;16:70–84.
190. Silverman EK, Weiss ST, Drazen JM, Chapman HA, Carey V, et al. Gender-related differences in severe, early-onset chronic obstructive pulmonary disease. Am J Respir Crit Care Med. 2000;162:2152–8.
191. Lahm T, Crisostomo PR, Markel TA, Wang M, Weil BR, et al. The effects of estrogen on pulmonary artery vasoreactivity and hypoxic pulmonary vasoconstriction: potential new clinical implications for an old hormone. Crit Care Med. 2008;36:2174–83.
192. Bolego C, Cignarella A, Sanvito P, Pelosi V, Pellegatta F, et al. The acute estrogenic dilation of rat aorta is mediated solely by selective estrogen receptor-alpha agonists and is abolished by estrogen deprivation. J Pharmacol Exp Ther. 2005;313:1203–8.
193. Douglas G, Cruz MN, Poston L, Gustafsson JA, Kublickiene K. Functional characterization and sex differences in small mesenteric arteries of the estrogen receptor-beta knockout mouse. Am J Physiol Regul Integr Comp Physiol. 2008;294:R112–20.
194. Lahm T, Crisostomo PR, Markel TA, Wang M, Wang Y, et al. Selective estrogen receptor-alpha and estrogen receptor-beta agonists rapidly decrease pulmonary artery vasoconstriction by a nitric oxide-dependent mechanism. Am J Physiol Regul Integr Comp Physiol. 2008;295:R1486–93.

195. Earley S, Resta TC. Estradiol attenuates hypoxia-induced pulmonary endothelin-1 gene expression. Am J Physiol Lung Cell Mol Physiol. 2002;283:L86–93.
196. Node K, Kitakaze M, Kosaka H, Minamino T, Funaya H, et al. Amelioration of ischemia- and reperfusion-induced myocardial injury by 17β-estradiol: role of nitric oxide and calcium-activated potassium channels. Circulation. 1997;96:1953–63.
197. Prakash YS, Togaibayeva AA, Kannan MS, Miller VM, Fitzpatrick LA, et al. Estrogen increases Ca2+ efflux from female porcine coronary arterial smooth muscle. Am J Physiol. 1999;276:H926–34.
198. Shimokawa H, Takeshita A. Rho-kinase is an important therapeutic target in cardiovascular medicine. Arterioscler Thromb Vasc Biol. 2005;25:1767–75.
199. Sakao S, Tanabe N, Tatsumi K. The estrogen paradox in pulmonary arterial hypertension. Am J Physiol Lung Cell Mol Physiol. 2010;299:L435–8.
200. Smith AM, Jones RD, Channer KS. The influence of sex hormones on pulmonary vascular reactivity: possible vasodilator therapies for the treatment of pulmonary hypertension. Curr Vasc Pharmacol. 2006;4:9–15.
201. Osipenko ON, Alexander D, MacLean MR, Gurney AM. Influence of chronic hypoxia on the contributions of non-inactivating and delayed rectifier K currents to the resting potential and tone of rat pulmonary artery smooth muscle. Br J Pharmacol. 1998;124:1335–7.
202. Millen J, MacLean MR, Houslay MD. Hypoxia-induced remodelling of PDE4 isoform expression and cAMP handling in human pulmonary artery smooth muscle cells. Eur J Cell Biol. 2006;85:679–91.
203. Xu DQ, Luo Y, Liu Y, Wang J, Zhang B, et al. Beta-estradiol attenuates hypoxic pulmonary hypertension by stabilizing the expression of p27kip1 in rats. Respir Res. 2010;11:182.
204. Xu D, Niu W, Luo Y, Zhang B, Liu M, et al. Endogenous estrogen attenuates hypoxia-induced pulmonary hypertension by inhibiting pulmonary arterial vasoconstriction and pulmonary arterial smooth muscle cells proliferation. Int J Med Sci. 2013;10:771–81.
205. Tofovic SP, Zhang X, Zhu H, Jackson EK, Rafikova O, et al. 2-Ethoxyestradiol is antimitogenic and attenuates monocrotaline-induced pulmonary hypertension and vascular remodeling. Vascul Pharmacol. 2008;48:174–83.
206. Lahm T, Albrecht M, Fisher AJ, Selej M, Patel NG, et al. 17beta-Estradiol attenuates hypoxic pulmonary hypertension via estrogen receptor-mediated effects. Am J Respir Crit Care Med. 2012;185:965–80.
207. Farha S, Asosingh K, Laskowski D, Licina L, Sekigushi H, et al. Pulmonary gas transfer related to markers of angiogenesis during the menstrual cycle. J Appl Physiol. 2007;103:1789–95.
208. Malamitsi-Puchner A, Sarandakou A, Tziotis J, Stavreus-Evers A, Tzonou A, et al. Circulating angiogenic factors during periovulation and the luteal phase of normal menstrual cycles. Fertil Steril. 2004;81:1322–7.
209. Demir R, Yaba A, Huppertz B. Vasculogenesis and angiogenesis in the endometrium during menstrual cycle and implantation. Acta Histochem. 2010;112:203–14.
210. English KM, Jones RD, Jones TH, Morice AH, Channer KS. Gender differences in the vasomotor effects of different steroid hormones in rat pulmonary and coronary arteries. Horm Metab Res. 2001;33:645–52.
211. Li HF, Zheng TZ, Li W, Qu SY, Zhang CL. Effect of progesterone on the contractile response of isolated pulmonary artery in rabbits. Can J Physiol Pharmacol. 2001;79:545–50.
212. Smith AM, Bennett RT, Jones TH, Cowen ME, Channer KS, et al. Characterization of the vasodilatory action of testosterone in the human pulmonary circulation. Vasc Health Risk Manag. 2008;4:1459–66.
213. Rowell KO, Hall J, Pugh PJ, Jones TH, Channer KS, et al. Testosterone acts as an efficacious vasodilator in isolated human pulmonary arteries and veins: evidence for a biphasic effect at physiological and supra-physiological concentrations. J Endocrinol Invest. 2009;32:718–23.
214. Farrukh IS, Peng W, Orlinska U, Hoidal JR. Effect of dehydroepiandrosterone on hypoxic pulmonary vasoconstriction: a Ca(2+)-activated K(+)-channel opener. Am J Physiol. 1998;274:L186–95.

215. Gupte SA, Li KX, Okada T, Sato K, Oka M. Inhibitors of pentose phosphate pathway cause vasodilation: involvement of voltage-gated potassium channels. J Pharmacol Exp Ther. 2002;301:299–305.
216. Gordon G, Mackow MC, Levy HR. On the mechanism of interaction of steroids with human glucose 6-phosphate dehydrogenase. Arch Biochem Biophys. 1995;318:25–9.
217. Tian WN, Braunstein LD, Pang J, Stuhlmeier KM, Xi QC, et al. Importance of glucose-6-phosphate dehydrogenase activity for cell growth. J Biol Chem. 1998;273:10609–17.
218. Simoncini T, Mannella P, Fornari L, Varone G, Caruso A, et al. Dehydroepiandrosterone modulates endothelial nitric oxide synthesis via direct genomic and nongenomic mechanisms. Endocrinology. 2003;144:3449–55.
219. Dessouroux A, Akwa Y, Baulieu EE. DHEA decreases HIF-1alpha accumulation under hypoxia in human pulmonary artery cells: potential role in the treatment of pulmonary arterial hypertension. J Steroid Biochem Mol Biol. 2008;109:81–9.
220. Dumas de La Roque E, Savineau JP, Metivier AC, Billes MA, Kraemer JP, et al. Dehydroepiandrosterone (DHEA) improves pulmonary hypertension in chronic obstructive pulmonary disease (COPD): a pilot study. Ann Endocrinol (Paris). 2012;73:20–5.
221. Paulin R, Meloche J, Jacob MH, Bisserier M, Courboulin A, et al. Dehydroepiandrosterone inhibits the Src/STAT3 constitutive activation in pulmonary arterial hypertension. Am J Physiol Heart Circ Physiol. 2011;301:H1798–809.
222. Alzoubi A, Toba M, Abe K, O'Neill KD, Rocic P, et al. Dehydroepiandrosterone restores right ventricular structure and function in rats with severe pulmonary arterial hypertension. Am J Physiol Heart Circ Physiol. 2013;304:H1708–18.
223. Straub RH. The complex role of estrogens in inflammation. Endocr Rev. 2007;28:521–74.
224. Gilliver SC. Sex steroids as inflammatory regulators. J Steroid Biochem Mol Biol. 2010;120:105–15.
225. Pierdominici M, Maselli A, Colasanti T, Giammarioli AM, Delunardo F, et al. Estrogen receptor profiles in human peripheral blood lymphocytes. Immunol Lett. 2010;132:79–85.
226. Cenci S, Weitzmann MN, Roggia C, Namba N, Novack D, et al. Estrogen deficiency induces bone loss by enhancing T-cell production of TNF-alpha. J Clin Invest. 2000;106:1229–37.
227. Lambert KC, Curran EM, Judy BM, Milligan GN, Lubahn DB, et al. Estrogen receptor alpha (ERalpha) deficiency in macrophages results in increased stimulation of CD4+ T cells while 17beta-estradiol acts through ERalpha to increase IL-4 and GATA-3 expression in CD4+ T cells independent of antigen presentation. J Immunol. 2005;175:5716–23.
228. Chiu L, Nishimura M, Ishii Y, Nieda M, Maeshima M, et al. Enhancement of the expression of progesterone receptor on progesterone-treated lymphocytes after immunotherapy in unexplained recurrent spontaneous abortion. Am J Reprod Immunol. 1996;35:552–7.
229. Mansour I, Reznikoff-Etievant MF, Netter A. No evidence for the expression of the progesterone receptor on peripheral blood lymphocytes during pregnancy. Hum Reprod. 1994;9:1546–9.
230. Hardy DB, Janowski BA, Corey DR, Mendelson CR. Progesterone receptor plays a major antiinflammatory role in human myometrial cells by antagonism of nuclear factor-kappaB activation of cyclooxygenase 2 expression. Mol Endocrinol. 2006;20:2724–33.
231. Piccinni MP, Giudizi MG, Biagiotti R, Beloni L, Giannarini L, et al. Progesterone favors the development of human T helper cells producing Th2-type cytokines and promotes both IL-4 production and membrane CD30 expression in established Th1 cell clones. J Immunol. 1995;155:128–33.
232. Huber SA, Kupperman J, Newell MK. Hormonal regulation of CD4(+) T-cell responses in coxsackievirus B3-induced myocarditis in mice. J Virol. 1999;73:4689–95.
233. Namazi MR. The Th1-promoting effects of dehydroepiandrosterone can provide an explanation for the stronger Th1-immune response of women. Iran J Allergy Asthma Immunol. 2009;8:65–9.
234. Yu CK, Liu YH, Chen CL. Dehydroepiandrosterone attenuates allergic airway inflammation in Dermatophagoides farinae-sensitized mice. J Microbiol Immunol Infect. 2002;35:199–202.

235. Suzuki T, Yu HP, Hsieh YC, Choudhry MA, Bland KI, et al. Estrogen-mediated activation of non-genomic pathway improves macrophages cytokine production following trauma-hemorrhage. J Cell Physiol. 2008;214:662–72.
236. Katayama ML, Federico MH, Brentani RR, Brentani MM. Eosinophil accumulation in rat uterus following estradiol administration is modulated by laminin and its integrin receptors. Cell Adhes Commun. 1998;5:409–24.
237. Hamano N, Terada N, Maesako K, Numata T, Konno A. Effect of sex hormones on eosinophilic inflammation in nasal mucosa. Allergy Asthma Proc. 1998;19:263–9.
238. Vasiadi M, Kempuraj D, Boucher W, Kalogeromitros D, Theoharides TC. Progesterone inhibits mast cell secretion. Int J Immunopathol Pharmacol. 2006;19:787–94.
239. Vliagoftis H, Dimitriadou V, Boucher W, Rozniecki JJ, Correia I, et al. Estradiol augments while tamoxifen inhibits rat mast cell secretion. Int Arch Allergy Immunol. 1992;98:398–409.
240. Tchernitchin AN, Barrera J, Arroyo P, Mena MA, Vilches K, et al. Degranulatory action of estradiol on blood eosinophil leukocytes in vivo and in vitro. Agents Actions. 1985;17:60–6.
241. Mayo JC, Sainz RM, Antolin I, Uria H, Menendez-Pelaez A, et al. Androgen-dependent mast cell degranulation in the Harderian gland of female Syrian hamsters: in vivo and organ culture evidence. Anat Embryol (Berl). 1997;196:133–40.
242. Gilroy RJ, Mangura BT, Lavietes MH. Rib cage and abdominal volume displacements during breathing in pregnancy. Am Rev Respir Dis. 1988;137:668–72.
243. Turner AF. The chest radiograph in pregnancy. Clin Obstet Gynecol. 1975;18:65–74.
244. Weinberger SE, Weiss ST, Cohen WR, Weiss JW, Johnson TS. Pregnancy and the lung. Am Rev Respir Dis. 1980;121:559–81.
245. Liberatore SM, Pistelli R, Patalano F, Moneta E, Incalzi RA, et al. Respiratory function during pregnancy. Respiration. 1984;46:145–50.
246. Yannone ME. Plasma progesterone levels in normal pregnancy, labor, and the puerperium. I. Method of assay. Am J Obstet Gynecol. 1968;101:1054–7.
247. Longcope C, Gorbach S, Goldin B, Woods M, Dwyer J, et al. The effect of a low fat diet on estrogen metabolism. J Clin Endocrinol Metab. 1987;64:1246–50.
248. Lakhani NJ, Sarkar MA, Venitz J, Figg WD. 2-Methoxyestradiol, a promising anticancer agent. Pharmacotherapy. 2003;23:165–72.
249. Orentreich N, Brind JL, Rizer RL, Vogelman JH. Age changes and sex differences in serum dehydroepiandrosterone sulfate concentrations throughout adulthood. J Clin Endocrinol Metab. 1984;59:551–5.
250. Mohr BA, Guay AT, O'Donnell AB, McKinlay JB. Normal, bound and nonbound testosterone levels in normally ageing men: results from the Massachusetts Male Ageing Study. Clin Endocrinol (Oxf). 2005;62:64–73.
251. Stricker R, Eberhart R, Chevailler MC, Quinn FA, Bischof P, et al. Establishment of detailed reference values for luteinizing hormone, follicle stimulating hormone, estradiol, and progesterone during different phases of the menstrual cycle on the Abbott ARCHITECT analyzer. Clin Chem Lab Med. 2006;44:883–7.

Chapter 3
Women and COPD

Catherine A. Meldrum and MeiLan K. Han

Abstract While historically COPD has been perceived as a disease of men, the past two decades have seen an increase in COPD prevalence, morbidity, and mortality in women. Total COPD deaths for women in the United States now surpass men. Unfortunately, women with COPD may also be more likely to go undiagnosed or misdiagnosed and are more likely to report diagnostic delay and insufficient access to physicians. The most important risk factor for COPD development in both men and women is tobacco smoke, but data suggest that women are both more susceptible to the effects of tobacco smoke and disproportionately represented in the subset of patients with COPD and no smoking history. Women in developing countries also experience more exposure to biomass smoke, thus increasing their risk for COPD. Women with COPD also report more severe dyspnea and poorer health status for the same level of tobacco exposure as well as experience more frequent exacerbations. From a biologic standpoint, sex hormone differences as well as genetic and epigenetic mechanisms have all been implicated in playing a role in COPD gender differences, but the degree to which biologic, psychological, and sociologic factors contribute to these noted gender differences remains difficult to completely resolve. Fortunately thanks to efforts of both the NIH and FDA, gender differences in COPD are an intense area of research and our understanding of this important arena continues to improve. This chapter focuses both on what we have come to understand about how gender influences disease development, diagnosis, presentation, and progression and on what we have yet to understand that will require further research.

C.A. Meldrum, PhD, RN
University of Michigan, Ann Arbor, MI, USA

M.K. Han, MD, MS (✉)
Department of Internal Medicine, Medical Director, Women's Respiratory Health Program, University of Michigan, Ann Arbor, MI, USA
e-mail: mrking@med.umich.edu

© Springer International Publishing Switzerland 2016
A.R. Hemnes (ed.), *Gender, Sex Hormones and Respiratory Disease*,
Respiratory Medicine, DOI 10.1007/978-3-319-23998-9_3

Introduction

For years, gender differences in pulmonary medicine have not traditionally been either an active area of research or a focus of most clinicians. Unfortunately, this approach led to a relative stagnation in our understanding the role that gender plays in pulmonary physiology and disease. However, in 1993, the U.S. Food and Drug Administration issued a guidance document, *Study and Evaluation of Gender Differences in Clinical Evaluation of Drugs*, recommending collection and analyses of data on sex-specific differences in the efficacy and safety drugs [1]. Then in 1994, the U.S. National Institutes of Health issued guidelines that sex and gender differences be evaluated in clinical trials to ensure safety and efficacy of drugs in the entire target population [2]. Fortunately, these policy changes have resulted in a significant increase in available data regarding how gender can influence all aspects of pulmonary disease, including chronic obstructive pulmonary disease (COPD) in particular.

COPD is defined as a progressive inflammatory disorder characterized by partially reversible airflow obstruction most frequently caused by chronic exposure to tobacco smoke.

Globally COPD is one of the most prevalent health conditions and a major cause of morbidity and mortality. It is estimated that over fifteen million people in the United States are affected by COPD [3, 4] with an estimated 210 million people affected worldwide [5]. While historically COPD has frequently been perceived as a disease of men, the past two decades have seen an increase in COPD prevalence, morbidity, and mortality in women [6]. By 2010, women accounted for 57.2 % of hospital discharges related to COPD [7]. Other gender differences in COPD have been reported ranging from differences in rate of diagnosis, risk factors, and the experience of this disease [8]. This chapter will focus both on what we have come to understand about how gender influences disease development, diagnosis, presentation, and progression and on what we have yet to understand that will require further research.

Risk Factors

By far the biggest risk factor for COPD, particularly in the developed world, is tobacco smoke exposure. In the United States, it is currently estimated that 18.1 % of those over age 18 or an estimated 42.1 million people smoke cigarettes [9]. This is actually a decrease compared to historical figures as can be seen in Fig. 3.1 where smoking rates (1974–2009) for both genders have for the most part decreased since 1974 [2]. In general, more men (20.1 %) in the United States smoke than women (14.5 %). A similar pattern, in general, is seen globally where it is estimated that one billion men and 250 million women smoke on a daily basis [10]. Fortunately, smoking prevalence in the United States has declined with current smoking rates among women in the United States at their lowest levels over the past 40 years [9].

Among young adults, however, the gender gap may be narrowing. Data from the National Survey on Drug Use and Health (NSDUH) presented in Fig. 3.2

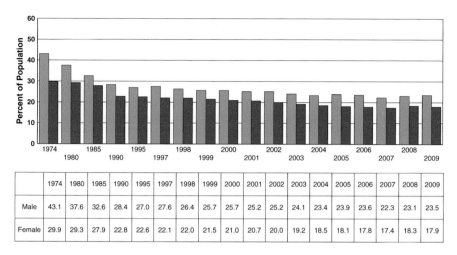

	1974	1980	1985	1990	1995	1997	1998	1999	2000	2001	2002	2003	2004	2005	2006	2007	2008	2009
Male	43.1	37.6	32.6	28.4	27.0	27.6	26.4	25.7	25.7	25.2	25.2	24.1	23.4	23.9	23.6	22.3	23.1	23.5
Female	29.9	29.3	27.9	22.8	22.6	22.1	22.0	21.5	21.0	20.7	20.0	19.2	18.5	18.1	17.8	17.4	18.3	17.9

Fig. 3.1 United States Smoking Rates (1974–2009) [9] Notes: (1) A current smoker is a person who has smoked at least 100 cigarettes and who now smokes. In 1992, the definition of a current smoker was modified to include persons who smoked every day or some days. (2) Because these estimates are based on a sample, they may differ from figures that would be obtained from a census of the population. Each data point reported is an estimate of the true population value and subject to sampling variability

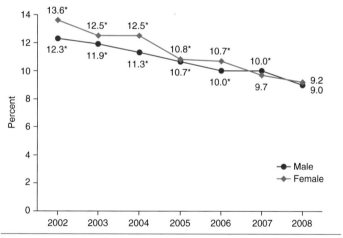

* Difference between this estimate and the 2008 estimate is statistically significant at the .05 level.
Source: 2002 to 2008 SAMHSA National Surveys on Drug Use and Health (NSDUHs).

Fig. 3.2 Past month cigarette use among youths (Aged 12–17 by Gender: 2002–2008)

demonstrate that despite a decline in cigarette use among youths, the decline has been more rapid for males resulting in very little gender difference in cigarette use in this age group as of 2008 [11]. Additionally alarming is the increased use of electronic cigarettes particularly among youth. Many of these products are marketed specifically for women, but the long-term health effects are unknown as well as the likelihood of conversion to other tobacco products.

Also not to be overlooked as a risk factor for COPD is "secondhand" or environmental tobacco smoke exposure [12]. The particle exposure from secondhand smoke mimics that of direct smoking; thus the inflammation and lung tissue damage is expected to be similar to that of direct smoking. Women are more frequently exposed to environmental tobacco smoke [13], particularly in the home [14]. Greater exposure for women may be due to the lag in smoking trends between men and women resulting in more nonsmoking women living with smoking men [13]. Of particular concern, women with low incomes may experience even greater exposure to environmental tobacco smoke [15]. Women with lower incomes may have less ability to limit or control exposure; one study, for instance, demonstrated that smoke-free laws had a greater impact on reducing smoke exposure in "medium-education" females as compared to "low-education" females [16].

For women in developing countries, biomass fuel which is used as a source of energy and cooking is a significant risk factor for COPD particularly in women. Multiple studies have now documented a relationship between biomass exposure and the development of respiratory disease in women [17]. A recent meta-analysis showed that this particular environmental exposure increased the risk of COPD in women 2.4 times more than other fuel types [17]. Other attributable environmental exposures that likely contribute to COPD development include exposures to fumes and biologic and mineral dusts. Biologic dusts include such things as animal dander, bacteria, pollen, and fungi. A recent study demonstrated that exposure to biologic dusts in particular increased risk of COPD in women but not in men [18].

Disease Prevalence

As tobacco is the primary risk factor for COPD in the developed world, generally the prevalence of COPD mirrors tobacco use with greater prevalence of COPD among men. However, it should also be pointed out that due largely to widespread underdiagnosis and underutilization of spirometry, prevalence estimates for COPD have been difficult to ascertain with certainty and vary widely due to differences in methodologies used to capture the data. The National Health Interview Study (NHIS) which is based upon self-report of chronic bronchitis or emphysema suggests the overall prevalence of COPD in the United States to be relatively stable from 1998 through 2009 with prevalence among women higher than men (Table 3.1) in all but the oldest age group [6]. Similarly, age-adjusted prevalence of COPD was also higher in women (7.3 %) than in men (5.7 %) in the Behavioral Risk Factor Surveillance Study (BRFSS) [19] whose methodology was also based upon self-report per telephone contact.

However, data from the National Health and Nutrition Examination Survey (NHANES) reported a lower overall prevalence in the United States of COPD in women (10.8 %) as opposed to men (17.4 %) [20]. This survey used a multistage, probability sampling design where selected individuals actually underwent confirmatory spirometry. It is likely this methodology is more robust than self-report. NHANES data corroborate other global data where a generally higher prevalence among men has also been demonstrated trending similarly with differences in smoking rates [21].

Table 3.1 Prevalence of COPD among adults aged 18 and over: United States 1998–2009

3-year period	Men	Women
1998–2000	4.4 (0.1)	6.7 (0.1)
2001–2003	4.6 (0.1)	6.7 (0.1)
2004–2006	4.3 (0.1)	6.3 (0.1)
2007–2009	4.1 (0.1)	6.1 (0.2)

Notes: COPD is chronic obstructive pulmonary disease. Age adjusted to the 2000 U.S. standard population
Sources: CDC/NCHS, Health Data Interactive and National Health Interview Study

Mortality

COPD is the third leading cause of death in the United States behind cancer and heart disease. Worldwide it is the fourth leading cause of morbidity and mortality, accounting for 5.8 % of all deaths [22]. It has been estimated that the annual deaths from COPD exceed lung cancer and breast cancer combined, accounting for 250 deaths per hour globally [22]. Trends in COPD death rates demonstrate a significant increase for both men and women who are current or former smokers, but the increase is most pronounced among current smokers [23] (Fig. 3.3). Unfortunately it is also projected that deaths from COPD will continue to increase by 30 % over the next 10 years [22].

With respect to gender differences in the United States, total deaths for women due to COPD have exceeded the number in men since 1999 (Table 3.2 and Fig. 3.4) [24]. However, the age-adjusted death rate for COPD is actually 1.3 times greater for men than women [25]. Figure 3.5 demonstrates the age-adjusted death rates for COPD by gender in the United States. The greater death *rate* due to COPD in men may reflect higher prevalence rates of COPD among men. The greater *total number* of COPD deaths for women may reflect more total women at the upper end of the age spectrum at risk for COPD death; women in general live longer [26] and may not be dying earlier of other causes as their male counterparts but rather living long enough to die of COPD.

Bias in Diagnosis

An important feature of this chronic disease is the high rate of underdiagnosis for both genders. It is estimated that in the United States alone over 14 million people remain undiagnosed [3]. Furthermore, spirometry remains highly underutilized with only about a third of individuals who have been given a diagnosis of COPD having undergone confirmatory spirometry which also opens the door for misdiagnosis [27]. Any person who has dyspnea, sputum production, chronic cough, family history of COPD, or a history of exposure to risk factors (tobacco smoke, occupational chemicals/dust, smoke from fuels, and home cooking) should be evaluated for COPD [28]. From a clinical standpoint, spirometry is required to make a

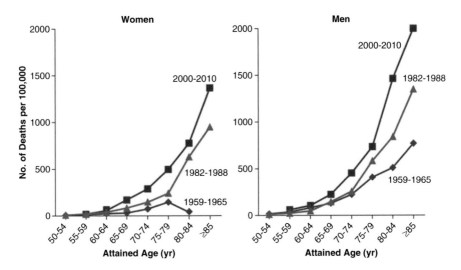

Fig. 3.3 Changes in rates of death from chronic obstructive pulmonary disease (COPD) over time among current female and male smokers in the three time periods [23]

Table 3.2 Number of COPD deaths by Gender in the United States, 1999–2009

Year	Men	Women
1999	60,795	58,729
2000	58,372	59,510
2001	58,218	60,526
2002	59,133	61,422
2003	59,321	63,062
2004	57,260	60,911
2005	61,120	65,929
2006	57,964	63,006
2007	59,961	64,516
2008	65,936	71,757
2009	63,899	70,066

Sources: Centers for Disease Control and Prevention, National Center for Health Statistics, CDC Wonder On-Line Database, compiled from Compressed Mortality File (1999–2009 Series 20 No. 20, 2012

diagnosis of airflow obstruction [29]. It is estimated that of those undiagnosed, the majority are those with mild to moderate disease where arguably interventions such as smoking cessation would have the most long-term impact [30, 31].

With respect to gender bias in diagnosis, several studies have attempted to address this question. The first was a survey of primary care physicians in North America where a prototypical history of cough and dyspnea in a smoker were presented [32]. Primary care physicians were surveyed for a likely diagnosis given history and physical examination results where half the surveys described the patient

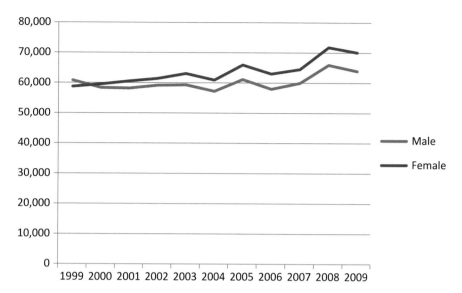

Fig. 3.4 COPD—Number of deaths by sex, 1999–2009 [106]

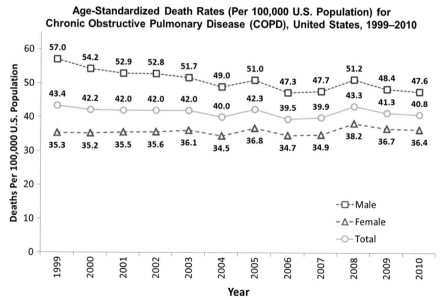

Fig. 3.5 Age-standardized death rates (Per 100,000 U.S. Population) for chronic obstructive pulmonary disease (COPD), United States, 1999–2010 [107]

as female and the other half as male. The likelihood of a correct COPD diagnosis was significantly greater for men than women (64.6 % vs. 49.9 %; $p=0.05$) with greater likelihood of misdiagnosis of asthma in women. Once survey respondents were provided with spirometry, the gender gap in misdiagnosis narrowed was still present. A similar follow-up survey study was conducted in Europe which also demonstrated increased misdiagnosis in women which disappeared when physicians were presented with spirometric data suggesting some improvement in physician gender bias [31]. A recent population-based survey in Spain also reported women (86.0 %) were 1.27 times more likely to be underdiagnosed than men (65.6 %) [33].

Survey data from the United States also suggest that women are also more likely to perceive a delay in diagnosis attributing lack of availability of providers and insurance issues [34]. If women are being underdiagnosed, there are several potential reasons. As smoking and COPD are generally more prevalent in men, as the studies presented suggest, physicians may be more likely to suspect a diagnosis of COPD in men. Gender differences in clinical presentation may also contribute to bias in the diagnosis [35–38]. While smoking is the most significant risk factor for COPD in the developed world, women make up the majority of individuals with COPD who are nonsmokers and as such may not match the risk profile that care providers typically look for [39]. Socioeconomic differences and access to health care could also play a role. These data underscore the need for increased patient and physician awareness as well as the importance of appropriate diagnostic testing in symptomatic patients.

Tobacco Susceptibility

While more men than women may smoke, data suggest that women may be more susceptible to the harmful effects of tobacco smoke [40–42]. The Lung Health Study demonstrated a more rapid decline in women who continued to smoke as compared to men [43]. A systematic review and meta-analysis concluded that women experience a greater rate of decline in lung function than men for a similar amount of tobacco exposure [44] (Fig. 3.6). Data from the National Emphysema Treatment Trial also demonstrated that women with similar severe lung function to their male counterparts had fewer pack-years of smoking history [38].

Several hypotheses have been offered as possible explanations for the increased susceptibility of women as compared to men to effects of tobacco smoke exposure. The lungs of women are relatively smaller than those of men, and thus each cigarette smoked may represent a higher relative "dose" for women. Some researchers have suggested that women may underreport tobacco use. However, this question has been examined. A meta-analysis of studies on tobacco reporting concluded that self-reported smoking data among women are generally accurate [45]. Secondhand smoke exposure and differences in cigarette brand preferences could also contribute to differences in susceptibility. Biological or hormonal differences between men and women have also been hypothesized to influence tobacco susceptibility [36, 37,

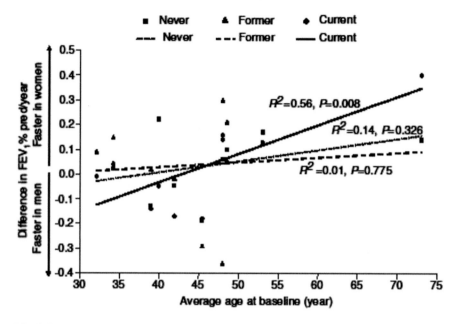

Fig. 3.6 Unweighted analysis of the relationship between age- and gender-related differences in the annual decline in FEV1 percentage predicted according to smoking status [44]

46, 47]. For instance, women have increased oxidative metabolism of several components of tobacco smoke. As a result, women may effectively experience a relatively higher and more prolonged exposure to oxidative substances that could accelerate the development of tobacco-related diseases, including lung cancer [48].

Disease Presentation

It is well established that the presence of cough, sputum production, and shortness of breath are classic symptoms of COPD, although increasing evidence suggests a difference in clinical symptom presentation by gender [49–51]. Most studies have found women to report more dyspnea than men despite similar lung function testing and fewer pack-years of smoking [35, 52, 53], although the data across studies are not completely consistent. The Confronting COPD International Survey demonstrated women were more likely to report severe dyspnea (OR, 1.30; 95 % CI, 1.10–1.54) despite significantly fewer pack-years of smoking, while reporting similar degrees of cough (OR, 84; 95 % CI, 0.72–0.98) [53]. In another prospective study of symptoms in male and female patients with mild to moderate COPD, similar proportions of men and women reported symptoms despite significantly greater pack-years of smoking in men [54]. Data from the international BREATHE study (Algeria, Egypt, Jordan, Lebanon, Morocco, Saudi Arabia, Syria, Tunisia, Turkey,

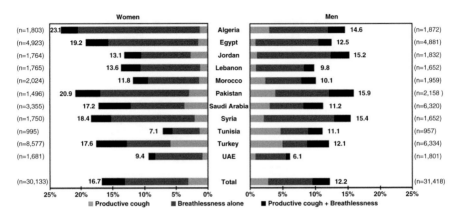

Fig. 3.7 Age-adjusted prevalence of respiratory symptoms by gender [55]

and United Arab Emirates) (Fig. 3.7) also reported that respiratory symptoms (productive cough and/or breathlessness) were more frequently observed in women than men [55]. On the contrary another study from the United States found no difference in severe shortness of breath experienced between genders and decreased reports of cough by women [34]. Differences in sputum production are also not consistent. Some studies have reported men having a higher rate of productive cough than women, while other cite no differences in sputum production reporting [53, 56, 57]. Some have suspected that differences in sputum production reporting may be related to willingness of women to report such symptoms.

Health-related quality of life (HRQOL) encompasses several dimensions including functional and symptom status, perception of health, biological/physical factors, and overall well-being [58]. It has been demonstrated that how one perceives HRQOL can impact health care outcomes [59]. Women tend to experience lower HRQOL than men as a result of COPD [52], even with similar lung function [35]. Gender differences have also been observed in the factors associated with decreased health-related quality of life. Chronic cough and sputum production, dyspnea, and oxygenation have been reported as significant predictors of a decreased health-related quality of life in women [8, 35], whereas exercise capacity, dyspnea, severity of lung hyperinflation, and comorbidities were reported as significant predictors of decreased health-related quality of life in men [35].

Other factors that may also contribute to this difference between genders include greater prevalence of anxiety and depression and increased frequency of COPD exacerbations among women [49, 52, 60–62]. Anxiety and depression are particularly pronounced in patients with COPD requiring hospitalization. Two studies of hospitalized patients with COPD recorded significantly higher anxiety scores in women than men [63, 64]. This is a particularly important issue as the risk of rehospitalization for patients with COPD has been demonstrated to be increased for patients with anxiety and low health status [65].

The experience of dyspnea encompasses physical, affective, and cognitive dimensions and the impact of dyspnea is a result not only by the degree of lung dysfunction but also the individual's emotional response and interpretation of that sensation [46]. Neurobiologic studies demonstrate women have greater intrinsic sensitivity to noxious somatic sensations such as dyspnea [40]. Gender differences in the laterality of prefrontal cortical processing of noxious stimuli have been demonstrated with neuroimaging studies [66]. The prefrontal cortex is involved in the cognitive modulation of emotion and therefore may play a role in gender differences in the interpretation of dyspnea.

Health Care Utilization and Management

The presence of a chronic disease is associated with expected increases in health care utilization. Several large trials have provided data regarding COPD exacerbations in men and women. The Understanding of the Potential Long-Term Impact of Tiotropium (UPLIFT) study followed nearly 6000 COPD patients over a 4-year time period treated with tiotropium versus placebo [67]. Overall exacerbation rates including moderate and severe events were higher for women as compared to men ($p < 0.001$; 95 % CI; 16–34 %) [67] (Fig. 3.8). The Toward a Revolution in COPD Health study (TORCH) evaluated the risk of death in over 6000 COPD patients over a 3-year time period treated with salmeterol and fluticasone, salmeterol alone, or fluticasone alone. Again, higher rates of exacerbations were noted in women, but similar rates of exacerbation-related hospitalizations were noted between genders [67]. COPDGene, a large observational study of approximately 10,000 patients,

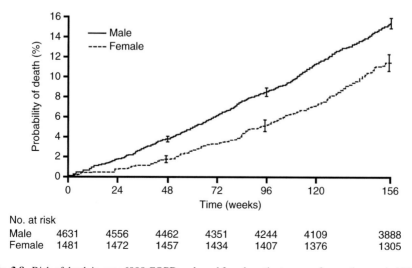

Fig. 3.8 Risk of death in over 6000 COPD male and female patients over a 3-year time period [49]

also reported increased rates of exacerbations in women as compared to men [68]. Additionally, there is a shorter time to one's first COPD exacerbation in women than men [49]. At this point, however, it is unknown whether these differences reflect a difference in disease biology, likelihood of reporting symptoms, or another factor such as differential presence of comorbidities. It has been hypothesized that diastolic dysfunction may play a role in COPD exacerbations [69], and it is well documented that diastolic heart failure, for instance, is more prevalent in women [70].

Interestingly, women's perception of health care management differs from that of men. Martinez et al. found that as compared to men, women were more likely to report that the amount of time spent with physician was insufficient and that it was difficult getting access to them when they need them [34]. The time in obtaining a diagnosis was perceived to be longer for women and they felt less educational information was provided to them by their physicians than men [34]. They were also more likely than men to seek out health information from other patients and online sources [34]. Despite this difference, however, both men and women were equally satisfied with their overall disease management.

Differences in Disease Biology and Phenotype

In theory, gender differences in COPD between men and women may result from biologic, social, or psychosocial factors, but teasing out the specific factor(s) for any particular aspect of the disease remains challenging. Sex hormone differences have been implicated as having a contributory role, and developmental data would suggest that sex hormones affect airway function [40]. Boys, for instance, have higher incidence of asthma than girls until age 15 [40]. Following that, the reverse occurs where the incidence rate is higher in girls than in boys until the perimenopause [40]. The change in asthma incidence in girls coincident with puberty and menopause suggests a potential role for sex hormones in airway function in asthma, but as of yet, teasing out a similar relationship in COPD has proven elusive. A cohort study evaluating the association between postmenopausal hormone use and new diagnoses of asthma or COPD reported an increased risk of asthma compared with non-hormone use but no difference in incidence of newly diagnosed COPD [71]. Thus, while sex hormones appear to play a role in asthma, their contribution to COPD pathogenesis and gender differences in COPD remain unclear.

Disease physiology may also differ between men and women with COPD. For instance, the National Emphysema Trial (NETT) reported that in a population of patients with severe emphysema, men were more likely than women to demonstrate bronchoreversibility [72]. However, the Lung Health Study found no difference in the frequency of bronchodilator response between men and women in a much milder patient population [73]. Therefore, the relationship between gender and bronchoreversibility in COPD may also be complicated by the amount of emphysema or overall disease severity.

Differences in radiographic type and distribution of lung abnormality between men and women with COPD have also been reported. The NETT reported that women had less severe overall emphysema, particularly in the periphery of the lung [74]. Histologic examination of resected tissue also suggested that the bronchioles in female patients had significantly thicker airway walls and smaller lumens. Interestingly, gender dimorphism in COPD was first suggested by Burrows et al. in 1987 when they hypothesized that there were two primary types of COPD: chronic asthmatic bronchitis and emphysema [75]. Burrows reported that in their cohort, those with chronic asthmatic bronchitis were more frequently female, whereas the emphysematous group were primarily male. More recent data from the COPDGene study also suggest that as compared to women, men in general had greater radiographically detected emphysema. However, in subjects with severe disease that would be more similar to the NETT patient population, no obvious differences in the amount of emphysema between men and women were seen although the distribution (peel versus core) in this study has not yet been examined. However, data from COPDGene did suggest that the wall area percent (wall thickness/total thickness) for subsegmental and subsubsegmental airways of women is greater than for men [37]. These phenotypic differences, if real, could potentially have important therapeutic implications.

Gender differences in genetic mechanisms in the pathogenesis of COPD may also exist. A study of early-onset COPD families found 71.4 % of those affected were women [76]. Furthermore, analysis of first-degree relatives of probands who were current or former smokers showed that female first-degree relatives had significantly greater lung function than their male first-degree relatives. These differences were only seen among current or ex-smokers, implying a genetic predisposition for smoking-related lung damage that is gender specific. Another study by the same group but in a different cohort again found that subjects with severe, early-onset COPD were predominantly female. A history of maternal respiratory disease was also present in many suggesting that mitochondrial DNA and X chromosome genes [77] could be playing a role and need to be further investigated.

Several studies over the past 10 years have also explored epigenetic mechanisms that contribute to COPD pathophysiology [78, 79] which certainly could play a role in gender differences in COPD. Hormone-induced DNA methylation and histone modification have been suggested by several lines of evidence, although this has not specifically yet been examined as a cause for gender differences in COPD [80]. Differences in gene expression, however, have been reported between men and women with COPD. Recently, sputum and blood were analyzed from participants in the ECLIPSE study, an observational cohort study in COPD [81]. The authors specifically examined genetic regulation pathways and determined that many genes important for mitochondrial functional, energy metabolism, and cellular response to pathogens show sex-specific regulatory connections [81]. These data suggest that many cellular functions may be under sex-specific regulatory control which could have very important implications ranging from disease pathogenesis to therapeutics.

Comorbidities in COPD

The importance of comorbidities in COPD is becoming increasingly recognized. Certain comorbid conditions such as cardiovascular disease and osteoporosis are more common in the COPD patient population. Other comorbidities such as overlap syndrome, the coexistence of COPD, and obstructive sleep apnea may not be more prevalent in COPD but are important as they may modify disease course [82]. Diabetes, hypertension, cardiovascular disease, and cancer have all been reported to increase the risk of death in COPD as well as significantly increase health care costs [83, 84, 85]. Certain comorbidities do appear to be more common in men versus women with COPD and therefore are worthy of discussion here. As was discussed earlier, anxiety and depression have been reported more frequently in women with COPD which may influence disease presentation and disease impact. In the general population, ischemic cardiac disease and systolic heart failure are in general more common in men while diastolic heart failure is more common in women [86]. In COPD specifically, a study of comorbidity in patients hospitalized for COPD also reported women to have a lower prevalence of ischemic heart disease but interestingly greater prevalence of heart failure, suggesting that diastolic dysfunction which is a more frequent cause of non-ischemic heart failure could be playing a greater role in women hospitalized with COPD [60]. Both ischemic heart disease and diastolic dysfunction could conceivably alter symptoms and quality of life or complicate or mimic exacerbations and thereby alter the presentation and clinical course for men versus women with COPD.

Osteoporosis is seen more frequently in women than men in the general population and even COPD is reported more frequently by women [87]. Intriguingly, data from the COPDGene study using CT scans to analyze bone mineral density recently demonstrated that male smokers had a small but significantly greater risk of low bone density and vertebral fractures as compared to female smokers [88]. Presence of COPD itself was also associated with lower bone mineral density. This study also showed an association between CT detected airway disease and higher bone density. It has also been previously demonstrated that there is an association between emphysema and lower bone density. Thus, it is possible that women with COPD may be more prone to an "airway disease, high bone density" disease phenotype and men to an "emphysema, low bone density" phenotype.

Therapeutic Implications

Tobacco Cessation

There is continued controversy as to whether there are gender differences in the ability to stop smoking. The US Surgeon General's report on women and smoking from 2001 concluded that women have more difficulty giving up smoking than men,

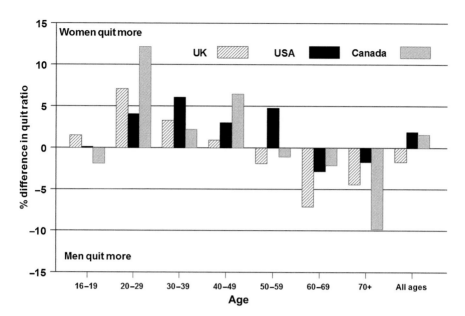

Fig. 3.9 Gender differences in quitting (female quit ratio–male quit ratio) by age group in the USA, Canada, and Britain [108]

both at short-term and long-term follow-up [89]. In studies using behavioral therapy, nicotine replacement, and bupropion, higher rates of tobacco cessation have been observed in men [43, 90–92]. However, the truth may be more complicated. In a study done in the United States, Canada, and United Kingdom using data from three majors surveys, it was found that younger women below the age of 50 were more likely to quit smoking than men, but after age 50 men were more likely to quit than women (Fig. 3.9).

Some theorize that gender differences exist because of the variance in seeking tobacco cessation assistance between men and women and therefore clinical trial results are not generalizable to the general population. According to the Centers for Disease Control (CDC), almost 70 % of United States adult smokers want to quit smoking. Women were most interested in quitting, had a higher past year quit attempt, and had a higher recent smoking cessation rate (Table 3.3).

Data from the National Health Interview Survey (United States, 2010) also support the claim than women have a higher prevalence of receiving information from a health provider on smoking cessation and using counseling and/or medication to assist in tobacco cessation (Table 3.4). Smoking is the most frequent cause of COPD in both genders, and consequently smoking cessation is the primary intervention to slow down the decline of lung function [93]. As discussed earlier, women may have more susceptibility to the effects of tobacco smoke so it is crucial for health care professionals to discuss smoking cessation with women as early as possible. Data from the Lung Health Study also suggest that smoking cessation may allow for a greater improvement in lung function especially in women [94]. However, recent

Table 3.3 Prevalence of interest in quitting,[a] past year quit attempt,[b] and recent smoking cessation[c] among adult smokers aged ≥18 years, by selected characteristics—National Health Interview Survey, United States, 2010

Characteristic	Interested in quitting		Past year quit attempt		Recent smoking cessation[d]	
	%	(95 % CI)	%	(95 % CI)	%	(95 % CI)
Overall	68.8	(67.2–70.5)	52.4	(50.7–54.0)	6.2	(5.4–7.0)
Sex						
Men	67.3	(65.0–69.6)	51.1	(48.8–53.4)	6.2	(5.1–7.2)
Women	70.7	(68.5–72.8)	53.8	(51.6–56.0)	6.3	(5.1–7.4)

Abbreviations: *CI* confidence interval
[a]Current smokers who reported that they wanted to stop smoking completely. Excludes 190 respondents whose smoking status was unknown
[b]Current smokers who reported that they stopped smoking for >1 day in the past 12 months because they were trying to quit smoking and former smokers who quit in the past year
[c]Former smokers who quit smoking in the past year for ≥6 months. Excludes 190 respondents whose smoking status was unknown
[d]Among current smokers who smoked for at least 2 years and former smokers who quit in the past year

Table 3.4 Prevalence of receiving a health professional's advice to quit smoking[a] and use of counseling[b] and medications[c] for cessation among adult smokers aged ≥18 years, by selected characteristics—National Health Interview Survey, United States, 2010

Characteristic	Received health professional's advice to quit		Used counseling		Used medication		Used counseling and/or medication	
	%	(95 % CI)	%	(95 % CI)	%	(95 % CI)	%	(95 % CI)
Overall	48.3	(46.5, 50.0)	5.9	(4.8, 7.1)	30.0	(28.2, 31.9)	31.7	(29.9, 33.6)
Sex								
Men	44.8	(42.2, 47.3)	5.3	(3.9, 6.8)	27.3	(24.5, 30.0)	28.8	(26.1, 31.6)
Women	51.7	(49.4, 54.1)	6.7	(5.0, 8.4)	33.2	(30.4, 36.1)	35.1	(32.0, 38.1)

Abbreviations: *CI* confidence interval
[a]Received advice from a medical doctor, dentist, or other health professional to quit smoking or quit using other kinds of tobacco among current smokers and those who quit in the last year who saw a doctor or other health professional in the past year. Excludes 190 respondents whose smoking status was unknown
[b]Used one-on-one counseling; a stop smoking clinic, class, or support group; and/or a telephone helpline or quitline in the past year among current smokers who tried to quit in the past year or used when stopped smoking among former smokers who quit in the past 2 years
[c]Used nicotine patch, nicotine gum or lozenge, nicotine-containing nasal spray or inhaler, varenicline (U.S. trade name Chantix), and/or bupropion (including trade names Zyban and Wellbutrin) in the past year among current smokers who tried to quit in the past year or used when stopped smoking among former smokers who quit in the past 2 years

evidence indicates differences between men and women in smoking treatment effectiveness and their biological response to nicotine [95, 96, 95]. Though some nicotine products appear to be equally effective for both genders, the reports on nicotine replacement therapy are inconsistent. Some report a less effectiveness in women though others found no gender differences in the outcomes [97, 98]. No significant gender differences in the efficacy of varenicline or bupropion have been reported.

Pharmacotherapeutics

Inhaled bronchodilators and bronchodilator/corticosteroid combinations are the mainstay of maintenance therapy for COPD. Based on available data to date, these classes of medications generally appear to work equally in men and women in terms of lung function improvement and exacerbation frequency reduction. The Euroscop study suggested that inhaled steroid use might improve phlegm production in men but not women [53]. The probability of respiratory deterioration when stopping inhaled steroids has also been suggested to be higher in woman than men with COPD [99]. No gender differences have been reported for other classes of therapeutics used in COPD including roflumilast, a PDE4 inhibitor recently approved for the treatment of COPD in those with chronic bronchitis and frequent exacerbations or azithromycin which was recently demonstrated to reduce the frequency of COPD exacerbations [100, 101].

Pulmonary Rehabilitation

Pulmonary rehabilitation has been thoroughly evaluated in numerous large clinical trials with the goals of reducing symptoms, increasing physical activity, and improving quality of life. Pulmonary rehabilitation participation has been reported as being similar between genders. Unfortunately, both men and women report similar health care management experiences with regard to the lack of access to these programs or the sheer existence of a program being available [34].

Oxygen Therapy

There may be differences in the frequency of oxygen prescriptions between men and women and its subsequent effect. In Sweden, oxygen prescriptions for women appear to be increasing at a more rapid rate than men [102]. In 2000 the rates for women who were prescribed oxygen therapy were 7.6 per 100,000 compared with 7.1 in men. There is conflicting data on long-term outcomes of women using oxygen. Machado et al. found survival to be significantly worse for female long-term oxygen therapy users than men [103]. On the contrary, others have found a greater

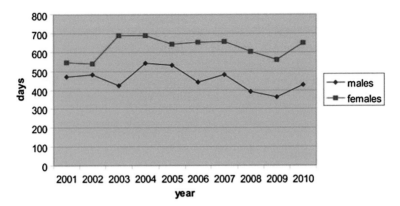

Fig. 3.10 Median survivals in patients with COPD receiving LTOT according to year of entrance for males and females, respectively [105]

survival in women prescribed oxygen compared to men [104]. More recent data (Fig. 3.10) from Denmark also support improved survival and a significant decreased risk of death (p = <0.001) in women using oxygen as compared to men [105]. Interestingly, compliance for using oxygen therapy as prescribed for men and women shows similar results [34]. The Long-Term Oxygen Treatment Trial, cosponsored by the National Institutes of Health and the Center for Medicare Services, will hopefully be able to shed light on this issue. While both men and women with COPD and severe hypoxia experience mortality benefit, it is not clear whether supplemental oxygen treatment in men or women provides long-term outcome improvements in those with more mild to moderate levels of hypoxemia.

Conclusions

There have been numerous interventional and observational studies done identifying gender differences in those with COPD. Given the increasing burden of COPD in women, it is critically important to understand the gender differences that exist within this disease. This remains, however, a challenging area of investigation as differences may be due to biologic, social, or psychologic factors. While we lack a full understanding of the mechanisms for these gender differences, a more gender-specific approach for COPD for treatment may be warranted.

Women may differ in the presentation of symptoms and the needs they have from their care providers. Gender-specific comorbidities and the differential impact of the disease itself on women must be addressed in order to improve the quality of life for women with COPD. It is well recognized that proper treatment can significantly improve the outcome of the disease. It is essential that future research help delineate the pathophysiology and treatment response in COPD taking into account gender as this could impact both pharmacological and non-pharmacological interventions.

References

1. Food and Drug Administration. Guideline for the study and evaluation of gender differences in the clinical evaluation of drugs. Fed Regist. 1993;58:39406–16.
2. National Institutes of Health. NIH Guidelines on the inclusion of women and minorities as subjects in clinical research. Fed Regist. 1994;59:14508–13.
3. Chronic Obstructive Pulmonary Disease Among Adults—United States, 2011. Morb Mortal Wkly Rep 2012;61(46):938–943.
4. Hoyert DL. Deaths: preliminary data for 2011. Natl Vital Stat Rep. 2012;61:1.
5. Aryal S, Diaz-Guzman E, Mannino DM. COPD and gender differences: an update. Transl Res. 2013;162:208–18.
6. Akinbami LJ. Chronic obstructive pulmonary disease among adults aged 18 and over in the United States, 1998–2009. Women (Oxford, England). 2013;6:8.
7. Centers for Disease Control and Prevention. National Center for Health Statistics. National Hospital Discharge Survey. In: Education ALARaH, ed. 2010.
8. Raherison C. Clinical characteristics and quality of life in women with COPD: an observational study. BMC Womens Health. 2014;14:31.
9. CDC. Current cigarette smoking among adults-US 2011. Morb Mortal Wkly Rep. 2012;61:5.
10. Fronczak A, Polańska K, Makowiec-Dabrowska T, Kaleta D. Smoking among women—strategies for fighting the tobacco epidemic. Przegl Lek. 2012;69:1103.
11. Garrett BE, Dube SR, Trosclair A, et al. Cigarette smoking—united states, 1965–2008. MMWR Surveill Summ. 2011;60:109–13.
12. Hemsing N. Women, environments and chronic disease: shifting the gaze from individual level to structural factors. Environ Health Insights. 2009;2:127–35.
13. Siegfried JM. Women and lung cancer: does oestrogen play a role? Lancet Oncol. 2001; 2:506–13.
14. Ernster V, Kaufman N, Nichter M, Samet J, Yoon S-Y. Women and tobacco: moving from policy to action. Bull World Health Organ. 2000;78:891–901.
15. Amos A, Greaves L, Nichter M, Bloch M. Women and tobacco: a call for including gender in tobacco control research, policy and practice. Tob Control. 2011;21:236–43.
16. Levy DT, Mumford EA, Compton C. Tobacco control policies and smoking in a population of low education women, 1992–2002. J Epidemiol Commun Health. 2006;60:20–6.
17. Po JYT, FitzGerald JM, Carlsten C. Respiratory disease associated with solid biomass fuel exposure in rural women and children: systematic review and meta-analysis. Thorax. 2011;66:232–9.
18. Matheson MC, Benke G, Raven J, et al. Biological dust exposure in the workplace is a risk factor for chronic obstructive pulmonary disease. Thorax. 2005;60:645–51.
19. Li C, Balluz LS, Ford ES, Okoro CA, Zhao G, Pierannunzi C. A comparison of prevalence estimates for selected health indicators and chronic diseases or conditions from the Behavioral Risk Factor Surveillance System, the National Health Interview Survey, and the National Health and Nutrition Examination Survey, 2007–2008. Prev Med. 2012;54:381–7.
20. Tilert T, Dillon C, Paulose-Ram R, Hnizdo E, Doney B. Estimating the U.S. prevalence of chronic obstructive pulmonary disease using pre- and post-bronchodilator spirometry: the National Health and Nutrition Examination Survey (NHANES) 2007–2010. Respir Res. 2013;14:103.
21. Landis SH. Continuing to Confront COPD International Patient Survey: methods, COPD prevalence, and disease burden in 2012–2013. Int J Chronic Obstructive Pulmon Dis. 2014;9:597.
22. WHO. World Health Statistics 2008: World Health Organization; 2008.
23. Thun MJ, Carter BD, Feskanich D, et al. 50-year trends in smoking-related mortality in the United States. N Engl J Med. 2013;368:351–64.
24. Centers for Disease Control and Prevention. Deaths from chronic obstructive pulmonary disease—United States, 2000–2005. MMWR Morb Mortal Wkly Rep. 2008;57:1229–32.

25. Ford ES, Croft JB, Mannino DM, Wheaton AG, Zhang X, Giles WH. COPD surveillance—United States, 1999–2011. Chest. 2013;144:284–305.
26. Olshansky SJ, Antonucci T, Berkman L, et al. Differences in life expectancy due to race and educational differences are widening, and many may not catch up. Health Aff. 2012;31: 1803–13.
27. Han MK, Kim MG, Mardon R, et al. Spirometry utilization for COPD: how do we measure up? Chest. 2007;132:403–9.
28. ATS/ERS Task Force. Standards for the diagnosis and management of patients with COPD [Internet]. Version 1.2. New York: American Thoracic Society; 2004 9-8-2003.
29. Zwar NA, Marks GB, Hermiz O, et al. Predictors of accuracy of diagnosis of chronic obstructive pulmonary disease in general practice. Med J Aust. 2011;195:168–71.
30. Hvidsten SC, Storesund L, Wentzel-Larsen T, Gulsvik A, Lehmann S. Prevalence and predictors of undiagnosed chronic obstructive pulmonary disease in a Norwegian adult general population. Clin Respir J. 2010;4:13–21.
31. Miravitlles M, Soriano JB, García-Río F, et al. Prevalence of COPD in Spain: impact of undiagnosed COPD on quality of life and daily life activities. Thorax. 2009;64:863–8.
32. Chapman KR, Tashkin DP, Pye DJ. Gender bias in the diagnosis of COPD. Chest. 2001;119:1691–5.
33. Ancochea J, Miravitlles M, García-Río F, et al. Underdiagnosis of chronic obstructive pulmonary disease in women: quantification of the problem, determinants and proposed actions. Arch Bronconeumol. 2013;49:223–9 (English Edition).
34. Martinez CH, Raparla S, Plauschinat CA, et al. Gender differences in symptoms and care delivery for chronic obstructive pulmonary disease. J Womens Health. 2012;21:1267–74.
35. de Torres JP. Gender associated differences in determinants of quality of life in patients with COPD: a case series study. Health Qual Life Outcomes. 2006;4:72.
36. de Torres JP, Casanova C, Cote CG, et al. Six-minute walking distance in women with COPD. COPD—J Chron Obstruct Pulmon Dis. 2011;8:300–5.
37. Kim YI, Schroeder J, Lynch D, et al. Gender differences of airway dimensions in anatomically matched sites on CT in smokers. COPD—J Chron Obstruct Pulmon Dis. 2011;8:285–92.
38. Varkey AB. Chronic obstructive pulmonary disease in women: exploring gender differences. Curr Opin Pulm Med. 2004;10:98–103.
39. Birring SS, Brightling CE, Bradding P, et al. Clinical, radiologic, and induced sputum features of chronic obstructive pulmonary disease in nonsmokers: a descriptive study. Am J Respir Crit Care Med. 2002;166:1078–83.
40. Becklake MR, Kauffmann F. Gender differences in airway behaviour over the human life span. Thorax. 1999;54:1119–38.
41. Langhammer A, Johnsen R, Holmen J, Gulsvik A, Bjermer L. Cigarette smoking gives more respiratory symptoms among women than among men The Nord-Trøndelag Health Study (HUNT). J Epidemiol Community Health. 2000;54:917–22.
42. Rennard S. Impact of COPD in North America and Europe in 2000: subjects' perspective of Confronting COPD International Survey. Eur Respir J. 2002;20:799–805.
43. Bjornson W. Gender differences in smoking cessation after 3 years in the Lung Health Study. Am J Publ Health (1971). 1995;85:223–30.
44. Gan W, Man S, Postma D, Camp P, Sin D. Female smokers beyond the perimenopausal period are at increased risk of chronic obstructive pulmonary disease: a systematic review and meta-analysis. Respir Res. 2006;7:52.
45. Patrick DL. The validity of self-reported smoking: a review and meta-analysis. Am J Publ Health (1971). 1994;84:1086–93.
46. Han MK, Postma D, Mannino DM, et al. Gender and chronic obstructive pulmonary disease. Am J Respir Crit Care Med. 2007;176:1179–84.
47. Kim DK, Hersh CP, Washko GR, et al. Epidemiology, radiology, and genetics of nicotine dependence in COPD. Respir Res. 2011;12:9.
48. Uppstad H, Osnes GH, Cole KJ, Phillips DH, Haugen A, Mollerup S. Sex differences in susceptibility to PAHs is an intrinsic property of human lung adenocarcinoma cells. Lung Cancer. 2011;71:264–70.

49. Celli B, Vestbo J, Jenkins CR, et al. Sex differences in mortality and clinical expressions of patients with chronic obstructive pulmonary disease. Am J Respir Crit Care Med. 2011;183: 317–22.
50. Lamprecht B, Vanfleteren LE, Studnicka M, et al. Sex-related differences in respiratory symptoms: results from the BOLD Study. Eur Respir J. 2013;42:858–60.
51. Vestbo J, Prescott E, Lange P. Association of chronic mucus hypersecretion with FEV1 decline and chronic obstructive pulmonary disease morbidity. Copenhagen City Heart Study Group. Am J Respir Crit Care Med. 1996;153:1530–5.
52. Di Marco F, Verga M, Reggente M, et al. Anxiety and depression in COPD patients: the roles of gender and disease severity. Respir Med. 2006;100:1767–74.
53. Watson L. Gender differences in the management and experience of Chronic Obstructive Pulmonary Disease. Respir Med. 2004;98:1207–13.
54. Watson L, Vonk JM, Löfdahl CG, et al. Predictors of lung function and its decline in mild to moderate COPD in association with gender: results from the Euroscop study. Respir Med. 2006;100:746–53.
55. Tageldin MA, Nafti S, Khan JA, et al. Distribution of COPD-related symptoms in the Middle East and North Africa: results of the BREATHE study. Respiratory Medicine. 2012;106 Suppl 2:S25–32.
56. Cydulka RK. Gender differences in emergency department patients with chronic obstructive pulmonary disease exacerbation. Acad Emerg Med. 2005;12:1173.
57. Martinez CH, Raparla S, Plaushinat CA, et al. Gender differences in the COPD Resource Network Needs Assessment Survey 2007. Am J Respir Crit Care Med. 2011;183:A1461.
58. Wilson IB. Linking clinical variables with health-related quality of life a conceptual model of patient outcomes. JAMA. 1995;273:59.
59. Schmier JK. The impact of asthma on health-related quality of life. J Asthma. 1998;35:585–97.
60. Almagro P, López García F, Cabrera FJ, et al. Comorbidity and gender-related differences in patients hospitalized for COPD. The ECCO study. Respir Med. 2010;104:253–9.
61. Ninot G. Stability of physical self: examining the role of chronic obstructive pulmonary disease. Revue européenne de psychologie appliquée. 2010;60:35–40.
62. Gift AG. Fatigue and other symptoms in patients with chronic obstructive pulmonary disease: do women and men differ? J Obstet Gynecol Neonatal Nurs. 1999;28:201.
63. Dowson C, Laing R, Barraclough R, et al. The use of the Hospital Anxiety and Depression Scale (HADS) in patients with chronic obstructive pulmonary disease: a pilot study. N Z Med J. 2001;114:447–9.
64. Gudmundsson G, Gislason T, Janson C, et al. Depression, anxiety and health status after hospitalisation for COPD: a multicentre study in the Nordic countries. Respir Med. 2006; 100:87–93.
65. Gudmundsson G, Gislason T, Janson C, et al. Risk factors for rehospitalisation in COPD: role of health status, anxiety and depression. Eur Respir J. 2005;26:414–9.
66. Paulson PE, Minoshima S, Morrow TJ, Casey KL. Gender differences in pain perception and patterns of cerebral activation during noxious heat stimulation in humans. Pain. 1998;76:223–9.
67. Tashkin D, Celli B, Kesten S, Lystig T, Decramer M. Effect of tiotropium in men and women with COPD: Results of the 4-year UPLIFT® trial. Respir Med. 2010;104:1495–504.
68. Han MK, Kazerooni EA, Lynch DA, et al. Chronic obstructive pulmonary disease exacerbations in the COPDGene study: associated radiologic phenotypes. Radiology. 2011;261:274–82.
69. Abusaid GH, Barbagelata A, Tuero E, Mahmood A, Sharma G. Diastolic dysfunction and COPD exacerbation. Postgrad Med. 2009;121:76–81.
70. Ferreira RG, Nicoara A, Phillips-Bute BG, Daneshmand M, Muehlschlegel JD, Swaminathan M. Diastolic dysfunction in patients undergoing cardiac surgery: the role of gender and age-gender interaction. J Cardiothorac Vasc Anesth. 2014;28:626–30.
71. Barr RG, Wentowski CC, Grodstein F, et al. Prospective study of postmenopausal hormone use and newly diagnosed asthma and chronic obstructive pulmonary disease. Arch Intern Med. 2004;164:379–86.

72. Martinez F, Criner G, Hoffman E, et al. Spirometric bronchoreversibility (SBR) in emphysema patients. Proc Am Thorac Soc. 2005;1:A635.
73. Anthonisen N, Lindgren P, Tashkin D, Kanner R, Scanlon P, Connett J. Bronchodilator response in the lung health study over 11 year. Eur Respir J. 2005;26:45–51.
74. Martinez FJ, Curtis JL, Sciurba F, et al. Sex differences in severe pulmonary emphysema. Am J Respir Crit Care Med. 2007;176:243–52.
75. Burrows B, Bloom JW, Traver GA, Cline MG. The course and prognosis of different forms of chronic airways obstruction in a sample from the general population. N Engl J Med. 1987;317:1309–14.
76. Silverman EK, Weiss ST, Drazen JM, et al. Gender-related differences in severe, early-onset chronic obstructive pulmonary disease. Am J Respir Crit Care Med. 2000;162:2152–8.
77. Foreman MG, Zhang L, Murphy J, et al. Early-onset chronic obstructive pulmonary disease is associated with female sex, maternal factors, and African American race in the COPDGene Study. Am J Respir Crit Care Med. 2011;184:414–20.
78. Vucic E, Thu K, Martinez V, et al. Lung tumors and non-malignant airways from patients with chronic lung inflammatory disease bear distinct genetic and epigenetic disruptions corresponding to metabolic processes involved in senescence and methylation. Cancer Metab. 2014;2:1–2.
79. Groen B, Brook P, Adcock I, Durham A. Late-breaking abstract: epigenetic inhibition of proliferation and inflammation in airway epithelium. Eur Respir J. 2014;44:2911.
80. Kaminsky Z, Wang SC, Petronis A. Complex disease, gender and epigenetics. Ann Med. 2006;38:530–44.
81. Glass K, Quackenbush J, Silverman EK, et al. Sexually-dimorphic targeting of functionally-related genes in COPD. BMC Syst Biol. 2014;8:118.
82. Marin JM, Soriano JB, Carrizo SJ, Boldova A, Celli BR. Outcomes in patients with chronic obstructive pulmonary disease and obstructive sleep apnea: The overlap syndrome. Am J Respir Crit Care Med. 2010;182:325–31.
83. Foster TS, Miller JD, Marton JP, Caloyeras JP, Russell MW, Menzin J. Assessment of the economic burden of COPD in the US: a review and synthesis of the literature. COPD: J Chron Obstruct Pulmon Dis. 2006;3:211–8.
84. Galizia G, Cacciatore F, Testa G, et al. Role of clinical frailty on long-term mortality of elderly subjects with and without chronic obstructive pulmonary disease. Aging Clin Exp Res. 2011;23:118–25.
85. Mannino DM, Thorn D, Swensen A, Holguin F. Prevalence and outcomes of diabetes, hypertension and cardiovascular disease in COPD. Eur Respir J. 2008;32:962–9.
86. Mehta PA, Cowie MR. Gender and heart failure: a population perspective. Heart (British Cardiac Society). 2006;92 Suppl 3:14–8.
87. Agusti A. Characterisation of COPD heterogeneity in the ECLIPSE cohort. Respir Res. 2010;11:122.
88. Jaramillo JD, Wilson C, Stinson DJ, et al. Reduced bone density and vertebral fractures in smokers: men and COPD patients at increased risk. Ann Am Thorac Soc. 2015;12:648–56.
89. Nusbaum ML, Gordon M, Nusbaum D, McCarthy MA, Vasilakis D. Smoke alarm: a review of the clinical impact of smoking on women. Prim Care Update Ob/Gyns. 2000;7:207–14.
90. Fortmann SP. Who shall quit? Comparison of volunteer and population-based recruitment in two minimal-contact smoking cessation studies. Am J Epidemiol. 1994;140:39–51.
91. Scharf D, Shiffman S. Are there gender differences in smoking cessation, with and without bupropion? Pooled-and meta-analyses of clinical trials of Bupropion SR. Addiction. 2004;99:1462–9.
92. Wetter DW. Gender differences in smoking cessation. J Consult Clin Psychol. 1999;67:555.
93. Pauwels RA, Buist AS, Calverley PMA, Jenkins CR, Hurd SS. Global strategy for the diagnosis, management, and prevention of chronic obstructive pulmonary disease. Am J Respir Crit Care Med. 2001;163:1256–76.
94. Connett JE, Murray RP, Buist AS, et al. Changes in smoking status affect women more than men: results of the Lung Health Study. Am J Epidemiol. 2003;157:973–9.

95. Lynch W. Biological basis of sex differences in drug abuse: preclinical and clinical studies. Psychopharmacology (Berlin, Germany). 2002;164:121–37.
96. Bierut LJ, Johnson EO, Saccone NL. A glimpse into the future—personalized medicine for smoking cessation. Neuropharmacology. 2014;76(Pt B):592–9.
97. Shiffman S. Nicotine patch and lozenge are effective for women. Nicotine Tob Res. 2005;7:119–27.
98. Wetter DW. Gender differences in response to nicotine replacement therapy: objective and subjective indexes of tobacco withdrawal. Exp Clin Psychopharmacol. 1999;7:135–44.
99. Schermer T, Hendriks A, Chavannes N, et al. Probability and determinants of relapse after discontinuation of inhaled corticosteroids in patients with COPD treated in general practice. Prim Care Respir J. 2004;13:48–55.
100. Albert RK, Connett J, Bailey WC, et al. Azithromycin for prevention of exacerbations of COPD. N Engl J Med. 2011;365:689–98.
101. Han MK, Tayob N, Murray S, et al. Predictors of chronic obstructive pulmonary disease exacerbation reduction in response to daily azithromycin therapy. Am J Respir Crit Care Med. 2014;189:1503–8.
102. Franklin KA, Gustafson T, Ranstam J, Ström K. Survival and future need of long-term oxygen therapy for chronic obstructive pulmonary disease—gender differences. Respir Med. 2007;101:1506–11.
103. Machado M-CL, Krishnan JA, Buist SA, et al. Sex differences in survival of oxygen-dependent patients with chronic obstructive pulmonary disease. Am J Respir Crit Care Med. 2006;174:524–9.
104. Crockett AJ. Survival on long-term oxygen therapy in chronic airflow limitation: from evidence to outcomes in the routine clinical setting. Int Med J. 2001;31:448–54.
105. Ringbaek TJ, Lange P. Trends in long-term oxygen therapy for COPD in Denmark from 2001 to 2010. Respir Med. 2014;108:511–6.
106. CDC. Chronic obstructive pulmonary disease among adults—United States, 2011. MMWR. 2012;61:938–43.
107. Age-Standardized Death rates (Per 100,000 U.S. Population) for Chronic Obstructive Pulmonary Disease (COPD), United States, 1999–2010. 2011. (Accessed February 12, 2015, 2015, at http://www.cdc.gov/copd/pdfs/graph_COPD_Death_Rates_United_States1999_2010.pdf.)
108. Jarvis MJ, Cohen JE, Delnevo CD, Giovino GA. Dispelling myths about gender differences in smoking cessation: population data from the USA, Canada and Britain. Tob Control. 2013;22:356–60.

Chapter 4
Sex, Gender, and Asthma

Dawn C. Newcomb

Abstract Asthma is a heterogeneous disease with a sexual dimorphism in prevalence that changes throughout life. As children, boys are more likely than girls to have asthma, but as adults women are more likely than men to have asthma. The prevalence of asthma in females increases around the age of menarche, suggesting a role for sex hormones in disease pathogenesis. In some women with asthma, increased symptoms are reported just prior to or during menstruation. Further, asthma symptoms during pregnancy and menopause also vary for women. In this chapter, we will discuss the findings from epidemiological, clinical, and molecular studies exploring the role of sex hormones and asthma. We will also discuss findings from animal models of asthma, focusing primarily on allergic asthma, and how these findings may be used to develop potential therapies or guide the personalized use of currently available asthma therapies.

Keywords Asthma • Allergic airway inflammation • Nonallergic inflammation • Innate and adaptive immune responses

Abbreviations

AHR	Airway hyperresponsiveness
AMΦ	Alveolar macrophage
APCs	Antigen-presenting cells
AR	Androgen receptor
BAL	Bronchoalveolar lavage
BMI	Body mass index
DCs	Dendritic cells
ER	Estrogen receptor

D.C. Newcomb, PhD (✉)
Division of Allergy, Pulmonary, and Critical Care Medicine, Department of Medicine,
Vanderbilt University Medical Center, T-1218 Medical Center North,
1161 21st Avenue South, Nashville, TN 37232, USA
e-mail: dawn.newcomb@vanderbilt.edu

© Springer International Publishing Switzerland 2016
A.R. Hemnes (ed.), *Gender, Sex Hormones and Respiratory Disease*,
Respiratory Medicine, DOI 10.1007/978-3-319-23998-9_4

FEV₁   Forced exhaled volume in one second
HDM   House dust mite
HRT   Hormone replacement therapy
IgE   Immunoglobulin E
IL   Interleukin
ILC2s   Group 2 innate lymphoid cells
ILC3s   Group 3 innate lymphoid cells
KO   Knockout
MHC   Major histocompatibility complex
NK   Natural killer cells
OVA   Ovalbumin
PR   Progesterone receptor
SARP   Severe Asthma Research Panel
TSLP   T helper (Th) thymic stromal lymphopoietin

Asthma is a multidimensional chronic disease that is characterized by reversible expiratory airflow limitation, airway hyperresponsiveness (AHR), and airway inflammation [1]. Asthma affects 5–10 % of the population in the United States and other developed countries, resulting in 300 million people worldwide having this disease [1]. A sex disparity, which changes with age, exists in asthma (Fig. 4.1) [2]. Before the age of 12, boys have an increased prevalence of asthma compared to girls [3], with approximately 11.9 % of boys having asthma compared to 7.5 % of girls having asthma [4]. The prevalence of asthma in adolescent girls increases at puberty, and as adults, 9.6 % of women have asthma compared to 6.3 % of men [4, 5]. This sex disparity in asthma is maintained until women approach menopause, when the prevalence in asthma declines [6].

Women with asthma also have increased asthma-related mortality and morbidity, more severe asthma phenotypes, less responsiveness to corticosteroid medications, and more fluctuations in asthma symptoms, corresponding to the menstrual cycle, compared to men with asthma [5, 7, 8]. As children, boys are twice as likely as girls

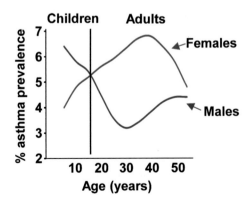

Fig. 4.1 Prevalence of asthma in females and males at various ages. Graph is adapted from Carey, M. et al. [2]

to be hospitalized for an asthma exacerbation (as reviewed in [9]). After the age of 15, however, girls and women are three times more likely than boys and men to be hospitalized for an asthma-related event [10–12]. The sex differences in hospitalizations of adult men and women with asthma are independent of controller medication use or length of time before seeking medical attention [9]. *Combined, these data suggest that asthma prevalence and the severity of asthma symptoms and exacerbations of asthma are increased in women compared to men. In this chapter, we will discuss the findings from epidemiological, clinical, and molecular studies exploring the role of sex hormones and asthma.*

Classifications Systems for Patients with Asthma

Asthma is a heterogeneous disease with many different phenotypes responsiveness to current therapies, and triggers for exacerbations [13]. Patients with asthma were classified as extrinsic (allergic) and intrinsic (nonallergic) based on clinical symptoms, IgE serum levels, atopy status, and age of onset [14]. Using this classification system, women had an increased prevalence in both allergic and nonallergic asthma compared to men. However, other phenotypic variables, such as forced expiratory volume in one second (FEV_1) pre- and post-bronchodilator, blood and sputum eosinophil and neutrophil counts, responsiveness to corticosteroids, age of onset, and asthma triggers, were not included when categorizing patients [14]. Not accounting for multiple variables resulted in patients with varying clinical symptoms, pathophysiology, and molecular markers being classified as having either allergic or nonallergic asthma. This categorization system created difficulty in determining the appropriate clinical trial populations for therapeutics targeting a specific mechanism for airway inflammation.

Recently a more sophisticated systems biology approach utilizing cluster modeling classification systems was used to categorize patients with asthma. Cluster analysis uses algorithms and a predefined set of asthma variables from patients with asthma and healthy controls to define asthma phenotypes [15–19]. Common variables used in these studies are shown in Table 4.1, and several groups have reported a female dominance in the clusters listed below [15–19]:

1. Early-onset atopic asthma
2. Later onset atopic asthma
3. Later onset asthma in obese individuals
4. More severe asthma with increased sputum neutrophils and decreased lung function

As denoted in the list above, cluster analysis statistical approaches have categorized women-dominated asthma phenotypes spread across the asthma spectrum; from early-onset mild, intermittent asthma to late-onset, severe asthma. To better understand these cellular and molecular variables used in cluster analysis studies, we will first review the basic immune mechanisms and cell types involved in asthma

Table 4.1 Variables used in cluster analysis studies for asthma [15–19]

Age of onset
Gender
BMI
Lung function testing
Allergies
Serum IgE levels
Sputum eosinophil and neutrophil counts
Medication use
Asthma symptom score questionnaires
Use of health care for asthma symptoms
Hospitalization for asthma

and then discuss findings from the literature. Defining the mechanisms and properly phenotyping patients will target patient populations that may benefit from various therapeutics when conducting clinical trials and designing treatment regiments.

Host Immune Responses in Asthma

Sir William Osler described asthma in the 1892 edition of Principles and Practice of Medicine as a disease with a genetic component, originating early in life that resulted in spasms of the bronchial muscles, swelling of bronchial mucous membrane, inflammation in bronchioles, and various circumstances that induced symptoms [20]. Approximately 70–80 % of patients with asthma are sensitized to allergens, pollen, dust mites, cockroach antigen, mold, etc., and asthma symptoms and exacerbations are increased with exposure to these allergens in these patients. However, other environmental stimuli, including viral infections, cigarette smoke, and air pollution, also may result in asthma symptoms through different innate and adaptive immune responses. *In this chapter, we will primarily discuss findings focused on the role of sex hormones in allergic asthma immunepathways(as shown in* Fig. 4.2*), but we will also introduce alternative, nonallergic immune pathways involved with asthma pathogenesis.*

The allergic airway immune response is characterized by increased CD4+ Th2 cells, eosinophils, mast cells, and basophils in the airway. Airway epithelial cells are the first point of contact for airway allergens, and airway epithelial cells are important for regulating antigen-presenting cells (APCs). APCs, including dendritic cells (DCs), alveolar macrophages (AMΦ), and B lymphocytes, engulf antigens and process them for presentation to the T cells, initiating the adaptive immune response [21, 22]. Antigens processed by APCs, through the endocytic pathway, are presented by major histocompatibility complex (MHC) class II molecules to CD4+ T lymphocytes. Naïve CD4+ T lymphocytes are activated when two events occur: (1) the antigen/MHC class II complex on the APC engages the T cell receptor, and (2) co-stimulation molecules, such as CD80 or CD86, on the APC bind to co-stimulation

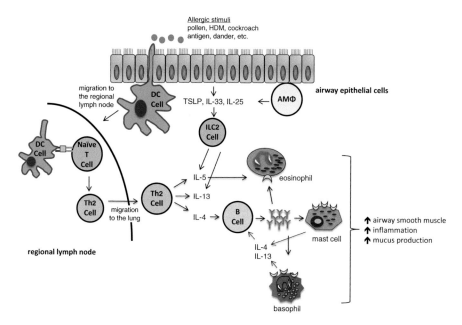

Fig. 4.2 Immune response to allergic stimuli resulting in increased AHR, allergic airway inflammation, and mucus production. Alveolar macrophage (*AMΦ*), dendritic cell (*DC*), house dust mite (*HDM*)

molecules, such as CD28, on the CD4+ T cells. DCs are the most potent APCs in activating naïve T cells [23, 24], and DCs also secrete chemokines that attract CD4+ Th2 differentiated cells and eosinophils to the lung [25].

Many cell types are involved in the allergic response, but the key cell types in initiating and amplifying the allergen-induced inflammatory cascade are the antigen-presenting DC and T helper 2 (Th2) lymphocytes. Th2 lymphocytes are CD4+ T cells that are differentiated from activated naïve T cells. Initiation of Th2 cell differentiation is not completely understood, but interleukin-4 (IL-4) is also required for Th2 cell differentiation [26, 27]. Th2 cells, as well as mast cells and basophils, secrete IL-4, and IL-4 is required for B lymphocytes to isotype switch antibody production to IgE [26, 27]. Th2 cells additionally produce a variety of other pro-allergic inflammatory cytokines such as IL-5, IL-9, IL-10, and IL-13. IL-5 is an important eosinophil regulatory factor and increases eosinophil maturation and proliferation [28]. IL-13 is a central mediator in AHR and also induces mucus hypersecretion from goblet (mucous) cells in the airway [27–29]. IL-9 is important for mast cell growth, T cell proliferation, IgE secretion from B cells, and mucus hypersecretion from goblet cells [30]. IL-10 is an anti-inflammatory cytokine that is secreted by Th2 cells as well as other cells, including T regulatory cells and Th17 cells. In summary, IL-4, IL-5, IL-9, and IL-13 are important for establishing the allergic airway response, and IL-10 is an important anti-inflammatory cytokine in the airway allergen immune response.

The allergic response to an aerosolized allergen is also characterized by antigen-specific immunoglobulin E (IgE) production by B lymphocytes whereupon IgE can bind to the high-affinity IgE receptor, FcεR1, on tissue mast cells and peripheral blood basophils. Antigen cross-linking of the antigen-specific IgE/FcεR1 complex ignites degranulation of the mast cells and basophils, causing release of soluble mediators, such as histamine and tryptase [13, 31]. Other mediators, including prostaglandins and leukotrienes, are also released in response to an allergen [32, 33]. Release of these mediators causes vasodilation and recruitment of inflammatory cells into the airway, including eosinophils and lymphocytes. Therefore, antigen cross-linking to FcεR1 is an important component of the immune response to allergens.

Recently a new cell type, group 2 innate lymphoid cells (ILC2), was described to be residing in the lung in small numbers and be important in airway immune responses. ILC2 are activated by IL-33, IL-25, and thymic stromal lymphopoietin (TSLP) which are secreted from airway epithelial cells and other immune cells, in response to allergens and other stimuli, such as infections with fungi, helminthes, and viruses [34–36]. ILC2 lack lineage markers for T cells, B cells, DCs, and macrophages [34, 37]. ILC2 express CD25 (IL-2Rα) and CD127 (IL-7Rα) as well as receptors for the ILC2 activating cytokines IL-25, IL-33, and/or TSLP [34, 36, 37]. Once activated, ILC2 quickly secrete large amounts of IL-13 and IL-5 compared to Th2 cells [37]. Therefore, while ILC2 are rare within the lung, ILC cytokine expression increases eosinophil infiltration into the lung and mucus production. *Collectively, the immune response toaerosolized allergenscauses an increase in airway inflammation, airway mucus hypersecretion by goblet cells (predominantly through IL-13), and increased airway smooth muscle constriction.*

Understanding the basic immune pathways in allergic asthma is a first step in determining the role of sex hormones on asthma. Another important step is determining the expression of estrogen receptors (ERs), progesterone receptors (PRs), and androgen receptors (ARs) on immune cells. Nuclear ERs, PRs, and ARs are readily expressed in inflammatory cells involved with asthma (as reviewed in [38]). Membrane-bound ERs are not found on T cells or cells of hematopoietic origin, but membrane-bound ERs are found on other cell types [38]. *Since sex hormone receptors are found on many different immune cells, sex hormones may affect several steps in allergic airway disease, including antigen uptake, antigen processing and presentation, adaptive immune effector function, antibody isotype switching to IgE, and mast cell degranulation. Throughout this chapter we will discuss the role of sex hormones in the allergic immune response.*

Changes in Sex Hormones during Puberty, Pregnancy, and Menopause Adversely Affect a Subset of Women with Asthma

As demonstrated in Fig. 4.1 the prevalence of asthma increases about the age of menarche, suggesting a role for sex hormones in asthma prevalence. Salam and colleagues reported girls who reached menarche prior to age 12 had a 2.08 higher risk for asthma compared to girls who reached menarche at age 12 or later [39].

These data suggest that ovarian hormones increase the risk for development of asthma. In the following subsections, we will discuss how various stages in life and fluctuations of hormones affect asthma prevalence and severity.

Pre- and Perimenstrual Asthma Symptoms

Twenty to thirty-five percent of women with asthma have pre- or perimenstrual worsening of asthma, but asthma exacerbations were independent of cyclic hormonal changes [40–44]. Estrogen and progesterone concentrations oscillate throughout with menstrual cycle, and these fluctuations in hormonal concentrations are thought to be potentially linked to changes in asthma symptoms. As shown in Fig. 4.3, estrogen concentrations peak on day 13 of a 28-day menstrual cycle, just prior to ovulation, and progesterone concentrations peak at days 22–24, four to six days prior to menses. Asthma symptoms are increased in the premenstrual phase of the cycle (days 25–28) when both estrogen and progesterone concentrations are low (Fig. 4.3). Clinical studies tracking asthma symptoms and peak expiratory flow rates in women through at least two menstrual cycles found increased symptoms and decreased peak flow rates in the morning during the premenstrual and perimenstrual phases of the cycle compared to other phases of the cycle [40, 43]. Women with premenstrual asthma symptoms had increased fractional exhaled nitric oxide (FeNO), a noninvasive measure of epithelial induced nitric oxide that correlates with eosinophilic inflammation [45], and eosinophils in the sputum in the premenstrual phase compared to the seventh day of their cycle [46]. However, no difference in the phase of the menstrual cycle of women requiring emergency department

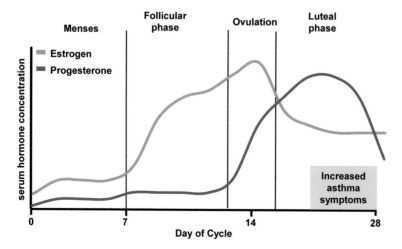

Fig. 4.3 Flucuations in estrogen and progesterone serum concentrations through a 28-day menstrual cycle. Estrogen and progesterone serum concentrations vary throughout the menstrual cycle

visits for asthma symptoms was reported [44]. *Combined, these studies suggest a subset of women with asthma have increased premenstrual asthma symptoms and decreased peak expiratory flow rates, but no change in asthma exacerbations during premenstrual phase of their cycle.*

Use of certain hormonal birth controls pills reduced the fluctuations of hormone levels and could potentially reduce pre- and perimenstrual asthma symptoms in women with asthma.

However, only a few studies, with small patient sizes, have been conducted to determine the effect of hormonal birth control medications on asthma symptoms through the menstrual cycle. One study followed 18 women with asthma through two menstrual cycles. Women not taking oral contraceptives ($n=9$) had increased AHR to adenosine monophosphate during the luteal phase and reduced diurnal peak expiratory flow rates. However, women taking oral contraceptives medications ($n=9$) did not have a significant increase in AHR to adenosine monophosphate or significant changes in morning and afternoon peak flow rates [47]. Another study followed 28 women with asthma for 12 weeks (2–4 menstrual cycles) and found no difference in asthma symptoms in women taking oral contraceptives versus women not taking oral contraceptives [48]. Therefore, additional studies, with larger patient populations that stratify different types of hormonal birth control medications, are needed to fully delineate if asthma symptoms are reduced in women taking hormonal contraceptives.

Pregnancy and Asthma

Asthma is a common chronic condition present during pregnancy with a 3.7–8.4 % prevalence among pregnant women [49]. Variations in asthma symptoms and asthma control during pregnancy are common. Two studies from the late 1980s reported that in pregnant women with asthma approximately one-third had decreased asthma symptoms, one-third had increased asthma symptoms, and one-third had no change in asthma symptoms [50, 51]. Since that time, there has been little improvement on predicting if asthma symptoms will increase, decrease, or remain the same in pregnant women. Researchers have shown that compared to women with mild asthma phenotypes, women with severe asthma were more likely to experience increased asthma symptoms later in the pregnancy, in the second and third trimesters [52]. Pregnant women with asthma were also more susceptible to respiratory viral infections, including rhinovirus and influenza, and viral infections increase asthma exacerbations [53, 54]. Variations in asthma symptoms and control in pregnant women are not fully understood, but are likely related to various phenotypes of asthma, hormonal changes during pregnancy, and adherence to asthma medications. Many pregnant women with asthma decide, either individually or as advised by their medical provider, to reduce or stop asthma medications to prevent adverse side effects on the fetus. However, National Heart, Lung, and Blood Institute and the Global Initiative for Asthma (GINA) guidelines indicate that pregnant women should maintain their current regimen of asthma medications, including inhaled corticosteroids, long-acting beta agonist, leukotriene modifiers, theophylline, and oral corticosteroids [55, 56]. Use of asthma medications during pregnancy was not associated with fetal abnormalities [57], and maintaining asthma control during pregnancy is important. More severe asthma, poorly controlled asthma, and asthma exacerbations during pregnancy are associated with increased risk for development of preeclampsia and gestational diabetes in the mother and preterm birth, low birth weight, and perinatal mortality for the baby [55, 57, 58].

Menopause and Asthma

As described above, ovarian hormones are associated with asthma. Therefore, one would predict that the decline in circulating ovarian hormones that occurs with menopause leads to decreased asthma in women. However, studies in menopausal women report variable findings, with asthma symptoms increasing, decreasing, or remaining the same when compared to premenopausal women or postmenopausal women on hormone replacement therapy (HRT) (as reviewed in [59]). The US Nurses' Health Study was a prospective study which followed 41,202 premeno-pausal women and 23,035 postmenopausal women from 1980 until 1990 [6]. Women were reclassified as pre- or postmenopausal every 2 years based on ques-tionnaire responses. At the end of the study, 582,135 person-years were documented with 726 new cases of asthma. The US Nurses' Health Study determined that post-menopausal women who never used HRT had a significant decrease in the risk of developing asthma compared to premenopausal women [6]. Further, postmeno-pausal women who used HRT had an increased age-adjusted risk for asthma com-pared to postmenopausal women who never used HRT [6]. The European Community Respiratory Healthy Surveys (ECRHS I) also conducted a study and reported no difference in self-reported asthma between premenopausal and post-menopausal women not taking HRT [60]. However, the ECRHSII cross-sectional study reported increased asthma symptoms in women during the menopause transi-tion (amenorrhea for 6+ months) compared to premenopausal women [61]. Further, the ECRHSII study reported increased asthma severity in women diagnosed with asthma during or after menopause [62]. *Combined, these studies suggest meno-pause and HRT are involved in asthma pathogenesis, but the mechanisms are not completely understood. Co-variables, including BMI, genetic factors, estrogenpro-ductionfrom adipose tissue, and insulin sensitivity, need to also be considered in future study design.*

Summary

Changes in circulating sex hormones occur throughout life for women and therefore it is challenging to design clinical studies that determine the roles of sex hormones in asthma pathogenesis. Further complicating clinical trials is sex hormones regu-late AHR, airway inflammation, and metabolism, important aspects in asthma pathogenesis. Therefore to define the mechanisms by which sex hormones regulate asthma pathogenesis researchers use asthma-like rodent (mainly mouse) models. We will discuss animal models of asthma in the next section.

Sex Hormones in Mouse Models of Asthma

Animal models which mimic asthma with increased airway inflammation, AHR, and mucus hypersecretion are vital for determining the mechanisms associated with asthma pathogenesis. Mouse models are used most readily due to reagent availability, knockout strains of mice, and genetically similar immune systems within inbred mouse strains. Sex differences and the role of sex hormones in mouse models of asthma have variable findings based on mouse strain, protocol used for inducing allergic airway inflammation, and endpoints analyzed. The subsections below describe the different findings in mice with regard to sex hormones at baseline (prior to inducing inflammation), during allergic airway inflammation, and during nonallergic airway inflammation.

Baseline AHR and Airway Physiology in Female and Male Mice

At baseline naïve mice have very few lymphocytes, neutrophils, and eosinophils in the bronchoalveolar lavage (BAL) fluid [63], and there is no sexual dimorphism in the percentages of baseline leukocytes in naïve mice [64]. However, baseline AHR is increased in male mice compared to female mice in both the BALB/c and C57BL/6 strains of mice [64]. ER-α-deficient mice (ER-α KO) have increased AHR compared to WT female mice [65, 66], and using an estrogen antagonist increased AHR compared to vehicle control [67]. Conversely, administering 17β-estradiol to male mice decreased AHR compared to vehicle control [67].

Researchers speculated that the increased AHR in male mice is due to male mice having decreased numbers of alveoli and decreased alveolar surface area compared to female mice [68]. To test this hypothesis, female mice were ovariectomized just after weaning (approximately 21 days) and similar alveolar structures were seen in ovariectomized female and male mice, suggesting sex hormones were important in the development of alveoli [68, 69]. Additional studies in ER-α and ER-β KO mice showed ER-α and ER-β signaling is required for fully developing alveolar structures in female mice, and that ER-β KO mice have decreased elastic recoil compared to WT female mice [69]. Increased numbers of alveoli and alveolar surface area may be responsible for the observed sex difference in AHR, and normalization for lung volume and size in a statistical model resulted in no difference in AHR between males and females.

Other factors including variations in vagal nerve-mediated pathways and smooth muscle contractility may also contribute to sex differences in AHR after stimulation.

Vagal nerve-mediated pathways are increased in response to methacholine and carbachol, chemicals known to increase smooth muscle contractility, in male mice compared to female mice [70]. Gonadectomized male mice also had similar vagal nerve responses as intact female mice, and restoring androgens to gonadectomized male mice increased the vagal nerve response and AHR to methacholine [70], suggesting androgens increased the vagal nerve response. However, no difference in ex vivo smooth muscle contractility assays to carbachol was reported in tracheal rings from male and female mice. Further, ER-α KO mice and WT female mice had similar smooth muscle contractility to carbachol [70]. *Combined, these results suggest sex hormones affect baseline AHR in mice independent of smooth muscle constriction.*

Dryness of the throat and vaginal dryness are symptoms reported by women during menopause. These symptoms suggest that sex hormones may affect mucous cell metaplasia and mucus production in the airway and the reproductive system. Therefore, researchers became interested in the role of estrogen and progesterone on mucus production in the nasal and airway epithelial cells. In 1975, Helmi and colleagues administered 10 μg/day ethynyl estradiol, a downstream hormone of the 17β-estradiol, to guinea pigs and measured mucous cell hyperplasia and metaplasia in nasal epithelial cells by histochemical staining. Guinea pigs administered ethynyl estradiol had increased mucous cell hyperplasia and metaplasia compared to vehicle-treated animals [71]. In vitro studies in human airway or nasal epithelial cells also showed that estrogen or progesterone increased mucus production and the expression of the mucus proteins, Muc5AC and Muc5B, compared to vehicle-treated cells [72, 73]. In summary, sex hormones regulate baseline airway responsiveness to methacholine as well as mucus production. Acknowledging baseline differences is vital for experiment design and interpretation of data as normalizing experimental results to percent baseline may not provide the most accurate interpretation of data.

Establishment of Allergic Airway Inflammation in Mice

During ongoing allergic airway inflammation the role of sex hormones varies based on the protocol used to induce allergic airway inflammation and the endpoint measured. The results discussed in the paragraphs below are summarized in Table 4.2. Two widely used models of allergic airway inflammation are: (1) ovalbumin (OVA) sensitization followed by OVA challenge and (2) exposure to house dust mite (HDM) antigen. Both these models increase airway inflammation, AHR, and mucus hypersecretion through a CD4+ Th2 cell-mediated mechanism. Female mice undergoing the OVA sensitized and challenged protocol or the HDM protocols had increased eosinophilic infiltration and IgE serum levels compared to male mice undergoing the same protocol [74–76]. Female mice with OVA-induced allergic airway inflammation also had significantly increased lung IL-4, IL-5, and IL-13 protein expression, mucous cell metaplasia, and airway remodeling compared to

Table 4.2 Summary of results for the role of sex hormones in mouse models of allergic airway inflammation

Protocol	Dominance by gender	Endpoints with increase	References
OVA sensitization and challenge	F>M	Infiltration of lymphocytes and eosinophils	[74–76]
		IL-13	
		Mucus	
		Airway remodeling	
		Serum IgE	
OVA sensitization and challenge	Castrated M>M	Infiltration of lymphocytes and eosinophils	[75]
		IL-13	
OVA sensitization and challenge	F > ovariex F	Airway inflammation	[77]
		AHR	
HDM	F>M	Serum IgE	[74]
		IL-4, IL-5, and IL-13 lung production	
OVA sensitization and challenge	ER-α KO > WT, ER-β KO	AHR	[66]

Admin administered, *F* female, *M* male, *ovariex* ovariectomized, *veh* vehicle

male mice [74–76]. Further, castration of male mice prior to OVA sensitization and challenge increased eosinophils and lymphocytes in the BAL fluid, mucous cell metaplasia, and airway inflammation compared to sham-operated mice [75]. However, an ovariectomy prior to OVA sensitization decreased OVA-induced airway inflammation and AHR compared to intact female BALB/c mice [77]. *These results suggest that ovarian sex hormones increased, while testosterone decreased, allergic airway inflammation, AHR, and mucous cell metaplasia.*

However, Carey and colleagues induced OVA-specific allergic airway inflammation with sensitization and challenge in WT, ER-α KO, and ER-β KO female C57BL/6 mice [66]. ER-α KO mice had a significant increase in AHR compared to WT and ER-β KO mice [66]. One potential explanation is AHR varies in different strains of mice, with C57BL/6 mice having decreased AHR compared to BALB/c mice [78]. Therefore, when interpreting these results, strain variations in AHR, allergic airway inflammation, and mucus production should be considered.

While OVA and HDM are two commonly used models for allergic airway inflammation, exposures to other stimuli, including tobacco smoke, also exacerbate allergic asthma symptoms. Seymour and colleagues determined the role of sex and progesterone in OVA-sensitized and challenged mice exposed to tobacco smoke from birth. Similar to the studies discussed previously, OVA-sensitized and challenged female mice in ambient air since birth had increased serum IgE levels, increased eosinophils, and increased IL-4, IL-5, and IL-13 protein expression in the lung compared to OVA-sensitized and challenged male mice in ambient air since birth [79]. Exposure to tobacco smoke since birth followed by OVA sensitization and challenge starting at 6 weeks of age increased OVA-specific IgE serum levels compared to OVA sensitization and challenge in female mice only. Cytokine expression of IL-4, IL-5, and IL-13 was significantly increased in male mice administered tobacco smoke followed by the OVA protocol compared to male mice in ambient airway undergoing the OVA protocol. Combined these data suggest gender differences exist in the allergic inflammatory response with ambient air or being exposed to tobacco smoke at birth. These data are very important for girls and boys exposed to secondhand smoke from birth who develop allergic airway inflammation.

Serum IgE levels were also increased in female mice compared to male mice after allergic sensitization and challenge [80]. Mast cells numbers in the uterine tissue of mice also fluctuate with the estrus cycle and estrogen and progesterone have been shown to cause mast cell degranulation [81]. Based on these findings, sex hormones were speculated to regulate mast cells during allergic airway inflammation. Estrogen treatment of bone marrow-derived mast cells increased degranulation, and this was inhibited in mast cells from ER-α KO mice. Further, in a human mast cell line (HMC-1), incubation with 17β-estradiol or progesterone significantly increased synthesis of β-tryptase, a serine proteinase found in the secretory granules of mast cells [81]. Combined these data suggest that sex hormones may be important for mast cell differentiation and degranulation and provide a piece to the puzzle of increased asthma prevalence and severity in women compared to men.

Sexual dimorphism exists in allergic asthma, but the mechanisms are not fully defined. Further research in mouse models and patients with allergic asthma is needed to determine the roles of sex hormones at the various steps in the immune response during allergic inflammation. Utilizing gonadectomized mice with restored sex hormones prior to initiation of allergic airway inflammation will aid in determining the mechanisms associated with the sex differences observed in asthma throughout life.

Other Triggers of Asthma and the Role of Sex Hormones on Immune Cells

Viral infections, environmental stimuli, obesity, stress, and exposure to toxins are additional stimuli that cause asthma exacerbation. Viral infections are the most frequent cause of asthma exacerbations, and therefore determining the role of sex hormones on viral-induced airway inflammation, AHR, and mucus production is important and remains largely unknown. Recent findings in either female mice or male mice showed increased IL-13 and IL-5 protein expression from ILC2 in response to influenza A or *Alternaria alternata*, a fungus known to cause airway inflammation [82]. Further, IL-17A protein expression from γδ T cells, Th17 cells, and ILC3 cells is reported to be increased in response to fungal or viral infections [83, 84]. Future experiments, incorporating mice of both sexes, gonadectomized mice, and mice deficient in estrogen signaling, are required to determine the role of sex hormones on ILC2, ILC3, γδ T cell, and Th17 cell cytokine expression and increased AHR, airway inflammation, and mucus production in mouse models.

Summary of Sex Hormones and Asthma

A gender disparity exists in asthma, and at puberty the prevalence of asthma increases in females compared to males. It is a very complicated, high-regulated process. Epidemiologic and clinical studies vary on the role of estrogen and progesterone in increasing asthma symptoms and severity, but the literature suggests that ovarian hormones increase asthma prevalence, symptoms, and severity. Accounting for sex differences in mouse models of asthma is the first step for determining the role of sex hormones in immune mechanisms associated with asthma. Further, designing clinical trials to include patients with various phenotypes of asthma, at the correct sex ratio, is important for determining if a therapeutic will work and if differential responses in asthma symptoms will be seen in women and men.

References

1. Prevention FtGSfAMa. Global Initiative for Asthma (GINA). http://www.ginasthma.org/. 2014 2014. Report No.
2. Carey MA, Card JW, Voltz JW, Arbes Jr SJ, Germolec DR, Korach KS, et al. It's all about sex: gender, lung development and lung disease. Trends Endocrinol Metab. 2007;18(8):308–13.
3. Almqvist C, Worm M, Leynaert B, Working group of GALENWPG. Impact of gender on asthma in childhood and adolescence: a GA2LEN review. Allergy. 2008;63(1):47–57.
4. Centers for Disease Control and Prevention, Vital Signs, May 2011. 2013.
5. Moorman JE, Zahran H, Truman BI, Molla MT. Current asthma prevalence—United States, 2006–2008. MMWR Surveill Summ. 2011;60(Suppl):84–6.
6. Troisi RJ, Speizer FE, Willett WC, Trichopoulos D, Rosner B. Menopause, postmenopausal estrogen preparations, and the risk of adult-onset asthma. A prospective cohort study. Am J Respir Crit Care Med. 1995;152(4 Pt 1):1183–8.
7. Gibbs CJ, Coutts II, Lock R, Finnegan OC, White RJ. Premenstrual exacerbation of asthma. Thorax. 1984;39(11):833–6.
8. Skobeloff EM, Spivey WH, Silverman R, Eskin BA, Harchelroad F, Alessi TV. The effect of the menstrual cycle on asthma presentations in the emergency department. Arch Intern Med. 1996;156(16):1837–40.
9. Kynyk JA, Mastronarde JG, McCallister JW. Asthma, the sex difference. Curr Opin Pulm Med. 2011;17(1):6–11.
10. Chen Y, Stewart P, Johansen H, McRae L, Taylor G. Sex difference in hospitalization due to asthma in relation to age. J Clin Epidemiol. 2003;56(2):180–7.
11. Hyndman SJ, Williams DR, Merrill SL, Lipscombe JM, Palmer CR. Rates of admission to hospital for asthma. BMJ. 1994;308(6944):1596–600.
12. Skobeloff EM, Spivey WH, St Clair SS, Schoffstall JM. The influence of age and sex on asthma admissions. JAMA. 1992;268(24):3437–40.
13. Borish L, Culp JA. Asthma: a syndrome composed of heterogeneous diseases. Ann Allergy Asthma Immunol. 2008;101(1):1–8.
14. Wenzel SE. Asthma phenotypes: the evolution from clinical to molecular approaches. Nat Med. 2012;18(5):716–25.
15. Moore WC, Meyers DA, Wenzel SE, Teague WG, Li H, Li X, et al. Identification of asthma phenotypes using cluster analysis in the Severe Asthma Research Program. Am J Respir Crit Care Med. 2010;181(4):315–23.
16. Haldar P, Pavord ID, Shaw DE, Berry MA, Thomas M, Brightling CE, et al. Cluster analysis and clinical asthma phenotypes. Am J Respir Crit Care Med. 2008;178(3):218–24.

17. Siroux V, Garcia-Aymerich J. The investigation of asthma phenotypes. Curr Opin Allergy Clin Immunol. 2011;11(5):393–9.
18. Wu W, Bleecker E, Moore W, Busse WW, Castro M, Chung KF, et al. Unsupervised phenotyping of Severe Asthma Research Program participants using expanded lung data. J Allergy Clin Immunol. 2014;133(5):1280–8.
19. Newby C, Heaney LG, Menzies-Gow A, Niven RM, Mansur A, Bucknall C, et al. Statistical cluster analysis of the British thoracic society severe refractory asthma registry: clinical outcomes and phenotype stability. PLoS One. 2014;9(7), e102987.
20. Osler W. The principles and practice of medicine: designed for the use of practitioners and students of medicine. New York: D. Appleton and Company; 1892. xvi, 2, 1079, 7, 8 p.
21. Corry DB, Kheradmand F. Induction and regulation of the IgE response. Nature. 1999;402(6760 Suppl):B18–23.
22. Holgate ST. The epidemic of allergy and asthma. Nature. 1999;402(6760 Suppl):B2–4.
23. Hammad H, Lambrecht BN. Dendritic cells and airway epithelial cells at the interface between innate and adaptive immune responses. Allergy. 2011;66(5):579–87.
24. Hammad H, Lambrecht BN. Dendritic cells and epithelial cells: linking innate and adaptive immunity in asthma. Nat Rev Immunol. 2008;8(3):193–204.
25. Lambrecht BN, Hammad H. Lung dendritic cells in respiratory viral infection and asthma: from protection to immunopathology. Annu Rev Immunol. 2012;30:243–70.
26. Abbas AK, Murphy KM, Sher A. Functional diversity of helper T lymphocytes. Nature. 1996;383(6603):787–93.
27. Wills-Karp M, Luyimbazi J, Xu X, Schofield B, Neben TY, Karp CL, et al. Interleukin-13: central mediator of allergic asthma. Science. 1998;282(5397):2258–61.
28. Wills-Karp M. Immunologic basis of antigen-induced airway hyperresponsiveness. Annu Rev Immunol. 1999;17:255–81.
29. Wills-Karp M. Interleukin-13 in asthma pathogenesis. Immunol Rev. 2004;202:175–90.
30. Goswami R, Kaplan MH. A brief history of IL-9. J Immunol. 2011;186(6):3283–8.
31. Busse WW, Lemanske Jr RF. Asthma. N Engl J Med. 2001;344(5):350–62.
32. Moore ML, Peebles Jr RS. Update on the role of prostaglandins in allergic lung inflammation: separating friends from foes, harder than you might think. J Allergy Clin Immunol. 2006;117(5):1036–9.
33. Kanaoka Y, Boyce JA. Cysteinyl leukotrienes and their receptors; emerging concepts. Allergy, Asthma & Immunol Res. 2014;6(4):288–95.
34. Halim TY, Krauss RH, Sun AC, Takei F. Lung natural helper cells are a critical source of Th2 cell-type cytokines in protease allergen-induced airway inflammation. Immunity. 2012;36(3):451–63.
35. Chang YJ, Kim HY, Albacker LA, Baumgarth N, McKenzie AN, Smith DE, et al. Innate lymphoid cells mediate influenza-induced airway hyper-reactivity independently of adaptive immunity. Nat Immunol. 2011;12(7):631–8.
36. Mjosberg JM, Trifari S, Crellin NK, Peters CP, van Drunen CM, Piet B, et al. Human IL-25- and IL-33-responsive type 2 innate lymphoid cells are defined by expression of CRTH2 and CD161. Nat Immunol. 2011;12(11):1055–62.
37. Scanlon ST, McKenzie AN. Type 2 innate lymphoid cells: new players in asthma and allergy. Curr Opin Immunol. 2012;24(6):707–12.
38. Bonds RS, Midoro-Horiuti T. Estrogen effects in allergy and asthma. Curr Opin Allergy Clin Immunol. 2013;13(1):92–9.
39. Salam MT, Wenten M, Gilliland FD. Endogenous and exogenous sex steroid hormones and asthma and wheeze in young women. J Allergy Clin Immunol. 2006;117(5):1001–7.
40. Agarwal AK, Shah A. Menstrual-linked asthma. J Asthma. 1997;34(6):539–45.
41. Eliasson O, Scherzer HH, DeGraff Jr AC. Morbidity in asthma in relation to the menstrual cycle. J Allergy Clin Immunol. 1986;77(1 Pt 1):87–94.
42. Hanley SP. Asthma variation with menstruation. Br J Dis Chest. 1981;75(3):306–8.
43. Shames RS, Heilbron DC, Janson SL, Kishiyama JL, Au DS, Adelman DC. Clinical differences among women with and without self-reported perimenstrual asthma. Ann Allergy, Asthma Immunol. 1998;81(1):65–72.

44. Brenner BE, Holmes TM, Mazal B, Camargo Jr CA. Relation between phase of the menstrual cycle and asthma presentations in the emergency department. Thorax. 2005;60(10):806–9.
45. Dweik RA, Boggs PB, Erzurum SC, Irvin CG, Leigh MW, Lundberg JO, et al. An official ATS clinical practice guideline: interpretation of exhaled nitric oxide levels (FENO) for clinical applications. Am J Respir Crit Care Med. 2011;184(5):602–15.
46. Oguzulgen IK, Turktas H, Erbas D. Airway inflammation in premenstrual asthma. J Asthma. 2002;39(6):517–22.
47. Tan KS, McFarlane LC, Lipworth BJ. Modulation of airway reactivity and peak flow variability in asthmatics receiving the oral contraceptive pill. Am J Respir Crit Care Med. 1997;155(4):1273–7.
48. Murphy VE, Gibson PG. Premenstrual asthma: prevalence, cycle-to-cycle variability and relationship to oral contraceptive use and menstrual symptoms. J Asthma. 2008;45(8):696–704.
49. Kwon HL, Belanger K, Bracken MB. Asthma prevalence among pregnant and childbearing-aged women in the United States: estimates from national health surveys. Ann Epidemiol. 2003;13(5):317–24.
50. Schatz M, Harden K, Forsythe A, Chilingar L, Hoffman C, Sperling W, et al. The course of asthma during pregnancy, post partum, and with successive pregnancies: a prospective analysis. J Allergy Clin Immunol. 1988;81(3):509–17.
51. Stenius-Aarniala B, Piirila P, Teramo K. Asthma and pregnancy: a prospective study of 198 pregnancies. Thorax. 1988;43(1):12–8.
52. Schatz M. Interrelationships between asthma and pregnancy: a literature review. J Allergy Clin Immunol. 1999;103(2 Pt 2):S330–6.
53. Forbes RL, Gibson PG, Murphy VE, Wark PA. Impaired type I and III interferon response to rhinovirus infection during pregnancy and asthma. Thorax. 2012;67(3):209–14.
54. Forbes RL, Wark PA, Murphy VE, Gibson PG. Pregnant women have attenuated innate interferon responses to 2009 pandemic influenza A virus subtype H1N1. J Infect Dis. 2012;206(5):646–53.
55. National Heart, Lung, and Blood Institute, National Asthma Education and Prevention Program Asthma and Pregnancy Working Group. NAEPP expert panel report. Managing asthma during pregnancy: recommendations for pharmacologic treatment-2004 update. J Allergy Clin Immunol. 2005;115(1):34–46.
56. (GINA) GIfA. Global Strategy for Asthma Management and Prevention. 2014.
57. Lim A, Stewart K, Konig K, George J. Systematic review of the safety of regular preventive asthma medications during pregnancy. Ann Pharmacother. 2011;45(7–8):931–45.
58. Murphy VE, Clifton VL, Gibson PG. Asthma exacerbations during pregnancy: incidence and association with adverse pregnancy outcomes. Thorax. 2006;61(2):169–76.
59. Ticconi C, Pietropolli A, Piccione E. Estrogen replacement therapy and asthma. Pulm Pharmacol Ther. 2013;26(6):617–23.
60. Gomez Real F, Svanes C, Bjornsson EH, Franklin KA, Gislason D, Gislason T, et al. Hormone replacement therapy, body mass index and asthma in perimenopausal women: a cross sectional survey. Thorax. 2006;61(1):34–40.
61. Real FG, Svanes C, Omenaas ER, Anto JM, Plana E, Jarvis D, et al. Lung function, respiratory symptoms, and the menopausal transition. J Allergy Clin Immunol. 2008;121(1):72–80. e3.
62. Balzano G, Fuschillo S, De Angelis E, Gaudiosi C, Mancini A, Caputi M. Persistent airway inflammation and high exacerbation rate in asthma that starts at menopause. Monaldi archives for chest disease = Archivio Monaldi per le malattie del torace/Fondazione clinica del lavoro, IRCCS [and] Istituto di clinica tisiologica e malattie apparato respiratorio, Universita di Napoli, Secondo ateneo. 2007;67(3):135–41.
63. Walters DM, Wills-Karp M, Mitzner W. Assessment of cellular profile and lung function with repeated bronchoalveolar lavage in individual mice. Physiol Genomics. 2000;2(1):29–36.
64. Card JW, Carey MA, Bradbury JA, DeGraff LM, Morgan DL, Moorman MP, et al. Gender differences in murine airway responsiveness and lipopolysaccharide-induced inflammation. J Immunol. 2006;177(1):621–30.

65. Card JW, Zeldin DC. Hormonal influences on lung function and response to environmental agents: lessons from animal models of respiratory disease. Proc Am Thorac Soc. 2009;6(7):588–95.
66. Carey MA, Card JW, Bradbury JA, Moorman MP, Haykal-Coates N, Gavett SH, et al. Spontaneous airway hyperresponsiveness in estrogen receptor-alpha-deficient mice. Am J Respir Crit Care Med. 2007;175(2):126–35.
67. Matsubara S, Swasey CH, Loader JE, Dakhama A, Joetham A, Ohnishi H, et al. Estrogen determines sex differences in airway responsiveness after allergen exposure. Am J Respir Cell Mol Biol. 2008;38(5):501–8.
68. Massaro GD, Mortola JP, Massaro D. Sexual dimorphism in the architecture of the lung's gas-exchange region. Proc Natl Acad Sci U S A. 1995;92(4):1105–7.
69. Massaro D, Massaro GD. Estrogen regulates pulmonary alveolar formation, loss, and regeneration in mice. Am J Physiol Lung Cell Mol Physiol. 2004;287(6):L1154–9.
70. Card JW, Voltz JW, Ferguson CD, Carey MA, DeGraff LM, Peddada SD, et al. Male sex hormones promote vagally mediated reflex airway responsiveness to cholinergic stimulation. Am J Physiol Lung Cell Mol Physiol. 2007;292(4):L908–14.
71. Helmi AM, El Ghazzawi IF, Mandour MA, Shehata MA. The effect of oestrogen on the nasal respiratory mucosa. An experimental histopathological and histochemical study. J Laryngol Otol. 1975;89(12):1229–41.
72. Tam A, Wadsworth S, Dorscheid D, Man SF, Sin DD. Estradiol increases mucus synthesis in bronchial epithelial cells. PLoS One. 2014;9(6), e100633.
73. Choi HJ, Chung YS, Kim HJ, Moon UY, Choi YH, Van Seuningen I, et al. Signal pathway of 17beta-estradiol-induced MUC5B expression in human airway epithelial cells. Am J Respir Cell Mol Biol. 2009;40(2):168–78.
74. Blacquiere MJ, Hylkema MN, Postma DS, Geerlings M, Timens W, Melgert BN. Airway inflammation and remodeling in two mouse models of asthma: comparison of males and females. Int Arch Allergy Immunol. 2010;153(2):173–81.
75. Hayashi T, Adachi Y, Hasegawa K, Morimoto M. Less sensitivity for late airway inflammation in males than females in BALB/c mice. Scand J Immunol. 2003;57(6):562–7.
76. Takeda M, Tanabe M, Ito W, Ueki S, Konnno Y, Chihara M, et al. Gender difference in allergic airway remodelling and immunoglobulin production in mouse model of asthma. Respirology. 2013;18(5):797–806.
77. Riffo-Vasquez Y, Ligeiro de Oliveira AP, Page CP, Spina D, Tavares-de-Lima W. Role of sex hormones in allergic inflammation in mice. Clin Exp Allergy. 2007;37(3):459–70.
78. Takeda K, Haczku A, Lee JJ, Irvin CG, Gelfand EW. Strain dependence of airway hyperresponsiveness reflects differences in eosinophil localization in the lung. Am J Physiol Lung Cell Mol Physiol. 2001;281(2):L394–402.
79. Seymour BW, Friebertshauser KE, Peake JL, Pinkerton KE, Coffman RL, Gershwin LJ. Gender differences in the allergic response of mice neonatally exposed to environmental tobacco smoke. Dev Immunol. 2002;9(1):47–54.
80. Melgert BN, Postma DS, Kuipers I, Geerlings M, Luinge MA, van der Strate BW, et al. Female mice are more susceptible to the development of allergic airway inflammation than male mice. Clin Exp Allergy. 2005;35(11):1496–503.
81. Jensen F, Woudwyk M, Teles A, Woidacki K, Taran F, Costa S, et al. Estradiol and progesterone regulate the migration of mast cells from the periphery to the uterus and induce their maturation and degranulation. PLoS One. 2010;5(12), e14409.
82. McSorley HJ, Blair NF, Smith KA, McKenzie AN, Maizels RM. Blockade of IL-33 release and suppression of type 2 innate lymphoid cell responses by helminth secreted products in airway allergy. Mucosal Immunol. 2014;7:1068–78.
83. Miossec P, Kolls JK. Targeting IL-17 and TH17 cells in chronic inflammation. Nat Rev Drug Discov. 2012;11(10):763–76.
84. Newcomb DC, Peebles Jr RS. Th17-mediated inflammation in asthma. Curr Opin Immunol. 2013;25(6):755–60.

Chapter 5
Sex Hormones, Sex, Gender, and Pulmonary Hypertension

Xinping (Peter) Chen and Eric D. Austin

Abstract Pulmonary arterial hypertension (PAH) is a devastating disease of the pulmonary vasculature resulting in right ventricular failure and death. PAH may occur as a primary disease or in association with a diverse range of diseases. While a skewed gender ratio with significantly more females diagnosed than males is common in PAH, other forms of PH more broadly do not have a pronounced sexual dimorphism. While more females are diagnosed with PAH, recent epidemiologic data suggest that survival among females is better than males, especially compared to older male patients. The mechanisms of the sex-related variations in phenotype are incompletely understood, but likely involve variation in response to parent compound sex hormones and their metabolites.

Introduction

Pulmonary hypertension (PH) is a progressive and devastating disease resulting in extreme elevation of pulmonary arterial pressure and subsequent right ventricular strain. Among its prominent subtypes is pulmonary arterial hypertension (PAH), which is characterized by pulmonary vascular remodeling of the distal pulmonary vasculature, ultimately leading to destruction and loss of the smallest pulmonary arteries [1]. Clinically, PAH results in reduced pulmonary arterial blood flow, increased pulmonary vascular resistance, and ultimately failure of the right heart [2]. PAH may occur as a primary disease or in association with a diverse range of diseases such as congenital heart disease, connective tissue disease (e.g., Scleroderma), and portal hypertension [3]. While a skewed gender ratio with

X. Chen, PhD
Department of Medicine, Division of Allergy, Pulmonary, and Critical Care Medicine,
Vanderbilt University School of Medicine, Nashville, TN, USA

E.D. Austin, MD, MSCI (✉)
Department of Pediatrics, Division of Allergy, Immunology, and Pulmonary Medicine,
Vanderbilt University School of Medicine, Suite DD-2205, Vanderbilt Medical Center North,
Nashville, TN 37232-2578, USA
e-mail: eric.austin@vanderbilt.edu

© Springer International Publishing Switzerland 2016
A.R. Hemnes (ed.), *Gender, Sex Hormones and Respiratory Disease*,
Respiratory Medicine, DOI 10.1007/978-3-319-23998-9_5

significantly more females diagnosed than males is common in PAH, other forms of PH more broadly do not have a pronounced sexual dimorphism [4–6]. Intriguingly, while more females are diagnosed with PAH, recent epidemiologic data from France and North America suggest that survival among females is better than males, especially compared to older male patients [7–9].

The apparent discrepancy between incidence and survival is one of several components of a prominent "estrogen paradox" in the PAH field [10]. While the term "estrogen paradox" could more broadly be designated a "sex paradox," its essence lies in several features, most prominent: (a) discrepancy between incidence and survival in human PAH according to sex; (b) the fact that the majority of animal models of PH suggest that female animals are less susceptible to develop PH for a variety of reasons including the fact that molecularly estrogens are antiproliferative and anti-inflammatory and also have physiologic effects consistent with improved right ventricular function and pulmonary vascular relaxation; and (c) many of the known molecular and physiologic effects of estrogens should be protective for the pulmonary vasculature.

Understanding the mechanistic details behind the "sex paradox" in PAH is crucial for many reasons, including not only improving clinical care but also due to the current National Institutes of Health (NIH) focus upon sex and gender equity in studies (NIH Press Release: September 23, 2014). Hopefully, in-depth understanding of the role of sex and sex hormones in PAH will stimulate novel therapeutic approaches to treat this devastating disease. This chapter briefly discusses the intersection of human, in vitro, and animal studies of pulmonary arterial hypertension and highlights the conflicting data concerning the "estrogen paradox" in PAH [10–13]. To comply with preferred national nomenclature, "sex" will be used to represent the status of "male" and "female" in lieu of the term "gender" [14].

Sex and the Epidemiology of PAH: Prevalent Cases Skew toward Females

PAH has been known as a female predominant disease for at least 65 years. Dresdale and colleagues initiated the modern medical descriptions of PAH (then known as primary pulmonary hypertension, PPH) in the 1950s as a disease seen more among females [15, 16]. Consistent with those reports, the NIH supported a Registry Study in the 1980s which supported the belief that PPH cases are more likely to be females [17]. While it is an accepted phenomenon, the true prevalence and incidence of PAH according to sex remains incompletely elucidated although many efforts to explore this further have been recently published or are under way [18]. It is important to recognize that most published studies to date have predominantly evaluated prevalent cases; this can inject bias because if sex-related effects influence survival, incidence and prevalence may not be equal.

Several recently published studies have contributed to our understanding of this issue, however, in larger populations. In North America, the Registry to Evaluate Early and Long-term PAH Disease Management (REVEAL)database studied over 2000 subjects in a large registry to describe clinical characteristics of PAH patients.

While designed to enroll prevalent and/or incident patients in the United States with WHO Group 1 PAH, the registry was biased toward prevalent cases due to overall rarity of PAH [19]. We learned from the REVEAL study that among prevalent cases of PAH (Group1 PH), the percentage of females is extremely high [7, 20]. Specifically, 79.5 % of the adult PAH patients were female in the initial reports, with the female-to-male ratio among IPAH patients 4.1:1. The NIH Registry had reported 1.7:1 in 1987, although this was a pre-therapy era with shorter survival than the current era [17]. As discussed below, survivor bias may skew prevalent case assessments.

In addition to PAH as a whole, the REVEAL Registry also demonstrated that in general the female predominance of prevalent cases is found across nearly all PAH subtypes (Table 5.1). But intriguingly, while females were more prevalent, REVEAL suggested that older males live shorter after diagnosis compared to younger males and to females [7]. As discussed next, data from France do not specifically replicate this finding, but do support the concept that males survive shorter after diagnosis than females.

In the early 2000s, French investigators enrolled 674 cases of PAH from 17 university hospitals across France over a 12-month period. They found a higher proportion of females among prevalent cases (67.1 % of prevalent cases) [6]. But, among new diagnoses (incident cases; $n = 121$) of PAH, the percentage of females was lower, at 57.0 % within that cohort ($n = 121$). While not a dramatic difference, the discrepancy in female predominance between incident and prevalent cases does suggest a survival benefit to being female over male consistent with the REVEAL data. Furthermore, in a follow-up study in France, those same investigators showed that heritable PAH (HPAH), idiopathic PAH (IPAH), and anorexigen-associated PAH all had improved survival for females compared to males [8, 9].

While the differences in survival according to sex remain unclear, it is known that survival in PAH is strongly influenced by the response and performance of the right ventricle to load stress [21]. While sex and sex hormone levels have been extensively studied in left heart failure, the role of sex hormones in right ventricular (RV) function irrespective of disease status is relatively understudied. Recently, some clues have emerged from the work of investigators of the Multi-Ethnic Study of

Table 5.1 Data from the REVEAL study: comparison of gender ratios observed in PAH patients with different types of WHO Group 1 PAH [20]

Type of Group 1 PAH	Number of patients (% female)	Ratio of females:males
All patients with Group 1 PAH	2525 (79.5 %)	3.9:1
IPAH	1166 (80.3 %)	4.1:1
Drugs/Toxins-PAH	134 (84.3 %)	5.4:1
CHD-PAH	250 (73.6 %)	2.8:1
CTD-PAH	639 (90.1)	9.1:1

Adapted from Badesch et al. Chest 2010;137;376–387

IPAH idiopathic PAH, *CHD* congenital heart disease, *CTD* connective tissue disease

Atherosclerosis (MESA) program. MESA is a multicenter prospective cohort study designed to investigate subclinical cardiovascular disease in White, African-American, Hispanic, and Chinese subjects [22]. While the MESA study is not specific to PAH (and in fact is a study of reportedly healthy subjects), its findings in postmenopausal women suggested that higher levels of circulating estradiol (one of the main "parent compound" estrogens) are associated with higher RV systolic function. In both healthy postmenopausal women and men, levels of androgens (testosterone and dehydroepiandrosterone) are associated with higher RV mass and larger RV volumes [23]. Among PAH patients, females had a higher RV ejection fraction at the time of diagnosis than male patients [24]. Thus, there is growing data to suggest that female sex may negatively influence pulmonary vascular disease pathogenesis, but positively influence right heart adaptation to the stress of pulmonary hypertension.

The Association Between Sex Hormones and Human PAH

The long-standing understanding that PAH is a disease influenced by sex suggests that factors related to genetic differences between the sexes (e.g., chromosomal differences, XX and XY) and/or hormonal variations contribute to disease pathogenesis and perhaps progression. There is a growing body of investigation exploring these possibilities.

Genetic Differences Related to the Sex Chromosomes To date, few studies have investigated sex chromosomal differences in humans. The X and Y chromosomes are vital contributors of genetic data to the human and other genomes. The X chromosome contributes about 155 million base pairs of DNA, representing approximately 5 % of the total DNA in cells. The Y chromosome contributes about 59 million base pairs of DNA, representing approximately 2 % of the total DNA in cells. Most genome-wide association studies have underinvestigated the contribution of sex chromosomes in all disease states due to the challenge of integrating the sex chromosomes using bioinformatics. There is a line of investigation suggestive that the presence of the Y chromosome is protective in hypoxia-associated mice models of PH, suggesting that genetic factors on the Y chromosome are relevant (ATS 2015 Conference: Am J Respir Crit Care Med 191;2015:A4100), which is an intriguing hypothesis.

Differences with Regard to Sex Hormones Unlike the sex chromosomes, which hopefully will prompt increased interest over time, there has been tremendous research interest in the sex hormones in the past decade. Traditionally, female sex hormones, in particular estrogens, have been perceived as protective of pulmonary vascular reactivity, inflammation, and remodeling. This has largely derived from animal model work on the disease over the past 30 years. In humans, it is notable that even for diseases with a global female predominance irrespective of PAH (e.g., connective tissue disease), the predominance of females among the subset of subjects with PAH is substantial. For example, the REVEAL study found that among PAH patients with connective tissue disease, nine females were represented for every one male [20]. Interestingly, unlike other forms of PAH, connective tissue disease-associated PAH is more often associated with older diagnosis, in particular postmenopausal women [20, 25]. The relationship between this finding and menopausal status could suggest that hormones are protective in connective tissue disease patients. In support of the hypothesis that female sex hormones are protective, a retrospective study of 61 scleroderma patients without echocardiographic evidence of pulmonary hypertension at the time of menopause demonstrated the development of PAH in the subsequent postmenopausal years among 20 patients was 0 % (mean duration of follow-up was 7.2 ± 3.5 years) for those using hormone replacement therapy; in contrast, 8 out of 41 patients (19.5 %) developed PAH after a similar period of time postmenopause (7.5 ± 3.9 years) but without any hormone replacement therapy [26]. This single study does suggest an association between hormone replacement therapy and protection among those with connective tissue disease, but certainly the topic requires further study.

There is more data to suggest that sex hormones, in particular estrogens, contribute in a detrimental manner to PAH. First, idiopathic and heritable PAH forms, as well as anorexigen-associated, are clinically known to manifest during or soon after pregnancy, and pharmacologic exposure to estrogens has been described in PAH patients although not systematically studied to date [27–30]. Most PAH clinicians caution patients to avoid pregnancy, in part due to the significant changes to blood volume and circulation. In addition, while the ramifications are unknown, there are significant increases in estrogens and progestins during pregnancy related to placental production [2]. Among female patients with portopulmonary PAH, genetic variations in estrogen signaling, as well as enhanced plasma estradiol levels, are associated with PAH [31]. Similarly, genetic variations in estrogen metabolism, as well as estrogen metabolite levels, are associated with heritable PAH in females due to mutations in bone morphogenetic protein receptor type 2 (*BMPR2*); recently, males with *BMPR2* gene mutations had similar irregularities in estrogen metabolites [32, 33].

From a broad epidemiologic perspective, there is a paucity of data concerning sex hormone exposures and PAH. However, a recent epidemiologic study sought to address this deficiency, using 88 patients attending the Eighth International Pulmonary Hypertension Association Conference. While lacking a control group for comparison, this study used sex hormone exposure questionnaires and found that 81 % of women with PAH reported prior use of any hormone therapy, with 70 % reporting exogenous hormone use for greater than 10 years. This supported an association of PAH with estrogen-containing compounds [34].

The Pulmonary Vasculature: Effects of Sex Hormones

Estrogens, progestins, and androgens have multiple effects on the pulmonary vasculature. Overall, it is difficult to label any one sex hormone as "detrimental" or "protective." On the contrary, the cell type, situation, and duration are likely highly important but still explain only a proportion of the variability. While this may not be the case for all forms of PH, for the PAH condition estrogens may be acutely protective but detrimental on a chronic basis. The data concerning other sex hormones is even more insufficiently elucidated.

Acutely, estrogens are likely protective for the pulmonary vasculature. Smooth muscle cell activation by estradiol results in vasodilation and attenuation of the vasoconstrictor response caused by various stimuli, including hypoxia. In the physiologic state, variations in estrogen levels (for example, as occurs in menstruating females) are associated with the degree of pulmonary artery vasoconstriction in response to hypoxia—hypoxic vasoconstriction is reduced with exposure to increased circulating estrogen levels [35]. While the precise mechanism may be multifactorial, estradiol appears to stimulate the release of compounds known to promote pulmonary artery relaxation, including prostacyclin and nitric oxide (NO) acutely [11].

While estrogens exert their effects by a multitude of manners, the canonical pathways of estradiol-induced vasorelaxation occur via binding to one of two estrogen receptors: ERα and ERβ [36, 37]. This has been shown largely via animal model work, such as in the Sprague–Dawley rat model. In this system, the acute vasodilatory effects of estradiol occur via acute ligand binding by estradiol to both estrogen receptor α (ERα) and estrogen receptor β (ERβ). In this model system, direct binding of both ERα and ERβ mediated arterial vasorelaxation [38]. But in addition to ERα and ERβ, growing data suggest that estrogens can both directly bind to DNA to influence transcription and non-genomically signal via the g-coupled protein receptor GPR30. GPR30-mediated signaling promotes vascular relaxation [39].

Despite the evidence that estrogens, or at least estradiol, acutely relax the pulmonary vasculature, there is concern that on a chronic basis they may be detrimental. In particular, estradiol promotes inappropriate pulmonary vascular proliferation and cell damage on a chronic basis in vitro. Much of this work has evolved from the sex hormone cancer literature, although there is growing evidence using lung vascular cells. For example, estradiol is a potent mitogen which promotes proliferation of pulmonary vascular smooth muscle cells and other cell types; estrogen antagonism by the drug tamoxifen blocks this effect [40]. In addition, estradiol may directly modify angiogenesis in a number of ways, including the alteration of endothelial cell migration and function via GPR30. Angiogenesis characterizes severe PAH in humans and this could be a feature accentuated by estrogens.

While much of the focus of sex hormones in PAH has centered upon estrogens, androgens likely modify pulmonary vascular cell function and growth, as well. Both testosterone and dehydroepiandrosterone (DHEA) appear protective via induction of vasodilatation in studies of pulmonary vascular smooth muscle cells via acute antagonism of calcium signaling with augmentation of potassium channel-mediated relaxation in male and female cells [41, 42]. In the setting of hypoxia, DHEA protects human pulmonary artery smooth muscle cells via reduction of hypoxia-inducible factor 1α, which is a vasoconstrictive agent in the pulmonary vasculature, suggesting a protective influence. Intriguingly, DHEA inhibits Src/STAT3 activation in the pulmonary artery smooth muscle cells of patients with PAH; while results of this activation are incompletely elucidated, upregulation of both *BMPR2* and miR-204 expression occurs and is relevant to pulmonary vascular homeostasis [43].

Overall, however, animal model data concerning the influence of androgens on the pulmonary hypertensive phenotype are mixed; for example, while male rodents are often more susceptible to most forms of experimental pulmonary hypertension, treatment with DHEA may be protective. As a result, a firm conclusion regarding the influence of androgens is difficult to provide at this time, pending additional animal studies which are currently under way [44].

Beyond Parent Compound Sex Hormones: Metabolites

While parent compound sex hormones likely play a role in pulmonary vascular homeostasis in health and disease, their metabolites likely contribute as well. The biology around the role of metabolites is even more incomplete, but of growing interest. Sex hormone metabolites likely mediate estrogenic and antiestrogenic effects on the pulmonary vasculature. In fact, inherent and iatrogenic variations in metabolism may account for the apparent contradictory influences of estrogens noted above. For example, while it appears that most parent compound estrogens (e.g., estradiol) are pro-proliferative on a chronic basis, not all estrogen metabolites share this impact. Depending on the estrogen metabolite, one can see disparate effects, and there may be variations according to cell type as with estradiol. The specifics of these differences have yet to be fully elucidated for parent compound sex hormones or their metabolites.

While androgens can be converted to estrogens, the metabolism of sex hormones is a complex process, largely mediated via the cytochrome P450 (CYP) family of enzymes both systemically and at a local level within the pulmonary vasculature (Fig. 5.1) [45, 46]. CYP1B1, for example, which oxidizes estradiol and estrone, is highly expressed in the lung and other organs [46]. Oxidation of estrogens also occurs by hydroxylation at the C-2, C-4, and C-16 position by CYP450 enzymes, followed by additional enzymatic reactions [47, 48]. It appears that "2-estrogens" are antimitogenic, while "16-estrogens" stimulate cellular proliferation by constitutively activating the estrogen receptors and this has been demonstrated in the pulmonary vasculature [46]. "16-estrogens" may also damage the genome directly via the formation of unstable DNA adducts [49, 50]. As a result, individuals who produce a higher ratio of "16-estrogens" compared to other estrogen metabolites may be at increased risk of diseases that result from both the mitogenic and genotoxic effects of estrogens [51–56].

Interest in the role of estrogens in PAH was redirected in the early 2000s due to the discovery by West et al. that *CYP1B1* expression associates with PAH among *BMPR2* mutation carriers. In fact, quantitative measures of *CYP1B1* expression showed tenfold lower expression levels in female patients compared to healthy *BMPR2* mutation carriers [57]. White and colleagues subsequently found enhanced CYP1B1 expression in the lungs of PAH patients without mutation [46].

As noted above, it was subsequently demonstrated that a specific urinary profile of estrogen metabolites is associated with PAH among female *BMPR2* mutation carriers. Specifically, PAH patients had significantly lower ratio of 2-hydroxyestrogens

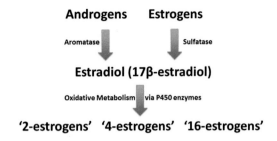

Fig. 5.1 Simplified schematic of sex hormones and estrogen metabolism. Sulfated estrogens, and androgens, are converted to parent compound estrogens including estradiol. Estradiol is metabolized by CYP450 enzyme activity into oxidized products, including those oxidized at the 2-, 4-, and 16-positions

(2-OHE$_{1/2}$): 16-α-hydroxyestrone (16-αOHE$_1$) compared to unaffected *BMPR2* mutation carriers [32]. In addition, certain functional polymorphisms in *CYP1B1* (a cytochrome P450 enzyme critical to estrogen metabolism) consistent with the urinary data are also associated with PAH in those subjects [32].

The influence of estrogen metabolites to PAH remains an area of active investigation. We and others believe that variations in estrogen metabolites influence the development of PAH, especially among those with an underlying disease risk. For example, estradiol and 16-αOHE$_1$ both downregulate BMPR2 expression in lymphocytes and lung vascular cells, which could amplify disease penetrance among *BMPR2* mutation carriers and/or create a new risk factor among those without mutation [32, 58]. In animal model studies, Bmpr2 mutant mice develop PAH at a much higher level of penetrance upon exposure to 16-αOHE$_1$ [33]. While estrogens reduced inflammatory cytokine expression acutely (a known beneficial effect of estrogens), they also amplified markers of pulmonary vascular injury. These included the alteration of genes related to thrombotic function, angiogenesis, planar polarity, and cellular metabolism [33]. Similarly, in a serotonin transporter (SERT)model of pulmonary hypertension known to amplify penetrance with female sex (in hypoxia, female mice that overexpress the serotonin transporter (SERT; SERT+ mice) exhibit PAH and exaggerated hypoxia-induced PAH, while male SERT+ mice do not [59, 60]); antagonism of ERα improves serotonin-dependent pulmonary hypertension and increases BMPR2 expression. In addition, ERα was found to be highly expressed pulmonary artery smooth muscle cells derived from PAH patients and increased in vitro via serotonin [61].

In contrast to the Bmpr2 and SERT murine data presented above, most animal models of pulmonary hypertension demonstrate a protective effect associated with female sex which appears to be mediated via parent compound estrogens, such as estradiol. The use of animal models to study pulmonary hypertension has been an area of controversy for many years. Admittedly, there is no perfect model and each animal model has advantages and drawbacks.

In most rodent models, including those which employ hypoxia and monocrotaline, and swine models (e.g., hypoxia), exposure to the insult of interest causes pulmonary hypertension to a much greater degree in male animals than females. The reasons for this are presently unclear [62–65]. Further complicating this, Sprague–Dawley rats exposed to monocrotaline develop pulmonary hypertension, but this is prevented and reversed with estradiol [66, 67]; however, ovariectomy of females promoted a pulmonary hypertensive phenotype [68]. Of particular interest given the data noted above that ERα promotes PAH, the beneficial effects of estrogen using the monocrotaline model appear to be mediated via ERβ specifically [66]. Further studies in additional animal models of PAH will be beneficial to help elucidate the complicated role of all sex hormones in the pathogenesis of PAH and explain the discrepancy between observations in humans and these animal models on the salutary or negative effects of estrogens.

The study of androgenic compounds, such as DHEA, is a logical consideration for pursuit using both animal models and cell-based studies. However, this is an area in need of expanded research. Some experimental pulmonary hypertension studies using male rates exposed to hypoxia and/or monocrotaline have shown improvement in the pulmonary hypertensive phenotype due to DHEA, and more studies are under way [43, 69, 70].

Conclusion

The female sex is associated with a higher incidence and prevalence of PAH in humans. The enhanced prevalence, and other recent findings, suggests that the female RV may be better suited to handle pulmonary hypertension for longer. But, the causes for this remain elusive. While sex hormones are increasingly implicated in the causation of PAH, the precise mechanisms require further study. Ultimately, precise understanding may result in important progress in solving this devastating disease via the development of novel therapeutic targets and prevention measures.

Sources of Support and Conflicts of Interest This work was supported in part by NIH grant K23 HL 098743 (PI: EDA). The authors have no potential conflicts of interest to disclose.

References

1. Tuder RM, Abman SH, Braun T, Capron F, Stevens T, Thistlethwaite PA, et al. Development and pathology of pulmonary hypertension. J Am Coll Cardiol. 2009;54(1 Suppl):S3–9.
2. McLaughlin VV, Archer SL, Badesch DB, Barst RJ, Farber HW, Lindner JR, et al. ACCF/AHA 2009 expert consensus document on pulmonary hypertension a report of the American College of Cardiology Foundation Task Force on Expert Consensus Documents and the American Heart Association developed in collaboration with the American College of Chest Physicians; American Thoracic Society, Inc.; and the Pulmonary Hypertension Association. J Am Coll Cardiol. 2009;53(17):1573–619.
3. Simonneau G, Robbins IM, Beghetti M, Channick RN, Delcroix M, Denton CP, et al. Updated clinical classification of pulmonary hypertension. J Am Coll Cardiol. 2009;54(1 Suppl):S43–54.

4. Badesch DB, Raskob GE, Elliott CG, Krichman AM, Farber HW, Frost AE, et al. Pulmonary arterial hypertension: baseline characteristics from the REVEAL registry. Chest. 2009;137:376–87.
5. Chin KM, Rubin LJ. Pulmonary arterial hypertension. J Am Coll Cardiol. 2008;51(16):1527–38.
6. Humbert M, Sitbon O, Chaouat A, Bertocchi M, Habib G, Gressin V, et al. Pulmonary arterial hypertension in France: results from a national registry. Am J Respir Crit Care Med. 2006;173(9):1023–30.
7. Benza RL, Miller DP, Gomberg-Maitland M, Frantz RP, Foreman AJ, Coffey CS, et al. Predicting survival in pulmonary arterial hypertension: insights from the Registry to Evaluate Early and Long-Term Pulmonary Arterial Hypertension Disease Management (REVEAL). Circulation. 2010;122(2):164–72.
8. Humbert M, Sitbon O, Yaici A, Montani D, O'Callaghan DS, Jais X, et al. Survival in incident and prevalent cohorts of patients with pulmonary arterial hypertension. Eur Respir J. 2010;36(3):549–55.
9. Humbert M, Sitbon O, Chaouat A, Bertocchi M, Habib G, Gressin V, et al. Survival in patients with idiopathic, familial, and anorexigen-associated pulmonary arterial hypertension in the modern management era. Circulation. 2010;122(20585011):156–63.
10. Tofovic SP. Estrogens and development of pulmonary hypertension: interaction of estradiol metabolism and pulmonary vascular disease. J Cardiovasc Pharmacol. 2010;56(6):696–708.
11. Lahm T, Crisostomo PR, Markel TA, Wang M, Weil BR, Novotny NM, et al. The effects of estrogen on pulmonary artery vasoreactivity and hypoxic pulmonary vasoconstriction: potential new clinical implications for an old hormone. Crit Care Med. 2008;36(7):2174–83.
12. de Jesus Perez VA. Making sense of the estrogen paradox in pulmonary arterial hypertension. Am J Respir Crit Care Med. 2011;184(6):629–30.
13. Lahm T, Tuder RM, Petrache I. Progress in solving the sex hormone paradox in pulmonary hypertension. Am J Physiol Lung Cell Mol Physiol. 2014;307(1):L7–26.
14. Institute of Medicine (U.S.). Committee on Understanding the Biology of Sex and Gender Differences., Wizemann TM, Pardue ML. Exploring the biological contributions to human health: does sex matter? Washington, DC: National Academy Press; 2001. Xx: 267.
15. Dresdale DT, Michtom RJ, Schultz M. Recent studies in primary pulmonary hypertension, including pharmacodynamic observations on pulmonary vascular resistance. Bull N Y Acad Med. 1954;30(3):195–207.
16. Dresdale DT, Schultz M, Michtom RJ. Primary pulmonary hypertension. I. Clinical and hemodynamic study. Am J Med. 1951;11(6):686–705.
17. Rich S, Dantzker DR, Ayres SM, Bergofsky EH, Brundage BH, Detre KM, et al. Primary pulmonary hypertension. A national prospective study. Ann Intern Med. 1987;107(2):216–23.
18. Brown LM, Chen H, Halpern S, Taichman D, McGoon MD, Farber HW, et al. Delay in recognition of pulmonary arterial hypertension: factors identified from the REVEAL Registry. Chest. 2011;140(1):19–26.
19. McGoon MD, Krichman A, Farber HW, Barst RJ, Raskob GE, Liou TG, et al. Design of the REVEAL registry for US patients with pulmonary arterial hypertension. Mayo Clin Proc. 2008;83(8):923–31.
20. Badesch DB, Raskob GE, Elliott CG, Krichman AM, Farber HW, Frost AE, et al. Pulmonary arterial hypertension: baseline characteristics from the REVEAL Registry. Chest. 2010;137(2):376–87.
21. D'Alonzo GE, Barst RJ, Ayres SM, Bergofsky EH, Brundage BH, Detre KM, et al. Survival in patients with primary pulmonary hypertension. Results from a national prospective registry. Ann Intern Med. 1991;115(5):343–9.
22. Bild DE, Bluemke DA, Burke GL, Detrano R, Diez Roux AV, Folsom AR, et al. Multi-ethnic study of atherosclerosis: objectives and design. Am J Epidemiol. 2002;156(9):871–81.
23. Ventetuolo CE, Ouyang P, Bluemke DA, Tandri H, Barr RG, Bagiella E, et al. Sex hormones are associated with right ventricular structure and function: the MESA-right ventricle study. Am J Respir Crit Care Med. 2011;183(5):659–67.

24. Kawut SM, Lima JA, Barr RG, Chahal H, Jain A, Tandri H, et al. Sex and race differences in right ventricular structure and function: the multi-ethnic study of atherosclerosis-right ventricle study. Circulation. 2011;123(22):2542–51.
25. Scorza R, Caronni M, Bazzi S, Nador F, Beretta L, Antonioli R, et al. Post-menopause is the main risk factor for developing isolated pulmonary hypertension in systemic sclerosis. Ann N Y Acad Sci. 2002;966:238–46.
26. Beretta L, Caronni M, Origgi L, Ponti A, Santaniello A, Scorza R. Hormone replacement therapy may prevent the development of isolated pulmonary hypertension in patients with systemic sclerosis and limited cutaneous involvement. Scand J Rheumatol. 2006;35(6):468–71.
27. Kleiger RE, Boxer M, Ingham RE, Harrison DC. Pulmonary hypertension in patients using oral contraceptives. A report of six cases. Chest. 1976;69(2):143–7.
28. Morse JH, Horn EM, Barst RJ. Hormone replacement therapy: a possible risk factor in carriers of familial primary pulmonary hypertension. Chest. 1999;116(3):847.
29. Irey NS, Manion WC, Taylor HB. Vascular lesions in women taking oral contraceptives. Arch Pathol. 1970;89(1):1–8.
30. Irey NS, Norris HJ. Intimal vascular lesions associated with female reproductive steroids. Arch Pathol. 1973;96(4):227–34.
31. Roberts KE, Fallon MB, Krowka MJ, Brown RS, Trotter JF, Peter I, et al. Genetic risk factors for portopulmonary hypertension in patients with advanced liver disease. Am J Respir Crit Care Med. 2009;179:835–42.
32. Austin ED, Cogan JD, West JD, Hedges LK, Hamid R, Dawson EP, et al. Alterations in oestrogen metabolism: implications for higher penetrance of familial pulmonary arterial hypertension in females. Eur Respir J. 2009;34(5):1093–9.
33. Fessel JP, Chen X, Frump A, Gladson S, Blackwell T, Kang C, et al. Interaction between bone morphogenetic protein receptor type 2 and estrogenic compounds in pulmonary arterial hypertension. Pulm Circ. 2013;3(3):564–77.
34. Sweeney L, Voelkel NF. Estrogen exposure, obesity and thyroid disease in women with severe pulmonary hypertension. Eur J Med Res. 2009;14(10):433–42.
35. Lahm T, Patel KM, Crisostomo PR, Markel TA, Wang M, Herring C, et al. Endogenous estrogen attenuates pulmonary artery vasoreactivity and acute hypoxic pulmonary vasoconstriction: the effects of sex and menstrual cycle. Am J Physiol Endocrinol Metab. 2007;293(3):E865–71.
36. Deroo BJ, Korach KS. Estrogen receptors and human disease. J Clin Invest. 2006;116(3):561–70.
37. Kumar V, Green S, Stack G, Berry M, Jin JR, Chambon P. Functional domains of the human estrogen receptor. Cell. 1987;51(6):941–51.
38. Lahm T, Crisostomo PR, Markel TA, Wang M, Wang Y, Tan J, et al. Selective estrogen receptor-{alpha} and estrogen receptor-{beta} agonists rapidly decrease pulmonary artery vasoconstriction by a nitric oxide-dependent mechanism. Am J Physiol Regul Integr Comp Physiol. 2008;295(5):R1486–93.
39. Kumar P, Wu Q, Chambliss KL, Yuhanna IS, Mumby SM, Mineo C, et al. Direct Interactions with G alpha i and G betagamma mediate nongenomic signaling by estrogen receptor alpha. Mol Endocrinol (Baltimore MD). 2007;21(6):1370–80.
40. Farhat MY, Vargas R, Dingaan B, Ramwell PW. In vitro effect of oestradiol on thymidine uptake in pulmonary vascular smooth muscle cell: role of the endothelium. Br J Pharmacol. 1992;107(3):679–83.
41. Jones RD, English KM, Pugh PJ, Morice AH, Jones TH, Channer KS. Pulmonary vasodilatory action of testosterone: evidence of a calcium antagonistic action. J Cardiovasc Pharmacol. 2002;39(6):814–23.
42. Smith AM, Bennett RT, Jones TH, Cowen ME, Channer KS, Jones RD. Characterization of the vasodilatory action of testosterone in the human pulmonary circulation. Vasc Health Risk Manag. 2008;4(6):1459–66.

43. Paulin R, Meloche J, Jacob MH, Bisserier M, Courboulin A, Bonnet S. Dehydroepiandrosterone inhibits the Src/STAT3 constitutive activation in Pulmonary Arterial Hypertension. Am J Physiol Heart Circ Physiol. 2011;301:H1798–809.
44. Dessouroux A, Akwa Y, Baulieu EE. DHEA decreases HIF-1alpha accumulation under hypoxia in human pulmonary artery cells: potential role in the treatment of pulmonary arterial hypertension. J Steroid Biochem Mol Biol. 2008;109(1–2):81–9.
45. Nebert DW, Russell DW. Clinical importance of the cytochromes P450. Lancet. 2002;360(9340):1155–62.
46. White K, Johansen AK, Nilsen M, Ciuclan L, Wallace E, Paton L, et al. Activity of the estrogen-metabolizing enzyme cytochrome P450 1B1 influences the development of pulmonary arterial hypertension. Circulation. 2012;126(9):1087–98.
47. Yager JD, Davidson NE. Estrogen carcinogenesis in breast cancer. N Engl J Med. 2006;354(3):270–82.
48. Nebert DW. Elevated estrogen 16 alpha-hydroxylase activity: is this a genotoxic or nongenotoxic biomarker in human breast cancer risk? J Natl Cancer Inst. 1993;85(23):1888–91.
49. Roy D, Cai Q, Felty Q, Narayan S. Estrogen-induced generation of reactive oxygen and nitrogen species, gene damage, and estrogen-dependent cancers. J Toxicol Environ Health B Crit Rev. 2007;10(4):235–57.
50. Bolton JL, Thatcher GR. Potential mechanisms of estrogen quinone carcinogenesis. Chem Res Toxicol. 2008;21(1):93–101.
51. Muti P, Bradlow HL, Micheli A, Krogh V, Freudenheim JL, Schunemann HJ, et al. Estrogen metabolism and risk of breast cancer: a prospective study of the 2:16alpha-hydroxyestrone ratio in premenopausal and postmenopausal women. Epidemiology. 2000;11(6):635–40.
52. Belous AR, Hachey DL, Dawling S, Roodi N, Parl FF. Cytochrome P450 1B1-mediated estrogen metabolism results in estrogen-deoxyribonucleoside adduct formation. Cancer Res. 2007;67(2):812–7.
53. Eliassen AH, Missmer SA, Tworoger SS, Hankinson SE. Circulating 2-hydroxy- and 16alpha-hydroxy estrone levels and risk of breast cancer among postmenopausal women. Cancer Epidemiol Biomarkers Prev. 2008;17(8):2029–35.
54. Kaaks R, Rinaldi S, Key TJ, Berrino F, Peeters PH, Biessy C, et al. Postmenopausal serum androgens, oestrogens and breast cancer risk: the European prospective investigation into cancer and nutrition. Endocr Relat Cancer. 2005;12(4):1071–82.
55. Missmer SA, Eliassen AH, Barbieri RL, Hankinson SE. Endogenous estrogen, androgen, and progesterone concentrations and breast cancer risk among postmenopausal women. J Natl Cancer Inst. 2004;96(24):1856–65.
56. Muti P, Westerlind K, Wu T, Grimaldi T, De Berry 3rd J, Schunemann H, et al. Urinary estrogen metabolites and prostate cancer: a case–control study in the United States. Cancer Causes Control. 2002;13(10):947–55.
57. West J, Cogan J, Geraci M, Robinson L, Newman J, Phillips JA, et al. Gene expression in BMPR2 mutation carriers with and without evidence of Pulmonary Arterial Hypertension suggests pathways relevant to disease penetrance. BMC Med Genomics. 2008;1(1):45.
58. Mair KM, Wright AF, Duggan N, Rowlands DJ, Hussey MJ, Roberts S, et al. Sex-dependent influence of endogenous estrogen in pulmonary hypertension. Am J Respir Crit Care Med. 2014;190(4):456–67.
59. MacLean MR, Deuchar GA, Hicks MN, Morecroft I, Shen S, Sheward J, et al. Overexpression of the 5-hydroxytryptamine transporter gene: effect on pulmonary hemodynamics and hypoxia-induced pulmonary hypertension. Circulation. 2004;109(17):2150–5.
60. White K, Dempsie Y, Nilsen M, Wright AF, Loughlin L, MacLean MR. The serotonin transporter, gender, and 17beta oestradiol in the development of pulmonary arterial hypertension. Cardiovasc Res. 2011;90(2):373–82.
61. Wright AF, Ewart MA, Mair K, Nilsen M, Dempsie Y, Loughlin L, et al. Oestrogen receptor alpha in pulmonary hypertension. Cardiovasc Res. 2015;106(2):206–16.
62. Moore LG, McMurtry IF, Reeves JT. Effects of sex hormones on cardiovascular and hematologic responses to chronic hypoxia in rats. Proc Soc Exp Biol Med. 1978;158(4):658–62.

63. Rabinovitch M, Gamble WJ, Miettinen OS, Reid L. Age and sex influence on pulmonary hypertension of chronic hypoxia and on recovery. Am J Physiol. 1981;240(1):H62–72.
64. McMurtry IF, Frith CH, Will DH. Cardiopulmonary responses of male and female swine to simulated high altitude. J Appl Physiol. 1973;35(4):459–62.
65. Hansmann G, Wagner RA, Schellong S, Perez VA, Urashima T, Wang L, et al. Pulmonary arterial hypertension is linked to insulin resistance and reversed by peroxisome proliferator-activated receptor-gamma activation. Circulation. 2007;115(10):1275–84.
66. Umar S, Iorga A, Matori H, Nadadur RD, Li J, Maltese F, et al. Estrogen rescues pre-existing severe pulmonary hypertension in rats. Am J Respir Crit Care Med. 2011;184:715–23.
67. Farhat MY, Chen MF, Bhatti T, Iqbal A, Cathapermal S, Ramwell PW. Protection by oestradiol against the development of cardiovascular changes associated with monocrotaline pulmonary hypertension in rats. Br J Pharmacol. 1993;110(2):719–23.
68. Ahn BH, Park HK, Cho HG, Lee HA, Lee YM, Yang EK, et al. Estrogen and enalapril attenuate the development of right ventricular hypertrophy induced by monocrotaline in ovariectomized rats. J Korean Med Sci. 2003;18(5):641–8.
69. Oka M, Karoor V, Homma N, Nagaoka T, Sakao E, Golembeski SM, et al. Dehydroepiandrosterone upregulates soluble guanylate cyclase and inhibits hypoxic pulmonary hypertension. Cardiovasc Res. 2007;74(3):377–87.
70. Bonnet S, Dumas-de-La-Roque E, Begueret H, Marthan R, Fayon M, Dos Santos P, et al. Dehydroepiandrosterone (DHEA) prevents and reverses chronic hypoxic pulmonary hypertension. Proc Natl Acad Sci USA. 2003;100(16):9488–93.

Chapter 6
Pulmonary Fibrosis

Andrew J. Bryant

Introduction

Pulmonary fibrosis is a broad term that describes a decreased ability of the lung to function in gas exchange due to thickening of the distal airways secondary to accumulation of extracellular matrix [1]. Unfortunately, patients often present with advanced illness, noting increasing shortness of breath and cough over a period of months to years. However, pulmonary fibrosis itself is a nonspecific term that can be associated with a number of underlying illnesses (such as connective tissue or autoimmune diseases) or occupational/environmental exposures (such as tobacco smoke) [2]. Pulmonary fibrosis can also be idiopathic, which actually represents the most commonly diagnosed form of the disease. This form of illness is primarily associated with aging, as are most diseases involving fibrosis, with only rare patients diagnosed prior to age of 60 or 65 years [3]. Unfortunately, there are currently only a few therapies for the treatment of pulmonary fibrosis, none of which are disease-modifying agents specific to the lung [4].

Not only does pulmonary fibrosis affect primarily the elderly population, it is also much more common in men than age-matched women. Currently, there is not enough literature detailing a cause of the gender bias—either a protective effect in women or a deleterious one in men—though the reason is most likely multifactorial and complex. There are known different exposures in men versus women, some occupational (coal or silica dust versus wood-burning stove) and others recreational (tobacco smoking). These differences are globally decreasing, as gender

A.J. Bryant, MD (✉)
Department of Medicine, Division of Pulmonary, Critical Care and Sleep Medicine,
University of Florida, 1600 SW Archer Road, M-452, 100225, Gainesville,
FL 36210-0225, USA
e-mail: Andrew.Bryant@medicine.ufl.edu

© Springer International Publishing Switzerland 2016
A.R. Hemnes (ed.), *Gender, Sex Hormones and Respiratory Disease*,
Respiratory Medicine, DOI 10.1007/978-3-319-23998-9_6

equality has led to more women in traditionally male-dominated fields of work, in addition to an equalization of predominantly young women who experiment with smoking tobacco.

In addition to these exogenous exposures, there are a myriad of potential endogenous risks for pulmonary fibrosis in women. This not only includes the increased risk of autoimmune-mediated systemic illness in women (such as rheumatism or sclerosis), but also some independent and intriguing protective factors associated with female sex hormones. The purpose of this chapter is to explore the role that gender plays in the development of pulmonary fibrosis, through first the host and then environment factors. The hope is that this will help in generating novel hypotheses for future study into this field, which has little in the way of disease treatment.

Part I. Host

Only a small amount of publications in the literature confer data regarding direct pathogenic effects of sex and gender on development of classically defined IPF. To this end, the first section of this chapter will focus mainly on autoimmune and connective tissue disease-associated interstitial lung disease. The next section will review potentially protective and deleterious factors that affect women with IPF.

Connective Tissue Disease (CTD)-Associated Interstitial Lung Disease (ILD)

CTD-associated ILD, a term that will be used interchangeably with collagen vascular disease associated ILD, is a form of autoimmune-mediated damage to the lung parenchyma. The disease is characterized as idiopathic interstitial pneumonias, with manifestations including nonspecific interstitial pneumonia (NSIP) or usual interstitial pneumonitis (UIP). It is commonly seen as a cause of morbidity and mortality complicating various autoimmune diseases, with prognosis dependent on the degree of underlying lung disease [5, 6]. Lung disease is believed to result from lung injury induced by a chronic inflammatory state, with resulting aberrant injury/repair mechanism [7]. Interestingly, in at least one study, patient with CTD-associated ILD had a worse clinical progression and outcome than a matched cohort of patients with IPF [8]. However, other studies suggest that CTD-associated ILD, even those associated with UIP features, fares better than those patients with IPF [9, 10]. This trend holds true despite no difference in the rate of decline of lung function [11], though there is potential for bias secondary to increased early detection of lung disease among those patients with CTD, and a reliable response to immunosuppressive therapy [12].

Autoimmune disease in general affects roughly 8 % of the general US population, of which nearly 80 % of patients are women [13]. In addition, women afflicted with autoimmune disease tend to have worse outcomes associated with illness, compared to male counterparts [14]. Given that the incidence of CTD increases correlating with women in the late teens and early-to-mid 40s, disease activity is thought to be associated with hormonal changes, menarche, and menopause, respectively. To this end, with increased lifetime "exposure" of menstruation—younger age at menarche—there is an increased risk of autoimmune disease. An excellent example is the twofold risk in development of systemic lupus erythematosus (SLE) in women with menarche occurring at less than 10 years (RR = 2.1, 95 % CI 1.4–3.2) [15]. The same phenomenon holds true for rheumatoid arthritis (RA), as well (RR = 1.6, 95 % CI 1.0–2.0) [16].

The following sections will serve to review several autoimmune diseases with associated ILD, and the implications of the role of gender in disease pathogenesis, prognosis, and mortality.

Scleroderma

Systemic sclerosis (SSc), or scleroderma, is the most commonly associated autoimmune disease with ILD, predominantly affecting women between the ages of 30 and 55 years of age [17]. Prevalence is estimated at between 50 and 300 cases per million population, with approximately 90 % of patients showing some degree of symptomatic or asymptomatic ILD [18].

Chest CT scan typically reveals an NSIP pattern, with bilateral lower lobe ground-glass opacities noted most often. However, disease has been shown to progress to lower lobe fibrosis with traction bronchiectasis, though UIP is rarely noted on histology [19]. Survival after diagnosis is typically 5–8 years, approximately 2–3 times that of patients diagnosed with IPF [20].

Multiple linkages have been postulated in the past linking SSc to a female predilection. Interestingly, per the above section on occupational exposure, SSc has been shown to be associated with vinyl chloride and silicon exposure. This stems mainly from literature, since disproven, linking SSc with breast augmentation and implants [21]. The initial large cohort study examined and found a spurious link between breast implantation (primarily silicon-based augmentation) and SSc in over 80,000 adult women of various ages. A subsequent meta-analysis showed no such association with either silicon or saline breast implants [22].

Another plausible biologic mechanism for female predominance of SSc involves the finding of fetal DNA in skin lesions of women diagnosed with the disease, suggesting an antimaternal graft-versus-host disease (GVHD)-like phenomenon, directed against the Y-chromosome [23]. This is also believed to be a class II HLA incompatibility problem, inducing host response, primarily T-cell related [24, 25].

Chimerism associated with SSc development in women is complicated by tobacco smoke exposure history in this patient population, with an increase in complicating vascular and lung disease noted in women with SSc who continue to smoke cigarettes [26]. Interestingly, the risk of lung disease is decreased among black versus Caucasian women, despite black females having an earlier age at diagnosis, again correlated to younger age of menarche [27].

Women not only have a greater prevalence of lung disease associated with SSc, they also have worse complications compared to male counterparts. In one epidemiologic study utilizing a US database, hospital rates for SSc were 4.5 times higher among women than men [28]. However, once hospitalized, the in-hospital mortality was 25 % less for women with degree of concomitant pulmonary fibrosis being the major predictor of poor or fatal outcome (OR 2.63, 95 % CI 1.98–3.49). The hospital data mirror outpatient information, which shows an increase in use of sick days or leaves of absence in women versus men with scleroderma and pulmonary fibrosis [29].

Though relatively rare, there is an increased risk of development of SSc-associated ILD complicated by pulmonary hypertension in women versus men [30]. Happily though the overall incidence of ILD/SSc and pulmonary hypertension is decreasing [31].

Rheumatoid Arthritis

RA is the most common of the CTDs, affecting nearly 1–2 % of the entire US population [32]. Pulmonary fibrosis often complicates RA, one of the more common extra-articular disorders associated with the disease [33]. Though still relatively uncommon, ILD is one of the leading causes of mortality in RA, second only to heart disease. Unfortunately, the prevalence of fibrosis is not well distinguished with variation estimated between 1 % and 58 % of patients. This is mainly based upon the heterogeneous nature and variable quality of studies examining the disease [34], as well as variation in the definition based upon clinical or radiologic terms. However, the most recent literature would suggest that ILD associated with RA afflicts nearly half of all patients with RA [35].

RA preferentially affects women in an approximate ratio of 3:1 (F:M) [36], and is one of several autoimmune diseases that is known to remit during pregnancy [37]. Women with RA tend to have worse disease activity than age-matched men [14]. Since RA tends to affect mainly premenopausal women, there is strong consideration that disease activity is mediated heavily by sex hormones, noting that male hormones (androgens, such as testosterone) tend to have a predominantly anti-inflammatory effect [38], and correlative studies have shown that men with decreased circulating levels of testosterone have increased severity of RA symptoms [39]. However, necessary studies documenting causality have not been performed, and thus there exists only a weak correlation between androgen expression and RA disease activity.

As noted above, a lower menarchal age and later menopause age have been associated with increased development of RA (RR 1.6, 95 % CI 1.1–2.4) [16]. There exists inconsistent evidence showing a protective role of oral contraceptive pill (OCP) use against the development of RA or ILD associated with RA [40].

Limited and conflicting data show that, at least in one small Austrian study, men may actually have an increased risk of lung disease associated with RA (including lung nodules and pleural based disease, $p=0.001$) [41]. This finding may be influenced by inherent gender bias in recruitment of RA and control patients [42]. Regardless, women with RA and ILD have more favorable outcomes in both morbidity (exercise tolerance) and mortality, compared to male counterparts [43]. A later study has reinforced the protective role of gender in RA-associated ILD, showing that female sex (HR 0.96) and a higher baseline diffusing capacity of the lung for carbon monoxide (DLCO, HR 0.96) were associated with better survival in the disease [8]. Indeed, women with RA-associated ILD uniformly have a better overall prognosis than age- and disease-matched men.

System Lupus Erythematosus

SLE is a chronic autoimmune disease that most commonly affects young women in a ratio of 6–10:1 (F:M), and women of color more so than Caucasians [44, 45]. When initially described in the literature, pulmonary complications were felt to be a late complication of SLE [46]. However, since as early as 1941 increased reports of early waxing and waning bronchopneumonitis were also described [47]. In a more recent autopsy series, 18 % of 120 subjects with SLE were found to have evidence of "interstitial pneumonitis" mixed with varying degrees of pleuritis and pleural effusion [48]. Radiographic features of ILD on high-resolution CT (HRCT) can be found in as many as 1/3 of all comers with SLE, though the vast majority of these patients are asymptomatic [49]. Most common pathologic and radiologic features of ILD associated with SLE are consistent with cellular or interstitial NSIP [50]. Concomitant diagnosis of pulmonary hypertension complicating parenchymal lung disease associated with SLE is wide ranging, though prevalent, affecting anywhere from 14 to 43 % of patients with SLE in the United States alone [51].

The LUpus in MInorities, NAture versus nurture (LUMINA)cohort—a well-known multiethnic cohort of US patients with SLE—was the first to note that in a small sampling of men diagnosed with SLE, patients were found to have a trend toward worse disease progression at time of diagnosis, and a more rapid decline in functional capability after diagnosis, though the majority of affected patients had disability related to lupus nephritis (63.5 % versus 52.1 %, $p=0.085$) [52, 53]. A similar cohort, The Grupo Latinoamericano de Estudio del Lupus (GLADEL), a 1997-initiated multinational prospective cohort of Latin American lupus centers, showed males had a higher rate of pulmonary disease (56.1 % vs 41.4 %, $p=0.002$), though the population of men was small, 123 of 1214 patients [54]. A final cohort from Greece showed—again—worse disease at the time of diagnosis in men, though this group did not demonstrate major organ difference effects between genders, except for renal disease [55].

As in other autoimmune diseases, the molecular mechanism for lupus-associated ILD is not well worked out; however, sex hormones are probably at least partly responsible, through hormone regulation and effects on cytokine and chemokine production [56]. For example, estrogen signals primarily through estrogen receptor (ER) α and β. Genetic deficiency of ERα in murine models of lupus results in a decrease in disease activity, and prolonged survival, while ERβ deficiency has no such effect [57]. ERα expression is most dense in immune cells, especially antigen-presenting cells (APCs), which may provide some clue in the autoimmune toler-ance, or lack thereof, displayed in patients with SLE. In this same vein, further studies have shown that sex hormone estrogen and prolactin are both capable of stimulating autoreactive B cells in blood from patients with SLE [58].

Sjogren's

Sjogren's similarly has a plausible, if not vague, connection to gender bias in devel-opment of underlying disease and associated ILD. Sjogren's syndrome is character-ized by autoimmune attack on secreting organs, affecting such processes as lacrimation and salivation, resulting in sicca symptoms such as dry mouth and cor-neal ulceration. It also breeds a characteristic mixed with alveolar and interstitial infiltrative lung disease on radiography [59], with histopathologic examination revealing findings consistent with NSIP or lymphocytic interstitial pneumonia (LIP), though there is frequently overlap with a UIP pattern [60].

There is little literature on the epidemiology, and none on the specific mecha-nism, of Sjogren's-associated ILD. The largest, most well done, study to date exam-ined 18 patients retrospectively identified over a 13-year period at one institution (1992–2004) [61]. The cohort had a median age of 62 years, 83 % of whom were women, and found that those patients with UIP pattern complicating Sjogren's tended to have a more rapid progression of lung disease, and decreased survival, upon diagnosis. Another study examining salivary gland biopsy in patients with ILD showed that in 54 % of women examined, there was evidence of Sjogren's-like disease, with "occult" ILD diagnosed by routine CT scanning [62]. Further studies are needed to both characterize patients with illness as well as animal models to aid in defining molecular mechanisms for disease development and progression.

Dermatomyositis/Polymyositis

As the entities name describe, dermatomyositis/polymyositis (DM/PM) are two closely related autoimmune diseases affecting muscle and soft tissues. DM/PM-associated ILD was first described by Mills and Matthews in 1956 [63], though it was not until 1974 that a study revealed epidemiologic associations with the ill-nesses. In this case series, DM/PM-associated ILD was described as affecting males and females equally, across a wide age gap (30–70 years of age). Upon histopatho-logic examination, most cases were shown to be consistent with "IPF," though the case definition was different from today's description of UIP [64]. A more recent case series, from the Mayo Clinic group, showed an even distribution of a more modern description of lung histopathology, ranging from organizing pneumonia, to

UIP, and diffuse alveolar damage (DAD) with hyaline membrane deposition [65]. The latter diagnosis was associated with a uniformly poor prognosis. This trend was found in a 2002 French study, which showed both a Hammon-Rich-like pattern and UIP heralded a worse prognosis in patients with DM/PM, requiring more aggressive therapy (e.g., immunosuppression) of the underlying disease [66]. A presentation associated with an NSIP pattern was found to respond well to immunosuppressive therapy in a separate Japanese study, where 11 out of 14 of these patients were female and had a moderate to severe impairment in pulmonary function testing [67].

Further evidence of a gender disparity in disease progression was shown by another Japanese group that studied the frequency of ILD (defined as "interstitial pneumonitis") complicating DM/PM in 53 adult patients from 1976 to 1993 [68]. In this cohort of patients, interstitial pneumonitis was found to complicate the course of illness in DM/PM predominantly in female patients (54.5 % versus 20 % men), though this may have been biased by a larger amount of women having imaging performed for evaluation of cancer in patients with DM.

Though a mechanism of disease is unknown, there is a gender pattern in differences of HLA-DRB1 allele that appears to influence the risk of development of ILD in patients with DM/PM [69]. This same genetic link may account for the difference in prognosis between men and women with DM/PM, whereupon women tend to have greater survival than age-matched male counterparts. This phenomenon has been demonstrated in a 2014 Italian study that reported a hazard ratio of 2.4 (95 % CI 1.0–5.6) [70]. These data shed light on an observed trend that men—especially men with DM/PM-associated ILD—tend to have worse morbidity and mortality than age-matched women with disease [71].

Mixed Connective Tissue Disease

Mixed CTD (MCTD; also known as Sharp's syndrome) is an overlapping CTD that shares elements with SLE, systemic sclerosis, RA, and polymyositis, with characteristically high levels of anti-U1RNP autoantibodies being pathognomonic for the disease [72, 73]. Pulmonary involvement is common in MCTD, affecting as many as 67 % of patients with ILD in one study, though not all patients were symptomatic with lung disease detected by HRCT screening [74]. There is some evidence that intensive immunosuppressive treatment for MCTD may also treat underlying pulmonary fibrosis, and associated pulmonary hypertension, though most disease appears to be both insidious and progressive without response to treatment [75].

There is little evidence with MCTD-associated ILD displaying a link between gender and disease presence or severity; however, one cohort study following patients at the University of Michigan found a majority female population with MCTD and ILD [76]. The same study found that ILD prevalence was greater in patients with a significant smoking history. Histopathology was most consistent with either UIP or emphysema pattern. Again, there was a greater treatment effect demonstrated in the MCTD-associated ILD group; however, overall prognosis was similar if not slightly worse than matched IPF controls.

List of Connective Tissue Disease (CTD)-associated Interstitial Lung Disease (ILD) with gender ratio and special features

Autoimmune disease	Female:Male ratio	Special features
Scleroderma	5:1	Computed tomography (CT) findings include nonspecific interstitial pattern (NSIP) bilateral ground-glass opacities (GGOs), with rare progression to usual Survival after diagnosis = 6–8 years
Rheumatoid Arthritis (RA)	3:1	Women with RA-associated ILD have improved survival with less functional decline than age-matched men with disease
Systemic Lupus Erythematosus (SLE)	9:1	CT findings are typically cellular or interstitial NSIP pattern, with parenchymal disease complicated by pulmonary hypertension (PH) in approximately 40 % of cases
Sjögren's Syndrome	6–10:1	Mixed alveolar and infiltrative interstitial lung disease consistent with NSIP or lymphocytic interstitial pneumonia (LIP), with frequent UIP pattern overlap that is associated with decreased survival
Dermatomyositis/ Polymyositis (DM/PM)	2:1	Organizing pneumonia, UIP, and diffuse alveolar damage (DAD) pattern with hyaline membrane deposition; women have decreased mortality compared to men with disease
Mixed CTD	2–3:1	Pulmonary involvement is common and predominantly UIP or emphysematous on CT scan, with slightly better prognosis than idiopathic pulmonary fibrosis (IPF)

Autoimmune Disease

Given the role of both exogenous and endogenous hormone fluctuations (from oral contraceptive pills (OCP) or pregnancy, for example) in autoimmune disease in women, it is worth briefly reviewing some of the specific effects that female sex hormones have on autoimmune regulation. There are multiple potential pragmatic benefits of hormone supplementation in women with CTD, including the importance of pregnancy planning [77, 78], and decreased bone loss in patients using glucocorticoids chronically [79]. However, the effect of sex hormones on disease activity continues to be debated.

For example, in one single-blind, non-placebo-controlled, randomized clinical trial, disease activity was compared in 162 patients who received either OCPs or an intrauterine device (IUD) for prophylaxis. There was no significant difference in disease activity noted, though patients with high disease activity and history of thrombosis were excluded [80]. Similar results were noted in a larger double-blind randomized controlled trial [81, 82]. This is compared to an older study that showed high flare rates (43 %) in OCP using groups compared to non-OCP using patients, though this was a retrospective cohort study [82]. This large UK study examining a cohort of female nurses reported increased incidence of autoimmune disease in hormone replacement users, though subsequent studies have not confirmed this trend [83]. One study elaborated on a potential biologic mechanism for protection, showing that endothelial inflammation is decreased in patients using hormone replacement therapy [84]. Pregnancy can likewise lead to improvement in some types of CTD, such as RA, in as many as 75 % of patients [85]. However, unfortunately disease relapse occurs in approximately 90 % of patients within 3 months of child delivery [86].

Idiopathic Pulmonary Fibrosis

IPF is the most common and severe form of idiopathic interstitial pneumonia. It is relentlessly progressive, leading to respiratory death within 2–5 years of diagnosis [87]. While historically there is some evidence that women have better improvement in response to steroid therapy, and thus a better overall prognosis, these older studies did not exclude ILD secondary to CTD, as described in the previous sections [88, 89]. Currently, there is agreement that IPF affects mainly an elderly male population [90], with more recent studies specifically excluding those patients with CTD or occult environmental exposure history, with special attention paid to young patients and women [91].

IPF is currently diagnosed predominantly with the use of high-resolution computed tomography (HRCT). Imaging typically reveals basilar predominant traction bronchiectasis, thickened interlobular septae, and subpleural honeycombing [2, 92]. However, if imaging is inconsistent with a diagnosis of IPF, conditions continue to exist where a patient requires surgical lung biopsy for definitive diagnosis, with histopathological examination revealing a UIP pattern [93, 94]. UIP in this setting is defined as microscopic honeycombing, fibroblastic foci, and a variegated pattern of chronic interstitial fibrosis, though this pattern can be seen in other diseases, as previously mentioned [95].

The current literature regarding mechanism of disease pathogenesis is clouded despite a flurry of recent activity on the subject. Especially as relates to gender predilection, there is little firm evidence regarding the mechanism of fibrosis in IPF; however, several theories do prevail. In this section, these ideas will be summarized, with emphasis finally on the role of sex hormones themselves in disease progression and severity.

Genetic Regulation

Familial forms of IPF do exist [96], though they are estimated to account for only approximately 5 % of overall cases of IPF. There are currently three main areas of IPF research that elucidate the genetic regulation of disease: [1] alteration in surfactant protein production, either SFTPC [97] or SFTPA2 ([98], [2]); telomerase mutations (TERT and TERC), the most common cause of familial IPF [99, 100]; and, finally, [3] mutations in the promoter region of MUC5B, identified recently as playing a role in IPF development in both familial and sporadic IPF, with the associated single nucleotide polymorphism (SNP) of MUC5B being found in 38 % of all IPF patients studied [101].

Surfactant Proteins

During lung development, it is known that the female fetal lung develops surfactant protein (SFTP) at an earlier time than the male lung, due to lack of androgen mediated decrease in SFTP [102]. The mechanism of this is believed due to chronic androgen exposure leading to an EGF-R mediated increase in TGF-β and subsequent decrease in SFTPB and SFTPC expression in type II alveolar epithelial cells (AECs) [103]. This phenomenon negatively regulates type II AEC maturation, with reverse cell reprogramming to a more immature cellular state [104]. Interestingly, an increase in production of SFTPA in those patients diagnosed with IPF portends a poor prognosis, with rapid decline in lung function, but this phenomenon is not recognized as being gender-specific [105].

Telomeres

Though several studies have examined the role of telomerase (TERT/TERC) mutation and subsequent telomere shortening in association with development of IPF, these studies have been for the most part sex matched and controlled, therefore rendering them difficult to glean information from regarding differences between men and women [106, 107]. Only one study has examined the role of sex hormones acting on the TERT gene [108]. This group began by noting that androgen therapy is often helpful in patients with disease of telomere dysfunction, such as dyskeratosis congenita. In this study, increased exposure of human cells from patients with telomerase dysfunction to estradiol correlated with increased telomerase activity and increased TERT mRNA production. Tamoxifen, an antagonist, caused the opposite effect, abolished by blocking signaling of estrogen receptor (ER)-A. It would thus be interesting to examine the finding in tissue provided by patients with IPF secondary to telomerase dysfunction, or even those with sporadic IPF.

MUC

Despite literature on correlation between MUC promoter regions and presence of IPF, little data exists on delineating the role of sex hormones in MUC-production or pathogenesis. The most relevant study examined decreased production of MUC2 in the gastrointestinal (GI) tract, showing a decreased response to GI injury in male versus female mice [109]. Whether this decrease, or alteration in function, exists in response to chronic lung injury, is unknown.

Alveolar Epithelium

In addition to heritable contributions to development of IPF, another prevailing theory regarding pathogenesis involves the type II AEC response to repetitive injury [110]. There are multiple hypotheses that lend credence to this line of thought.

Unfolded Protein Response (UPR)/Endoplasmic Reticulum (ER)-Stress

While a detailed description is beyond the scope of this chapter, in short the UPR is a method by which the cell has developed to handle misfolded proteins, either from genetic mutations (such as a change in SFTP), or viral infection [111]. It is an adaptive response to cell injury of most any type that halts production, or augments, of proteins to facilitate proper folding and functioning, with the aid of cellular chaperoning. An accumulation of misfolded proteins leads to the phenomenon of ER-stress, and apoptosis [112]. In IPF, increased ER-stress has been shown to be integral to fibrotic remodeling in type II AECs. Using mice with mutated, and misfolded, SFTPC in type II AECs, mice were given a "second hit" with intratracheal bleomycin, exposing the vulnerable epithelium to fibrotic remodeling [113].

No current literature is available that links UPR or ER-stress to gender-related development or progression of IPF, however a few studies are suggestive of a link. The first study showed that female mice were protected against development of insulin-resistance in inflammatory-cell associated obesity [114]. Though not mediated directly by ER-stress, the authors did show a decrease in UPR marker Gp78, suggesting that female sex was protective against progression of the UPR. In a similar fashion, dextrose-induced ER-stress and superoxide production was shown to be attenuated in vascular endothelial cells exposed to increased levels of estradiol [115]. These studies are provocative for pathogenic mechanisms and potential therapies, as detailed in the final section of the chapter.

Epithelial-Mesenchymal Transition

Since AEC hypertrophy and phenotypic alteration to a "fibroblast-like" state is an important phenomenon believed to be involved in development of UIP and IPF [116], a large amount of literature has focused on the crosstalk between epithelial and mesenchymal cells, and the hotly debated topic of EMT [117]. Little has been studied in the way of EMT related to IPF and gender, however the cancer literature provides several potential provocative avenues for future research.

An example is the role of estrogen receptors in EMT. ER-β has been shown to be protective against tumor cells with EMT features (down-regulation of E-cadherin and nuclear β-catenin activation) [118]. The picture quickly becomes complicated though, with competing literature demonstrating that proliferation of tumor cells producing ER-α is correlated with an increase in mesenchymal markers [119]. This may, in part, explain why functional studies have shown worse outcome associated with EMT in females versus males. One example is a study examining podocyte injury in rats via EMT-related fibrogenesis – female rats displayed increase injury and nephrosis, compared to control males [120].

Innate Immunity

The interaction between alveolar macrophages and AECs in coordinating fibroblast recruitment and activation is an active area of research in the field of pulmonary fibrosis. Innate immune cell marker CCL2 has been implicated in the development of IPF, via an alteration of macrophage polarization to a pro-inflammatory phenotype [121]. Similarly, macrophage major mediator LPA and receptor LPAR1 have been shown to be necessary for the development of pulmonary fibrosis in animal models [122].

Extrapolating data again from inflammation-mediated obesity research, increased levels of macrophage activation marker MCP-1 were found in male versus female patients, resulting in increased pancreatic islet cell destruction and fibrosis, and subsequent insulin resistance [123]. A similar phenomenon may be protect female versus male patients with pulmonary fibrosis, thought more studies are needed to explore this hypothesis fully.

Integrin

The physiologic process that accompanies and coordinates wound repair is known to be deranged in fibroblasts isolated from patients with IPF. Normally cell-to-cell communicating proteins, called integrins, coordinate repair through interaction with the extracellular matrix (ECM) and effecter inflammatory cells such as circulating monocytes [124]. However, this feedback mechanism that prevents aberrant wound repair is often turned off in IPF patient samples [125].

Again, while no literature exists on alteration in integrin signaling and gender together influencing the development of pulmonary fibrosis, an association can be extrapolated from existing data. For example, one study has previously demonstrated increased integrin receptor signaling on circulating antigen presenting cells (APCs) after injury in men versus women [126]. Somewhat contradicting this concept is the finding that downstream pro-fibrotic mediators have been found to result in worsened lung fibrosis in estradiol-supplemented rats, in a bleomycin-model of pulmonary fibrosis [127]. Specifically, these investigators found increased transcriptional levels of procollagen I and TGF-β1—these levels were subsequently decreased after ovariectomy in similarly treated rats. However, other similar studies have drawn the polar opposite conclusion [128], suggesting that the true link is more complicated than appears and requires further study.

MicroRNA (miRNA)

Exciting new research in the field of pulmonary fibrosis has focused on the role of "noncoding" or miRNA. This product can change the biologic response of a cell through regulation of mRNA transcription and translation via the RNA interference pathway [129]. Inhibition of several miRNAs (let-7d [130], miR21 [131], miR200 [132], and miR17~92 [133]) has been shown to decrease the profibrotic phenotype of fibroblasts from patients with IPF, as well as in the murine bleomycin model of pulmonary fibrosis.

Interestingly, maternally imprinted miR154 has been shown to be upregulated in pulmonary fibrosis, thought to suggest a reversion to the fetal lung phenotype, a common theme in the IPF literature [134]. While, again, almost no studies have explicitly studied the role of miRNA in gender related to IPF pathogenesis, there is a small body of literature that links gender and miRNA regulation. One such study showed that in addition to noncoding RNA regulation by age, gender was shown to influence a number of miRNA, both production and activity, in human platelets. While there was no immediate or specific therapy offered by the report, it does stress the importance of sex consideration in future studies that examine microRNA and the link to IPF [135].

Epigenetics

Noncoding RNA can be placed in a larger category of epigenetic marks that represent heritable changes that have no effect on sequence of DNA, yet play a crucial role in genetic expression, influenced by aging, diet, and—importantly—environment. Other examples of epigenetic regulation include DNA methylation (hyper- or hypo-) and modification of histone tails [136].

The regulatory nature of epigenetic phenomenon in IPF is relatively novel. A recently published early DNA methylation study convincingly displays evidence that large numbers of CpG motifs (targets for methylation) are differentially methylated in lung samples from patients with IPF versus normal controls [137, 138]. Increased physical activity in women has been linked to a decrease in hypomethylation of several anti-inflammatory genes, resulting in increased suppression of the resulting baseline inflammatory milieu [139]. This applies mainly to the concept of aging, of which fibrosis is often an accompanying complication.

Sex Hormones

Despite strong epidemiological evidence of gender trends in the prevalence of IPF, showing a male predilection and a worse overall prognosis of those men versus age-matched women, there is little data regarding the role of traditional sex hormones in IPF development of progression. One study, in particular, examines the sex-specific genetic expression patterns by disease severity in ex vivo lung tissue samples [140]. There was no change in typical sex hormones, androgens and associated estrogens or progresterone. Only two genes, CH3L1 and MMP7, showed an interaction between sex and IPF severity, with men having worse prognosis associated with up-regulation of these two genes. Interestingly, MMP7 is known to be involved in ECM degradation and wound healing, providing a plausible link to other proposed mechanisms of IPF development, discussed previously [141].

Finally, one other study examined the role of dehydroepiandrosterone (DHEA) as a potential mechanism in the development of IPF [142]. DHEA is an endogenous steroid hormone that functions as a biologic intermediate for several androgens and estrogen sex hormones. The study showed that DHEA supplementation caused a decrease in TGF-β1-induced collagen production, as well as fibroblast to myofibroblast differentiation. Thus, DHEA supplementation, facilitating an increase in predominantly estrogen intermediate sex hormones had an inverse relationship to profibrotic mediators and pulmonary fibrosis. Given the importance of sex hormones to other lung diseases, especially pulmonary hypertension, this finding would appear to be a reasonable base for further exploration, defining the link between IPF and gender, protective or otherwise.

Part II. Environment

Tobacco Smoke

Epidemiology of Tobacco Use in Women

Thus, a large number of endogenous factors have a known and potentially enormous effect on the development of IPF in women, as well as men. However this is not the only influence on disease pathogenesis. For the remainder of this chapter, focus will be shifted from the effect of host factors in the development of IPF, to the influence of environment on disease pathogenesis. According to the most recent Centers for Disease Control and Prevention survey collected in 2012, over 42 million people currently smoke tobacco-related products in the United States alone, accounting for greater than 18 % of adults greater than 18 years of age (www.cdc.gov/tobacco). Though overall prevalence has decreased from 2005 (20.9 % of adults at that time), tobacco-related death is estimated to account for over 400,000 deaths per year, or more than one out of every five recorded deaths (http://www.cdc.gov/mmwr/index2014.html). While men continue to be more likely to smoke than women (20.5 % versus 15.8 % of polled Americans), there is evidence that women are increasing their tobacco consumption worldwide, with an increase to 20 % of all women estimated by 2025 (approximately 530 million women) (http://www.cdc.gov/brfss/annual_data/annual_2013.html). Most alarming is that despite inroads being made in anti-tobacco efforts in adolescent boys, there is a plateau seen in young women from 2005 to 2012, with evidence for increased use of cigarettes as casual smokers and an increased designation as a current daily smoker (18 % of girls versus 12 %

of boys) (http://www.cdc.gov/nchs/products/nhsr.htm). This is evidenced by an increased use of smoking on at least 20 days of the month (8 %, versus 6 % of young men). This trend is especially sustained in women with low income, represented by a minority group, and those who have a lower level of education.

Tobacco Use and IPF

Though the exact nature of the relationship between tobacco smoke and IPF is controversial, cigarette use is a known and validated risk factor for development and progression of IPF, with a near linear relationship described between amount of lifetime tobacco smoke exposure and decreased survival after diagnosis of IPF [143]. This increase in mortality is especially true as related to the relatively novel recognized entity of combined pulmonary fibrosis and emphysema (CPFE), which has an even worse prognosis than that described with isolated interstitial lung disease (less than 20 % survival at 2 years), and a four to five-fold increase in developing co-morbid pulmonary hypertension associated with chronic lung disease [144]. While the majority of patients with CPFE represented in the literature have been elderly men, there is an increasing incidence of women noted.

Familial and idiopathic IPF are known to have increased prevalence among ever-smokers, as evidenced by a study that showed an increase in disease development from 34.1 % to 67.3 % ($p < 0.0001$) with history of smoking [96]. However, it is worth noting that this estimate is at odds with data from an older study that showed better prognosis in patients diagnosed with IPF who were current smokers [145], though the article notes that the effect may have been influenced by smokers seeking earlier medical care than non-smokers. The latter point was supported by another study that showed better survival in non-smokers, with a noted "healthy smoker effect" (selection and survival bias intrinsic to previous trials study designs) leading to appearance of improved survival in smokers [146].

There exist biologically plausible mechanisms by which tobacco smoke may influence the development of IPF, strengthening the above correlations. The most thoroughly described mechanism involves cigarette-smoke induced oxidative stress that impairs the function of histone deacetylase (HDAC)-2 activity, contributing to post-translational modification of inflammatory gene regulators, leading to an increase in the chronic inflammatory state, and eventual fibrosis [147–149]. This line of research, and thus dedicated therapeutics targeting the described pathways, are still in their infancy. Thus, tobacco cessation remains the most heavily recommended treatment and prevention strategy.

Sociocultural Influence on Tobacco Use

There exist many hurdles to tobacco cessation that are unique to women. A major concern documented since the latter days of the women's liberation movement has been the increased use of tobacco amongst women [150]. A concern from the late 1960s forward was that the appropriate equalization of rights between men and women in the work place and beyond would have an untoward side effect of equalizing use of products such as alcohol and cigarettes [151]. Advertising companies recognized this trend early, utilizing magazine and television advertisements to equate cigarette smoking with social attractiveness and stressing the utility of smoking to maintain low weight to female viewers [152]. This trend occurred in tandem with the pervasive thought that cigarette use represented a wholesome/healthy outdoor activity and was a status symbol representing increased free time and media exposure [153]. Television and print ads also began to successfully target households in a lower socioeconomic class, with an increase in tobacco use noted in such households since the early 1990s [154]. Such exposure focused on the notion of cigarette use for young women as liberating, sophisticated, attractive, glamorous and – importantly – slim [155]. However, there was also an elegant campaign directed at older women as well, focusing on the pleasurable aspects of cigarette use, stressing tobacco's role in relaxation from day-to-day responsibilities and burdens [156].

Biologic Influence on Tobacco Use

Beyond sociologic influences on a woman's hindrance to tobacco cessation, there exist biologic mechanisms that have been hypothesized to influence continued cigarette use. In its simplest form, the menstrual cycle itself has been found to influence smoking behavior [157], with an association found between the luteal phase of menstruation and increased craving for tobacco, ultimately, cigarette use [158]. In previously published survey data, women described a greater relief of "negative feelings" associated with the intake of nicotine, though subsequent studies have shown this correlation to be weak or nonexistent [159]. However, at least one study demonstrated that progesterone treatment in the early follicular phase of the menstrual cycle can attenuate cravings, and aid in tobacco cessation attempts [160].

From a similar pharmacologic standpoint, estrogen has also been shown to have an effect on cigarette smoking behavior. Estrogen supplementation, either through an oral contraceptive pill or pregnancy, may act as a non-competitive nicotine receptor antagonist leading to an alteration in nicotine pharmacokinetics, rendering a decrease in nicotine "effectiveness" and a need to smoke more cigarettes to achieve the same neuropsychological effects [161–163]. This phenomenon has been demonstrated in a rat model of tobacco use, where the female animal was more likely to self-administer nicotine during the estrogen peak of the estrous cycle [164].

The effect of progesterone and estrogen on addiction may partially explain why women require a shorter duration of exposure to nicotine in tobacco smoke in order to become addicted [165], though some of this effect may be due to susceptibility to external cues. The consideration of the effect of psychological disease similarly must be considered—patients with untreated depression and anxiety, of which women make up a majority, have increased use of tobacco products compared to treated control patients [166].

Environmental Risk Factors

Occupational Exposure

While metal, silica, and wood dust are consistently identified environmental risk factors for development of IPF in jobs historically conducted solely by men (ship-building, car manufacturing and furniture building) [167, 168], women do have independent known exposures that contribute to development and progression of pulmonary fibrosis. For example, in one study, women who practiced the profession of hairdressing were noted to have an increased odds ratio of development of IPF (3.6, 95 % CI 0.9–13.9), presumably secondary to exposure to noxious inhalants [169]. In addition, rural work exposure to vegetable and animal dust is noted to be a risk factor for development of pulmonary fibrosis in women, greater than men [170]. Importantly, this domiciliary exposure also extends to wood fire exposure, even in developed countries [171].

Biomass Fuel

The vast majority of wood, or biomass, fuel exposure in women occurs globally, where it remains the most commonly used means of cooking and preparing food [172, 173]. Though some would argue that the lung disease that develops in response to this exposure is independent from a diagnosis of IPF—most categorizing the illness as a pneumoconiosis or hypersensitivity pneumonitis—the risk factor can cause a progressive chronic lung disease marked respiratory failure and development of cor pulmonale, at least similar to IPF [174, 175]. While the disease has been alternately referred to within the past several years as "hut lung" (a mixed-dust pneumoconiosis) in the literature [176], there exists reasonable evidence from studies that the exploration of occupational exposures, such as biomass fuel and food preparation remains a problem even outside of rural and underdeveloped areas. However, there is controversy regarding the occupational distribution that begs for larger and longer duration observational trials [177].

Conclusion

The role of gender in IPF therefore appears to protect against the development of disease in women. However, the pathogenesis of IPF involves a complex interplay between the environment and host, one that may ultimately see an equalization of men and women with disease, especially with rising rates of women that smoke tobacco. This is further complicated by the fact that over the years, many female patients who would have been previously diagnosed with IPF have been re-classified as having ILD associated with autoimmune disease and CTD. This diagnostic bias may also play a role in the previously held belief that women responded to therapy for IPF better than their male counterparts, as many of these patients likely had an underlying CTD that was responsive to immunosuppressive therapy for their "IPF".

In the most recent epidemiologic studies, IPF does seem to occur in women at a lower rate than men, and exploration of potential causes for this finding are important for both prognostic reasons, as well as hypothesis-generating concepts for future potential therapies. Potential areas of future research include not only mechanistic pathways involving basic molecular biology targets, but also epigenetic contributions to IPF that deal with differential DNA methylation or noncoding RNA. None of these studies would obviate the need for further research into tempering addiction to cigarette smoke exposure, or legislation to regulate air quality control, both necessary to decrease all manner of lung diseases. To that end, future research should also focus on defining specific phenotypes of women with IPF, examining cohorts for common comorbidities—such as concurrent or associated pulmonary hypertension, for example—in an effort to better classify and study these groups of illnesses. It is with this improvement in classification, either in men or women that we can begin to make inroads into treating fatal lung diseases, such as IPF.

References

1. Blackwell TS, Tager AM, Borok Z, Moore BB, Schwartz DA, Anstrom KJ, Bar-Joseph Z, Bitterman P, Blackburn MR, Bradford W, Brown KK, Chapman HA, Collard HR, Cosgrove GP, Deterding R, Doyle R, Flaherty KR, Garcia CK, Hagood JS, Henke CA, Herzog E, Hogaboam CM, Horowitz JC, King Jr TE, Loyd JE, Lawson WE, Marsh CB, Noble PW, Noth I, Sheppard D, Olsson J, Ortiz LA, O'Riordan TG, Oury TD, Raghu G, Roman J, Sime PJ, Sisson TH, Tschumperlin D, Violette SM, Weaver TE, Wells RG, White ES, Kaminski N, Martinez FJ, Wynn TA, Thannickal VJ, Eu JP. Future directions in idiopathic pulmonary fibrosis research. An NHLBI workshop report. Am J Respir Crit Care Med. 2014;189:214–22.
2. Noble PW, Barkauskas CE, Jiang D. Pulmonary fibrosis: patterns and perpetrators. J Clin Invest. 2012;122:2756–62.
3. Faner R, Rojas M, Macnee W, Agusti A. Abnormal lung aging in chronic obstructive pulmonary disease and idiopathic pulmonary fibrosis. Am J Respir Crit Care Med. 2012;186:306–13.
4. Ahluwalia N, Shea BS, Tager AM. New therapeutic targets in idiopathic pulmonary fibrosis. Aiming to rein in runaway wound-healing responses. Am J Respir Crit Care Med. 2014;190:867–78.
5. Wells AU, Denton CP. Interstitial lung disease in connective tissue disease—mechanisms and management. Nat Rev Rheumatol. 2014;10:728–39.
6. Vij R, Strek ME. Diagnosis and treatment of connective tissue disease-associated interstitial lung disease. Chest. 2013;143:814–24.
7. Hsu E, Shi H, Jordan RM, Lyons-Weiler J, Pilewski JM, Feghali-Bostwick CA. Lung tissues in patients with systemic sclerosis have gene expression patterns unique to pulmonary fibrosis and pulmonary hypertension. Arthritis Rheum. 2011;63:783–94.
8. Kim EJ, Elicker BM, Maldonado F, Webb WR, Ryu JH, Van Uden JH, Lee JS, King Jr TE, Collard HR. Usual interstitial pneumonia in rheumatoid arthritis-associated interstitial lung disease. Eur Respir J. 2010;35:1322–8.

9. Wells AU, Hansell DM, Rubens MB, Cullinan P, Haslam PL, Black CM, Du Bois RM. Fibrosing alveolitis in systemic sclerosis. Bronchoalveolar lavage findings in relation to computed tomographic appearance. Am J Respir Crit Care Med. 1994;150:462–8.
10. Park JH, Kim DS, Park IN, Jang SJ, Kitaichi M, Nicholson AG, Colby TV. Prognosis of fibrotic interstitial pneumonia: idiopathic versus collagen vascular disease-related subtypes. Am J Respir Crit Care Med. 2007;175:705–11.
11. Strand MJ, Sprunger D, Cosgrove GP, Fernandez-Perez ER, Frankel SK, Huie TJ, Olson AL, Solomon J, Brown KK, Swigris JJ. Pulmonary function and survival in idiopathic vs secondary usual interstitial pneumonia. Chest. 2014;146:775–85.
12. Fischer A, du Bois R. Interstitial lung disease in connective tissue disorders. Lancet. 2012;380:689–98.
13. Fairweather D, Frisancho-Kiss S, Rose NR. Sex differences in autoimmune disease from a pathological perspective. Am J Pathol. 2008;173:600–9.
14. Sokka T, Toloza S, Cutolo M, Kautiainen H, Makinen H, Gogus F, Skakic V, Badsha H, Peets T, Baranauskaite A, Geher P, Ujfalussy I, Skopouli FN, Mavrommati M, Alten R, Pohl C, Sibilia J, Stancati A, Salaffi F, Romanowski W, Zarowny-Wierzbinska D, Henrohn D, Bresnihan B, Minnock P, Knudsen LS, Jacobs JW, Calvo-Alen J, Lazovskis J, Pinheiro Gda R, Karateev D, Andersone D, Rexhepi S, Yazici Y, Pincus T, Group Q-R. Women, men, and rheumatoid arthritis: analyses of disease activity, disease characteristics, and treatments in the QUEST-RA study. Arthritis Res Ther. 2009;11:R7.
15. Costenbader KH, Feskanich D, Stampfer MJ, Karlson EW. Reproductive and menopausal factors and risk of systemic lupus erythematosus in women. Arthritis Rheum. 2007;56:1251–62.
16. Karlson EW, Mandl LA, Hankinson SE, Grodstein F. Do breast-feeding and other reproductive factors influence future risk of rheumatoid arthritis? Results from the Nurses' Health Study. Arthritis Rheum. 2004;50:3458–67.
17. Herzog EL, Mathur A, Tager AM, Feghali-Bostwick C, Schneider F, Varga J. Review: interstitial lung disease associated with systemic sclerosis and idiopathic pulmonary fibrosis: how similar and distinct? Arthritis Rheumatol. 2014;66:1967–78.
18. Gabrielli A, Avvedimento EV, Krieg T. Scleroderma. N Engl J Med. 2009;360:1989–2003.
19. Solomon JJ, Olson AL, Fischer A, Bull T, Brown KK, Raghu G. Scleroderma lung disease. Eur Respir Rev. 2013;22:6–19.
20. Altman RD, Medsger Jr TA, Bloch DA, Michel BA. Predictors of survival in systemic sclerosis (scleroderma). Arthritis Rheum. 1991;34:403–13.
21. Sanchez-Guerrero J, Colditz GA, Karlson EW, Hunter DJ, Speizer FE, Liang MH. Silicone breast implants and the risk of connective-tissue diseases and symptoms. N Engl J Med. 1995;332:1666–70.
22. Janowsky EC, Kupper LL, Hulka BS. Meta-analyses of the relation between silicone breast implants and the risk of connective-tissue diseases. N Engl J Med. 2000;342:781–90.
23. Artlett CM, Smith JB, Jimenez SA. Identification of fetal DNA and cells in skin lesions from women with systemic sclerosis. N Engl J Med. 1998;338:1186–91.
24. Famularo G, De Simone C. Systemic sclerosis from autoimmunity to alloimmunity. South Med J. 1999;92:472–6.
25. Lian X, Xiao R, Hu X, Kanekura T, Jiang H, Li Y, Wang Y, Yang Y, Zhao M, Lu Q. DNA demethylation of CD40l in CD4+ T cells from women with systemic sclerosis: a possible explanation for female susceptibility. Arthritis Rheum. 2012;64:2338–45.
26. Harrison BJ, Silman AJ, Hider SL, Herrick AL. Cigarette smoking as a significant risk factor for digital vascular disease in patients with systemic sclerosis. Arthritis Rheum. 2002;46:3312–6.
27. Mayes MD, Lacey Jr JV, Beebe-Dimmer J, Gillespie BW, Cooper B, Laing TJ, Schottenfeld D. Prevalence, incidence, survival, and disease characteristics of systemic sclerosis in a large US population. Arthritis Rheum. 2003;48:2246–55.
28. Chung L, Krishnan E, Chakravarty EF. Hospitalizations and mortality in systemic sclerosis: results from the Nationwide Inpatient Sample. Rheumatology. 2007;46:1808–13.

29. Sandqvist G, Scheja A, Eklund M. Working ability in relation to disease severity, everyday occupations and well-being in women with limited systemic sclerosis. Rheumatology. 2008;47:1708–11.
30. Hachulla E, de Groote P, Gressin V, Sibilia J, Diot E, Carpentier P, Mouthon L, Hatron PY, Jego P, Allanore Y, Tiev KP, Agard C, Cosnes A, Cirstea D, Constans J, Farge D, Viallard JF, Harle JR, Patat F, Imbert B, Kahan A, Cabane J, Clerson P, Guillevin L, Humbert M, Itiner AIRSSG. The three-year incidence of pulmonary arterial hypertension associated with systemic sclerosis in a multicenter nationwide longitudinal study in France. Arthritis Rheum. 2009;60:1831–9.
31. Bauer PR, Schiavo DN, Osborn TG, Levin DL, St Sauver J, Hanson AC, Schroeder DR, Ryu JH. Influence of interstitial lung disease on outcome in systemic sclerosis: a population-based historical cohort study. Chest. 2013;144:571–7.
32. Anaya JM, Diethelm L, Ortiz LA, Gutierrez M, Citera G, Welsh RA, Espinoza LR. Pulmonary involvement in rheumatoid arthritis. Semin Arthritis Rheum. 1995;24:242–54.
33. Roschmann RA, Rothenberg RJ. Pulmonary fibrosis in rheumatoid arthritis: a review of clinical features and therapy. Semin Arthritis Rheum. 1987;16:174–85.
34. Frank ST, Weg JG, Harkleroad LE, Fitch RF. Pulmonary dysfunction in rheumatoid disease. Chest. 1973;63:27–34.
35. Gabbay E, Tarala R, Will R, Carroll G, Adler B, Cameron D, Lake FR. Interstitial lung disease in recent onset rheumatoid arthritis. Am J Respir Crit Care Med. 1997;156:528–35.
36. Lockshin MD. Sex differences in autoimmune disease. Orthop Clin North Am. 2006;37:629–33.
37. Nelson JL, Hughes KA, Smith AG, Nisperos BB, Branchaud AM, Hansen JA. Maternal-fetal disparity in HLA class II alloantigens and the pregnancy-induced amelioration of rheumatoid arthritis. N Engl J Med. 1993;329:466–71.
38. Cutolo M, Seriolo B, Villaggio B, Pizzorni C, Craviotto C, Sulli A. Androgens and estrogens modulate the immune and inflammatory responses in rheumatoid arthritis. Ann N Y Acad Sci. 2002;966:131–42.
39. Spector TD, Perry LA, Tubb G, Silman AJ, Huskisson EC. Low free testosterone levels in rheumatoid arthritis. Ann Rheum Dis. 1988;47:65–8.
40. Hannaford PC, Kay CR, Hirsch S. Oral contraceptives and rheumatoid arthritis: new data from the Royal College of General Practitioners' oral contraception study. Ann Rheum Dis. 1990;49:744–6.
41. Popp W, Rauscher H, Ritschka L, Braun O, Scherak O, Kolarz G, Zwick H. Prediction of interstitial lung involvement in rheumatoid arthritis. The value of clinical data, chest roentgenogram, lung function, and serologic parameters. Chest. 1992;102:391–4.
42. Rajasekaran BA, Shovlin D, Lord P, Kelly CA. Interstitial lung disease in patients with rheumatoid arthritis: a comparison with cryptogenic fibrosing alveolitis. Rheumatology. 2001;40:1022–5.
43. Young A, Koduri G, Batley M, Kulinskaya E, Gough A, Norton S, Dixey J. Early Rheumatoid Arthritis Study g. Mortality in rheumatoid arthritis. Increased in the early course of disease, in ischaemic heart disease and in pulmonary fibrosis. Rheumatology. 2007;46:350–7.
44. Swigris JJ, Fischer A, Gillis J, Meehan RT, Brown KK. Pulmonary and thrombotic manifestations of systemic lupus erythematosus. Chest. 2008;133:271–80.
45. Siegel M, Lee SL. The epidemiology of systemic lupus erythematosus. Semin Arthritis Rheum. 1973;3:1–54.
46. Sante LR, Wyatt JP. Roentgenological and pathological observations in antigenic pneumonitis, its relationship to the collagen diseases. Am J Roentgenol Radium Ther. 1951;66:527–45.
47. Klemperer PPA, Baehr G. Pathology of disseminated lupus erythematosus. Arch Pathol. 1941;569–631.
48. Haupt HM, Moore GW, Hutchins GM. The lung in systemic lupus erythematosus. Analysis of the pathologic changes in 120 patients. Am J Med. 1981;71:791–8.

49. Bankier AA, Kiener HP, Wiesmayr MN, Fleischmann D, Kontrus M, Herold CJ, Graninger W, Hubsch P. Discrete lung involvement in systemic lupus erythematosus: CT assessment. Radiology. 1995;196:835–40.
50. Tansey D, Wells AU, Colby TV, Ip S, Nikolakoupolou A, du Bois RM, Hansell DM, Nicholson AG. Variations in histological patterns of interstitial pneumonia between connective tissue disorders and their relationship to prognosis. Histopathology. 2004;44:585–96.
51. Winslow TM, Ossipov MA, Fazio GP, Simonson JS, Redberg RF, Schiller NB. Five-year follow-up study of the prevalence and progression of pulmonary hypertension in systemic lupus erythematosus. Am Heart J. 1995;129:510–5.
52. Andrade RM, Alarcon GS, Fernandez M, Apte M, Vila LM, Reveille JD, Group LS. Accelerated damage accrual among men with systemic lupus erythematosus: XLIV. Results from a multiethnic US cohort. Arthritis Rheum. 2007;56:622–30.
53. Schwartzman-Morris J, Putterman C. Gender differences in the pathogenesis and outcome of lupus and of lupus nephritis. Clin Dev Immunol. 2012;2012:604892.
54. Garcia MA, Marcos JC, Marcos AI, Pons-Estel BA, Wojdyla D, Arturi A, Babini JC, Catoggio LJ, Alarcon-Segovia D. Male systemic lupus erythematosus in a Latin-American inception cohort of 1214 patients. Lupus. 2005;14:938–46.
55. Voulgari PV, Katsimbri P, Alamanos Y, Drosos AA. Gender and age differences in systemic lupus erythematosus. A study of 489 Greek patients with a review of the literature. Lupus. 2002;11:722–9.
56. Nussinovitch U, Shoenfeld Y. The role of gender and organ specific autoimmunity. Autoimmun Rev. 2012;11:A377–385.
57. Cunningham M, Gilkeson G. Estrogen receptors in immunity and autoimmunity. Clin Rev Allergy Immunol. 2011;40:66–73.
58. Shoenfeld Y, Tincani A, Gershwin ME. Sex gender and autoimmunity. J Autoimmun. 2012;38:J71–73.
59. Lohrmann C, Uhl M, Warnatz K, Ghanem N, Kotter E, Schaefer O, Langer M. High-resolution CT imaging of the lung for patients with primary Sjogren's syndrome. Eur J Radiol. 2004;52:137–43.
60. Ito I, Nagai S, Kitaichi M, Nicholson AG, Johkoh T, Noma S, Kim DS, Handa T, Izumi T, Mishima M. Pulmonary manifestations of primary Sjogren's syndrome: a clinical, radiologic, and pathologic study. Am J Respir Crit Care Med. 2005;171:632–8.
61. Parambil JG, Myers JL, Lindell RM, Matteson EL, Ryu JH. Interstitial lung disease in primary Sjogren's syndrome. Chest. 2006;130:1489–95.
62. Fischer A, Swigris JJ, du Bois RM, Groshong SD, Cool CD, Sahin H, Lynch DA, Gillis JZ, Cohen MD, Meehan RT, Brown KK. Minor salivary gland biopsy to detect primary Sjogren syndrome in patients with interstitial lung disease. Chest. 2009;136:1072–8.
63. Mills ES, Mathews WH. Interstitial pneumonitis in dermatomyositis. J Am Med Assoc. 1956;160:1467–70.
64. Frazier AR, Miller RD. Interstitial pneumonitis in association with polymyositis and dermatomyositis. Chest. 1974;65:403–7.
65. Tazelaar HD, Viggiano RW, Pickersgill J, Colby TV. Interstitial lung disease in polymyositis and dermatomyositis. Clinical features and prognosis as correlated with histologic findings. Am Rev Respir Dis. 1990;141:727–33.
66. Marie I, Hachulla E, Cherin P, Dominique S, Hatron PY, Hellot MF, Devulder B, Herson S, Levesque H, Courtois H. Interstitial lung disease in polymyositis and dermatomyositis. Arthritis Rheum. 2002;47:614–22.
67. Arakawa H, Yamada H, Kurihara Y, Nakajima Y, Takeda A, Fukushima Y, Fujioka M. Nonspecific interstitial pneumonia associated with polymyositis and dermatomyositis: serial high-resolution CT findings and functional correlation. Chest. 2003;123:1096–103.
68. Nambu Y, Mouri M, Toga H, Ohya N, Iwata T, Kobashi Y. Gender and underlying diseases affect the frequency of the concurrence of adult polymyositis/dermatomyositis and interstitial pneumonia. Chest. 1994;106:1931–2.

69. Furuya T, Hakoda M, Tsuchiya N, Kotake S, Ichikawa N, Nanke Y, Nakajima A, Takeuchi M, Nishinarita M, Kondo H, Kawasaki A, Kobayashi S, Mimori T, Tokunaga K, Kamatani N. Immunogenetic features in 120 Japanese patients with idiopathic inflammatory myopathy. J Rheumatol. 2004;31:1768–74.

70. Chen IJ, Jan Wu YJ, Lin CW, Fan KW, Luo SF, Ho HH, Liou LB, Tsai WP, Chen JY, Yang CH, Kuo CF, Yu KH. Interstitial lung disease in polymyositis and dermatomyositis. Clin Rheumatol. 2009;28:639–46.

71. Danieli MG, Gambini S, Pettinari L, Logullo F, Veronesi G, Gabrielli A. Impact of treatment on survival in polymyositis and dermatomyositis. A single-centre long-term follow-up study. Autoimmun Rev. 2014;13:1048–54.

72. Sharp GC, Irvin WS, Tan EM, Gould RG, Holman HR. Mixed connective tissue disease—an apparently distinct rheumatic disease syndrome associated with a specific antibody to an extractable nuclear antigen (ENA). Am J Med. 1972;52:148–59.

73. Distler JH, Manger B, Spriewald BM, Schett G, Distler O. Treatment of pulmonary fibrosis for twenty weeks with imatinib mesylate in a patient with mixed connective tissue disease. Arthritis Rheum. 2008;58:2538–42.

74. Bodolay E, Szekanecz Z, Devenyi K, Galuska L, Csipo I, Vegh J, Garai I, Szegedi G. Evaluation of interstitial lung disease in mixed connective tissue disease (MCTD). Rheumatology. 2005;44:656–61.

75. Wiener-Kronish JP, Solinger AM, Warnock ML, Churg A, Ordonez N, Golden JA. Severe pulmonary involvement in mixed connective tissue disease. Am Rev Respir Dis. 1981;124:499–503.

76. Kocheril SV, Appleton BE, Somers EC, Kazerooni EA, Flaherty KR, Martinez FJ, Gross BH, Crofford LJ. Comparison of disease progression and mortality of connective tissue disease-related interstitial lung disease and idiopathic interstitial pneumonia. Arthritis Rheum. 2005;53:549–57.

77. Lateef A, Petri M. Hormone replacement and contraceptive therapy in autoimmune diseases. J Autoimmun. 2012;38:J170–176.

78. Urowitz MB, Gladman DD, Farewell VT, Stewart J, McDonald J. Lupus and pregnancy studies. Arthritis Rheum. 1993;36:1392–7.

79. Ramsey-Goldman R, Dunn JE, Huang CF, Dunlop D, Rairie JE, Fitzgerald S, Manzi S. Frequency of fractures in women with systemic lupus erythematosus: comparison with United States population data. Arthritis Rheum. 1999;42:882–90.

80. Sanchez-Guerrero J, Uribe AG, Jimenez-Santana L, Mestanza-Peralta M, Lara-Reyes P, Seuc AH, Cravioto MD. A trial of contraceptive methods in women with systemic lupus erythematosus. N Engl J Med. 2005;353:2539–49.

81. Petri M, Kim MY, Kalunian KC, Grossman J, Hahn BH, Sammaritano LR, Lockshin M, Merrill JT, Belmont HM, Askanase AD, McCune WJ, Hearth-Holmes M, Dooley MA, Von Feldt J, Friedman A, Tan M, Davis J, Cronin M, Diamond B, Mackay M, Sigler L, Fillius M, Rupel A, Licciardi F, Buyon JP, Trial O-S. Combined oral contraceptives in women with systemic lupus erythematosus. N Engl J Med. 2005;353:2550–8.

82. Sanchez-Guerrero J, Liang MH, Karlson EW, Hunter DJ, Colditz GA. Postmenopausal estrogen therapy and the risk for developing systemic lupus erythematosus. Ann Intern Med. 1995;122:430–3.

83. Cooper GS, Dooley MA, Treadwell EL, St Clair EW, Gilkeson GS. Hormonal and reproductive risk factors for development of systemic lupus erythematosus: results of a population-based, case–control study. Arthritis Rheum. 2002;46:1830–9.

84. Lekakis J, Papamichael C, Mavrikakis M, Voutsas A, Stamatelopoulos S. Effect of long-term estrogen therapy on brachial arterial endothelium-dependent vasodilation in women with Raynaud's phenomenon secondary to systemic sclerosis. Am J Cardiol. 1998;82:1555–7. A1558.

85. Ostensen M, Villiger PM. The remission of rheumatoid arthritis during pregnancy. Semin Immunopathol. 2007;29:185–91.

86. Beretta L, Caronni M, Origgi L, Ponti A, Santaniello A, Scorza R. Hormone replacement therapy may prevent the development of isolated pulmonary hypertension in patients with systemic sclerosis and limited cutaneous involvement. Scand J Rheumatol. 2006;35:468–71.

87. Martinez FJ, Safrin S, Weycker D, Starko KM, Bradford WZ, King Jr TE, Flaherty KR, Schwartz DA, Noble PW, Raghu G, Brown KK, Group IPFS. The clinical course of patients with idiopathic pulmonary fibrosis. Ann Intern Med. 2005;142:963–7.

88. Turner-Warwick M, Burrows B, Johnson A. Cryptogenic fibrosing alveolitis: clinical features and their influence on survival. Thorax. 1980;35:171–80.

89. de Cremoux H, Bernaudin JF, Laurent P, Brochard P, Bignon J. Interactions between cigarette smoking and the natural history of idiopathic pulmonary fibrosis. Chest. 1990;98:71–6.

90. American Thoracic Society. Idiopathic pulmonary fibrosis: diagnosis and treatment International consensus statement. American Thoracic Society (ATS), and the European Respiratory Society (ERS). Am J Respir Crit Care Med. 2000;161:646–64.

91. Coultas DB, Zumwalt RE, Black WC, Sobonya RE. The epidemiology of interstitial lung diseases. Am J Respir Crit Care Med. 1994;150:967–72.

92. Noble PW, Homer RJ. Back to the future: historical perspective on the pathogenesis of idiopathic pulmonary fibrosis. Am J Respir Cell Mol Biol. 2005;33:113–20.

93. Hunninghake GW, Zimmerman MB, Schwartz DA, King Jr TE, Lynch J, Hegele R, Waldron J, Colby T, Muller N, Lynch D, Galvin J, Gross B, Hogg J, Toews G, Helmers R, Cooper Jr JA, Baughman R, Strange C, Millard M. Utility of a lung biopsy for the diagnosis of idiopathic pulmonary fibrosis. Am J Respir Crit Care Med. 2001;164:193–6.

94. Raghu G, Mageto YN, Lockhart D, Schmidt RA, Wood DE, Godwin JD. The accuracy of the clinical diagnosis of new-onset idiopathic pulmonary fibrosis and other interstitial lung disease: a prospective study. Chest. 1999;116:1168–74.

95. Churg A, Muller NL, Flint J, Wright JL. Chronic hypersensitivity pneumonitis. Am J Surg Pathol. 2006;30:201–8.

96. Steele MP, Speer MC, Loyd JE, Brown KK, Herron A, Slifer SH, Burch LH, Wahidi MM, Phillips 3rd JA, Sporn TA, McAdams HP, Schwarz MI, Schwartz DA. Clinical and pathologic features of familial interstitial pneumonia. Am J Respir Crit Care Med. 2005;172:1146–52.

97. Thomas AQ, Lane K, Phillips 3rd J, Prince M, Markin C, Speer M, Schwartz DA, Gaddipati R, Marney A, Johnson J, Roberts R, Haines J, Stahlman M, Loyd JE. Heterozygosity for a surfactant protein C gene mutation associated with usual interstitial pneumonitis and cellular nonspecific interstitial pneumonitis in one kindred. Am J Respir Crit Care Med. 2002;165:1322–8.

98. Wang Y, Kuan PJ, Xing C, Cronkhite JT, Torres F, Rosenblatt RL, DiMaio JM, Kinch LN, Grishin NV, Garcia CK. Genetic defects in surfactant protein A2 are associated with pulmonary fibrosis and lung cancer. Am J Hum Genet. 2009;84:52–9.

99. Armanios MY, Chen JJ, Cogan JD, Alder JK, Ingersoll RG, Markin C, Lawson WE, Xie M, Vulto I, Phillips 3rd JA, Lansdorp PM, Greider CW, Loyd JE. Telomerase mutations in families with idiopathic pulmonary fibrosis. N Engl J Med. 2007;356:1317–26.

100. Tsakiri KD, Cronkhite JT, Kuan PJ, Xing C, Raghu G, Weissler JC, Rosenblatt RL, Shay JW, Garcia CK. Adult-onset pulmonary fibrosis caused by mutations in telomerase. Proc Natl Acad Sci U S A. 2007;104:7552–7.

101. Seibold MA, Wise AL, Speer MC, Steele MP, Brown KK, Loyd JE, Fingerlin TE, Zhang W, Gudmundsson G, Groshong SD, Evans CM, Garantziotis S, Adler KB, Dickey BF, du Bois RM, Yang IV, Herron A, Kervitsky D, Talbert JL, Markin C, Park J, Crews AL, Slifer SH, Auerbach S, Roy MG, Lin J, Hennessy CE, Schwarz MI, Schwartz DA. A common MUC5B promoter polymorphism and pulmonary fibrosis. N Engl J Med. 2011;364:1503–12.

102. Nielsen HC. Androgen receptors influence the production of pulmonary surfactant in the testicular feminization mouse fetus. J Clin Invest. 1985;76:177–81.

103. Dammann CE, Ramadurai SM, McCants DD, Pham LD, Nielsen HC. Androgen regulation of signaling pathways in late fetal mouse lung development. Endocrinology. 2000;141:2923–9.

104. Provost PR, Simard M, Tremblay Y. A link between lung androgen metabolism and the emergence of mature epithelial type II cells. Am J Respir Crit Care Med. 2004;170:296–305.
105. Kinder BW, Brown KK, McCormack FX, Ix JH, Kervitsky A, Schwarz MI, King Jr TE. Serum surfactant protein-A is a strong predictor of early mortality in idiopathic pulmonary fibrosis. Chest. 2009;135:1557–63.
106. Amsellem V, Gary-Bobo G, Marcos E, Maitre B, Chaar V, Validire P, Stern JB, Noureddine H, Sapin E, Rideau D, Hue S, Le Corvoisier P, Le Gouvello S, Dubois-Rande JL, Boczkowski J, Adnot S. Telomere dysfunction causes sustained inflammation in chronic obstructive pulmonary disease. Am J Respir Crit Care Med. 2011;184:1358–66.
107. Diaz de Leon A, Cronkhite JT, Yilmaz C, Brewington C, Wang R, Xing C, Hsia CC, Garcia CK. Subclinical lung disease, macrocytosis, and premature graying in kindreds with telomerase (TERT) mutations. Chest. 2011;140:753–63.
108. Calado RT, Yewdell WT, Wilkerson KL, Regal JA, Kajigaya S, Stratakis CA, Young NS. Sex hormones, acting on the TERT gene, increase telomerase activity in human primary hematopoietic cells. Blood. 2009;114:2236–43.
109. Wallace JL, Vong L, Dharmani P, Srivastava V, Chadee K. Muc-2-deficient mice display a sex-specific, COX-2-related impairment of gastric mucosal repair. Am J Pathol. 2011;178:1126–33.
110. King Jr TE, Pardo A, Selman M. Idiopathic pulmonary fibrosis. Lancet. 2011;378:1949–61.
111. Walter P, Ron D. The unfolded protein response: from stress pathway to homeostatic regulation. Science. 2011;334:1081–6.
112. Ron D, Walter P. Signal integration in the endoplasmic reticulum unfolded protein response. Nat Rev Mol Cell Biol. 2007;8:519–29.
113. Lawson WE, Cheng DS, Degryse AL, Tanjore H, Polosukhin VV, Xu XC, Newcomb DC, Jones BR, Roldan J, Lane KB, Morrisey EE, Beers MF, Yull FE, Blackwell TS. Endoplasmic reticulum stress enhances fibrotic remodeling in the lungs. Proc Natl Acad Sci U S A. 2011;108:10562–7.
114. Li L, Hossain MA, Sadat S, Hager L, Liu L, Tam L, Schroer S, Huogen L, Fantus IG, Connelly PW, Woo M, Ng DS. Lecithin cholesterol acyltransferase null mice are protected from diet-induced obesity and insulin resistance in a gender-specific manner through multiple pathways. J Biol Chem. 2011;286:17809–20.
115. Haas MJ, Raheja P, Jaimungal S, Sheikh-Ali M, Mooradian AD. Estrogen-dependent inhibition of dextrose-induced endoplasmic reticulum stress and superoxide generation in endothelial cells. Free Radic Biol Med. 2012;52:2161–7.
116. Hyde DM, King Jr TE, McDermott T, Waldron Jr JA, Colby TV, Thurlbeck WM, Flint WM, Ackerson L, Cherniack RM. Idiopathic pulmonary fibrosis. Quantitative assessment of lung pathology. Comparison of a semiquantitative and a morphometric histopathologic scoring system. Am Rev Respir Dis. 1992;146:1042–7.
117. Chapman HA. Epithelial-mesenchymal interactions in pulmonary fibrosis. Annu Rev Physiol. 2011;73:413–35.
118. Goulioumis AK, Fuxe J, Varakis J, Repanti M, Goumas P, Papadaki H. Estrogen receptor-beta expression in human laryngeal carcinoma: correlation with the expression of epithelial-mesenchymal transition specific biomarkers. Oncol Rep. 2009;22:1063–8.
119. Pinhal CS, Lopes A, Torres DB, Felisbino SL, Rocha Gontijo JA, Boer PA. Time-course morphological and functional disorders of the kidney induced by long-term high-fat diet intake in female rats. Nephrol Dial Transplant. 2013;28:2464–76.
120. Hung YC, Chang WC, Chen LM, Chang YY, Wu LY, Chung WM, Lin TY, Chen LC, Ma WL. Non-genomic estrogen/estrogen receptor alpha promotes cellular malignancy of immature ovarian teratoma in vitro. J Cell Physiol. 2014;229:752–61.
121. Baran CP, Opalek JM, McMaken S, Newland CA, O'Brien Jr JM, Hunter MG, Bringardner BD, Monick MM, Brigstock DR, Stromberg PC, Hunninghake GW, Marsh CB. Important roles for macrophage colony-stimulating factor, CC chemokine ligand 2, and mononuclear phagocytes in the pathogenesis of pulmonary fibrosis. Am J Respir Crit Care Med. 2007;176:78–89.

122. Tager AM, LaCamera P, Shea BS, Campanella GS, Selman M, Zhao Z, Polosukhin V, Wain J, Karimi-Shah BA, Kim ND, Hart WK, Pardo A, Blackwell TS, Xu Y, Chun J, Luster AD. The lysophosphatidic acid receptor LPA1 links pulmonary fibrosis to lung injury by mediating fibroblast recruitment and vascular leak. Nat Med. 2008;14:45–54.
123. Ruige JB, Bekaert M, Lapauw B, Fiers T, Lehr S, Hartwig S, Herzfeld de Wiza D, Schiller M, Passlack W, Van Nieuwenhove Y, Pattyn P, Cuvelier C, Taes YE, Sell H, Eckel J, Kaufman JM, Ouwens DM. Sex steroid-induced changes in circulating monocyte chemoattractant protein-1 levels may contribute to metabolic dysfunction in obese men. J Clin Endocrinol Metab. 2012;97:E1187–1191.
124. Xia H, Diebold D, Nho R, Perlman D, Kleidon J, Kahm J, Avdulov S, Peterson M, Nerva J, Bitterman P, Henke C. Pathological integrin signaling enhances proliferation of primary lung fibroblasts from patients with idiopathic pulmonary fibrosis. J Exp Med. 2008;205:1659–72.
125. Tian B, Lessan K, Kahm J, Kleidon J, Henke C. beta 1 integrin regulates fibroblast viability during collagen matrix contraction through a phosphatidylinositol 3-kinase/Akt/protein kinase B signaling pathway. J Biol Chem. 2002;277:24667–75.
126. Lefevre N, Corazza F, Duchateau J, Desir J, Casimir G. Sex differences in inflammatory cytokines and CD99 expression following in vitro lipopolysaccharide stimulation. Shock. 2012;38:37–42.
127. Gharaee-Kermani M, Hatano K, Nozaki Y, Phan SH. Gender-based differences in bleomycin-induced pulmonary fibrosis. Am J Pathol. 2005;166:1593–606.
128. Voltz JW, Card JW, Carey MA, Degraff LM, Ferguson CD, Flake GP, Bonner JC, Korach KS, Zeldin DC. Male sex hormones exacerbate lung function impairment after bleomycin-induced pulmonary fibrosis. Am J Respir Cell Mol Biol. 2008;39:45–52.
129. Booton R, Lindsay MA. Emerging role of MicroRNAs and long noncoding RNAs in respiratory disease. Chest. 2014;146:193–204.
130. Pandit KV, Corcoran D, Yousef H, Yarlagadda M, Tzouvelekis A, Gibson KF, Konishi K, Yousem SA, Singh M, Handley D, Richards T, Selman M, Watkins SC, Pardo A, Ben-Yehudah A, Bouros D, Eickelberg O, Ray P, Benos PV, Kaminski N. Inhibition and role of let-7d in idiopathic pulmonary fibrosis. Am J Respir Crit Care Med. 2010;182:220–9.
131. Liu G, Friggeri A, Yang Y, Milosevic J, Ding Q, Thannickal VJ, Kaminski N, Abraham E. miR-21 mediates fibrogenic activation of pulmonary fibroblasts and lung fibrosis. J Exp Med. 2010;207:1589–97.
132. Yang S, Banerjee S, de Freitas A, Sanders YY, Ding Q, Matalon S, Thannickal VJ, Abraham E, Liu G. Participation of miR-200 in pulmonary fibrosis. Am J Pathol. 2012;180:484–93.
133. Dakhlallah D, Batte K, Wang Y, Cantemir-Stone CZ, Yan P, Nuovo G, Mikhail A, Hitchcock CL, Wright VP, Nana-Sinkam SP, Piper MG, Marsh CB. Epigenetic regulation of miR-17~92 contributes to the pathogenesis of pulmonary fibrosis. Am J Respir Crit Care Med. 2013;187:397–405.
134. Milosevic J, Pandit K, Magister M, Rabinovich E, Ellwanger DC, Yu G, Vuga LJ, Weksler B, Benos PV, Gibson KF, McMillan M, Kahn M, Kaminski N. Profibrotic role of miR-154 in pulmonary fibrosis. Am J Respir Cell Mol Biol. 2012;47:879–87.
135. Simon LM, Edelstein LC, Nagalla S, Woodley AB, Chen ES, Kong X, Ma L, Fortina P, Kunapuli S, Holinstat M, McKenzie SE, Dong JF, Shaw CA, Bray PF. Human platelet microRNA-mRNA networks associated with age and gender revealed by integrated plateletomics. Blood. 2014;123:e37–45.
136. Yang IV, Schwartz DA. Epigenetic control of gene expression in the lung. Am J Respir Crit Care Med. 2011;183:1295–301.
137. Rabinovich EI, Selman M, Kaminski N. Epigenomics of idiopathic pulmonary fibrosis: evaluating the first steps. Am J Respir Crit Care Med. 2012;186:473–5.
138. Sanders YY, Ambalavanan N, Halloran B, Zhang X, Liu H, Crossman DK, Bray M, Zhang K, Thannickal VJ, Hagood JS. Altered DNA methylation profile in idiopathic pulmonary fibrosis. Am J Respir Crit Care Med. 2012;186:525–35.

139. Ross CM. A possible epigenetic explanation for the relationship between physical activity and exceptional health among older women. Arch Intern Med. 2010;170:1087.
140. McGee SP, Zhang H, Karmaus W, Sabo-Attwood T. Influence of sex and disease severity on gene expression profiles in individuals with idiopathic pulmonary fibrosis. Int J Mol Epidemiol Genet. 2014;5:71–86.
141. Abbas A, Aukrust P, Russell D, Krohg-Sorensen K, Almas T, Bundgaard D, Bjerkeli V, Sagen EL, Michelsen AE, Dahl TB, Holm S, Ueland T, Skjelland M, Halvorsen B. Matrix metalloproteinase 7 is associated with symptomatic lesions and adverse events in patients with carotid atherosclerosis. PLoS One. 2014;9, e84935.
142. Mendoza-Milla C, Valero Jimenez A, Rangel C, Lozano A, Morales V, Becerril C, Chavira R, Ruiz V, Barrera L, Montano M, Pardo A, Selman M. Dehydroepiandrosterone has strong antifibrotic effects and is decreased in idiopathic pulmonary fibrosis. Eur Respir J. 2013;42:1309–21.
143. Samara KD, Margaritopoulos G, Wells AU, Siafakas NM, Antoniou KM. Smoking and pulmonary fibrosis: novel insights. Pulm med. 2011;2011:461439.
144. Cottin V, Nunes H, Brillet PY, Delaval P, Devouassoux G, Tillie-Leblond I, Israel-Biet D, Court-Fortune I, Valeyre D, Cordier JF, Groupe d'Etude et de Recherche sur les Maladies Orphelines P. Combined pulmonary fibrosis and emphysema: a distinct underrecognised entity. Eur Respir J. 2005;26:586–93.
145. King Jr TE, Tooze JA, Schwarz MI, Brown KR, Cherniack RM. Predicting survival in idiopathic pulmonary fibrosis: scoring system and survival model. Am J Respir Crit Care Med. 2001;164:1171–81.
146. Antoniou KM, Hansell DM, Rubens MB, Marten K, Desai SR, Siafakas NM, Nicholson AG, du Bois RM, Wells AU. Idiopathic pulmonary fibrosis: outcome in relation to smoking status. Am J Respir Crit Care Med. 2008;177:190–4.
147. Barnes PJ, Adcock IM, Ito K. Histone acetylation and deacetylation: importance in inflammatory lung diseases. Eur Respir J. 2005;25:552–63.
148. Coward WR, Watts K, Feghali-Bostwick CA, Jenkins G, Pang L. Repression of IP-10 by interactions between histone deacetylation and hypermethylation in idiopathic pulmonary fibrosis. Mol Cell Biol. 2010;30:2874–86.
149. Coward WR, Watts K, Feghali-Bostwick CA, Knox A, Pang L. Defective histone acetylation is responsible for the diminished expression of cyclooxygenase 2 in idiopathic pulmonary fibrosis. Mol Cell Biol. 2009;29:4325–39.
150. Van Reek J, Drop MJ. Cigarette smoking in the USA: sociocultural influences. Rev Epidemiol Sante Publique. 1986;34:168–73.
151. Hanson MJ. Sociocultural and physiological correlates of cigarette smoking in women. Health Care Women Int. 1994;15:549–62.
152. Steele JR, Raymond RL, Ness KK, Alvi S, Kearney I. A comparative study of sociocultural factors and young adults' smoking in two Midwestern communities. Nicotine Tob Res. 2007;9 Suppl 1:S73–82.
153. Sieminska A, Jassem E. The many faces of tobacco use among women. Med Sci Monit. 2014;20:153–62.
154. Greaves L, Hemsing N. Women and tobacco control policies: social-structural and psychosocial contributions to vulnerability to tobacco use and exposure. Drug Alcohol Depend. 2009;104 Suppl 1:S121–130.
155. Gilpin EA, Farkas AJ, Emery SL, Ake CF, Pierce JP. Clean indoor air: advances in California, 1990–1999. Am J Public Health. 2002;92:785–91.
156. Anderson SJ, Glantz SA, Ling PM. Emotions for sale: cigarette advertising and women's psychosocial needs. Tob Control. 2005;14:127–35.
157. Allen SS, Bade T, Center B, Finstad D, Hatsukami D. Menstrual phase effects on smoking relapse. Addiction. 2008;103:809–21.
158. Marks JL, Hair CS, Klock SC, Ginsburg BE, Pomerleau CS. Effects of menstrual phase on intake of nicotine, caffeine, and alcohol and nonprescribed drugs in women with late luteal phase dysphoric disorder. J Subst Abuse. 1994;6:235–43.

159. Allen SS, Hatsukami D, Christianson D, Nelson D. Symptomatology and energy intake during the menstrual cycle in smoking women. J Subst Abuse. 1996;8:303–19.
160. Sofuoglu M, Babb DA, Hatsukami DK. Progesterone treatment during the early follicular phase of the menstrual cycle: effects on smoking behavior in women. Pharmacol Biochem Behav. 2001;69:299–304.
161. Benowitz NL, Lessov-Schlaggar CN, Swan GE, Jacob 3rd P. Female sex and oral contraceptive use accelerate nicotine metabolism. Clin Pharmacol Ther. 2006;79:480–8.
162. Dempsey D, Jacob 3rd P, Benowitz NL. Accelerated metabolism of nicotine and cotinine in pregnant smokers. J Pharmacol Exp Ther. 2002;301:594–8.
163. Perkins KA. Smoking cessation in women. Special considerations. CNS Drugs. 2001;15:391–411.
164. Donny EC, Caggiula AR, Rowell PP, Gharib MA, Maldovan V, Booth S, Mielke MM, Hoffman A, McCallum S. Nicotine self-administration in rats: estrous cycle effects, sex differences and nicotinic receptor binding. Psychopharmacology (Berl). 2000;151:392–405.
165. Westermeyer J, Boedicker AE. Course, severity, and treatment of substance abuse among women versus men. Am J Drug Alcohol Abuse. 2000;26:523–35.
166. Fiorentine R, Anglin MD, Gil-Rivas V, Taylor E. Drug treatment: explaining the gender paradox. Subst Use Misuse. 1997;32:653–78.
167. Iwai K, Mori T, Yamada N, Yamaguchi M, Hosoda Y. Idiopathic pulmonary fibrosis. Epidemiologic approaches to occupational exposure. Am J Respir Crit Care Med. 1994;150:670–5.
168. Hoagland H. Cultural and environmental changes affecting health and medicine. J Lancet. 1966;86:530–6.
169. Baumgartner KB, Samet JM, Coultas DB, Stidley CA, Hunt WC, Colby TV, Waldron JA. Occupational and environmental risk factors for idiopathic pulmonary fibrosis: a multicenter case–control study. Collaborating Centers. Am J Epidemiol. 2000;152:307–15.
170. Baumgartner KB, Samet JM, Stidley CA, Colby TV, Waldron JA. Cigarette smoking: a risk factor for idiopathic pulmonary fibrosis. Am J Respir Crit Care Med. 1997;155:242–8.
171. Scott J, Johnston I, Britton J. What causes cryptogenic fibrosing alveolitis? A case–control study of environmental exposure to dust. BMJ. 1990;301:1015–7.
172. de Koning HW, Smith KR, Last JM. Biomass fuel combustion and health. Bull World Health Organ. 1985;63:11–26.
173. Perez-Padilla R, Regalado J, Vedal S, Pare P, Chapela R, Sansores R, Selman M. Exposure to biomass smoke and chronic airway disease in Mexican women. A case–control study. Am J Respir Crit Care Med. 1996;154:701–6.
174. Padmavati S, Pathak SN. Chronic cor pulmonale in Delhi: a study of 127 cases. Circulation. 1959;20:343–52.
175. Sandoval J, Salas J, Martinez-Guerra ML, Gomez A, Martinez C, Portales A, Palomar A, Villegas M, Barrios R. Pulmonary arterial hypertension and cor pulmonale associated with chronic domestic woodsmoke inhalation. Chest. 1993;103:12–20.
176. Mukhopadhyay S, Gujral M, Abraham JL, Scalzetti EM, Iannuzzi MC. A case of hut lung: scanning electron microscopy with energy dispersive x-ray spectroscopy analysis of a domestically acquired form of pneumoconiosis. Chest. 2013;144:323–7.
177. Harris JM, Cullinan P, McDonald JC. Occupational distribution and geographic clustering of deaths certified to be cryptogenic fibrosing alveolitis in England and Wales. Chest. 2001;119:428–33.

Chapter 7
Sex-Specific Differences in Lung Cancer

Laura P. Stabile and Timothy F. Burns

Abstract Lung cancer is the leading cause of cancer deaths for both men and women in the United States. Lung cancer exceeded breast cancer as the primary cause of female cancer deaths in 1987 and now kills more women than the next two most common cancers in females (breast and colorectal) combined. The rate of lung cancer diagnoses for men has declined in the last 30 years; however, lung cancer incidence has risen for women. Whether or not women have an increased risk of lung cancer remains controversial. There is, however, no debate to the fact that the biology of lung cancer differs between the sexes. Here we review the explanations for the observed sex differences in lung cancer presentation, including disparities in clinical characteristics, genetic factors and hormonal influences, as well as variations in incidence rates, outcomes, and therapeutic response. Finally, the current status and future implications for pharmacological blockade of the estrogen pathway for lung cancer treatment are discussed.

Keywords Lung cancer • NSCLC • SCLC • Estrogen • Hormones • Aromatase • Estrogen receptor • EGFR • ALK • HPV • Anti-estrogen • Aromatase inhibitor • Tobacco • Never-smoking lung cancer

Abbreviations

AC	Adenocarcinoma
AI	Aromatase inhibitor
AI	Aromatase inhibitor, ER, estrogen receptor

L.P. Stabile, PhD (✉)
Department of Pharmacology & Chemical Biology, University of Pittsburgh
Cancer Institute, Hillman Cancer Center Research Pavilion,
2.32b, 5117 Centre Avenue, Pittsburgh, PA 15213-1863, USA
e-mail: stabilela@upmc.edu

T.F. Burns, MD, PhD
Department of Medicine, Division of Hematology-Oncology, University of Pittsburgh
Cancer Institute, Hillman Cancer Center Research Pavilion, 2.18e, 5117 Centre Avenue,
Pittsburgh, PA 15213-1863, USA
e-mail: burnstf@upmc.edu

© Springer International Publishing Switzerland 2016
A.R. Hemnes (ed.), *Gender, Sex Hormones and Respiratory Disease*,
Respiratory Medicine, DOI 10.1007/978-3-319-23998-9_7

ALK	Anaplastic lymphoma kinase
CBR	Clinical benefit rate
CYP1A1	Cytochrome P450 1A1
DRC	DNA repair capacity
EGFR	Epidermal growth factor receptor
ER	Estrogen Receptor
GRPR	Gastrin-releasing peptide receptor
GSTM1	Glutathione S-transferase M1
HPV	Human papillomavirus
IGFR-1	Insulin-like growth factor-1 receptor
NSCLC	Non-small cell lung cancer
PFS	Progression-free survival
PR	Partial response
RR	Response rate
SCC	Squamous cell carcinoma
SCLC	Small cell lung cancer
SERM	Selective estrogen receptor modulator
TKI	Tyrosine kinase inhibitor
VEGFR	Vascular endothelial growth factor receptor

Lung Cancer and Smoking Incidence among Males and Females

Lung cancer is the leading cause of cancer death in the United States and worldwide. In 2014, an estimated 224,210 new cases will be diagnosed and 159,260 deaths will occur in the United States alone. Almost half of these cases (108,210) and deaths (72,330) will occur in women, making lung cancer the second leading cause of cancer in women and by far the leading cause of cancer death in women. Each year, lung cancer kills more women than the next two most common causes (breast and colorectal cancer) of cancer death combined. Furthermore, the lifetime risk of developing a lung cancer is 1/16 for women compared to a lifetime risk of 1/13 for men [1]. Although not the only cause of lung cancer, the vast majority of lung cancers are due to cigarette smoking in both men and women.

Approximately 90 % of lung cancer deaths in men and 80 % of lung cancer deaths in women have been linked to tobacco use [2]. Currently, the Center for Disease Control estimates that 42.1 million people or 18.1 % of the US adult population are current smokers [3]. Cigarette smoking remains more common among men (20.5 %) than women (15.8 %). This current prevalence of female smoking is a product of a dramatic cultural shift in the social acceptance of female smoking during the last century. Prior to the Second World War and the entry of a large number of women into the workforce, only a small percentage of women smoked; however, this percentage peaked in 1965 at 33 %. The level of smoking in women

remained elevated until the late 1970s and started slowing declining in the 1980s
[4]. In contrast, although greater than half of American males smoked prior to 1965,
the prevalence of male smoking significantly decreased during the next two decades.
These epidemiological trends are reflected in the sharp increase in female lung cancer deaths between 1965 and 1995 compared to all other cancer types and the continued plateau into this century with only a recent decline in deaths ([1] and Fig.
7.1). In comparison, the incidence of male lung cancer deaths peaked in the 1980s
and has declined significantly since 1990. Recent studies have further examined the
large increase in lung cancer deaths and one study in particular which examined
deaths from lung cancer over a 50-year period (1959–2010) demonstrated a 16.8-
fold increase in lung cancer deaths in women [5]. Remarkably, half of these deaths
occurred in the last 20 years. Importantly, they found that in a contemporary cohort

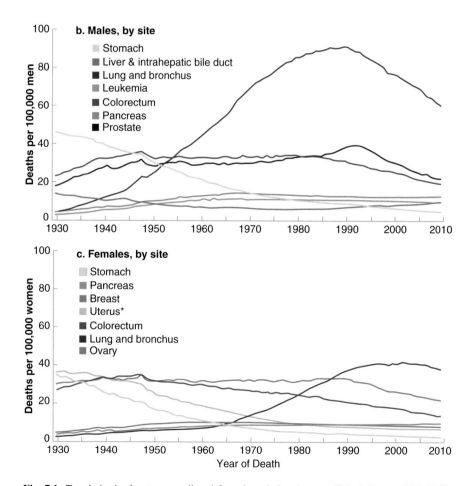

Fig. 7.1 Trends in death rates overall and for selected sites by sex, United States, 1930–2010.
(Reprinted with permission from Siegel et al. [1])

that the risk of death from lung cancer in current smokers was essentially the same in men and women compared to those who never smoked.

Although the risk of death from lung cancer in current smokers appears to be similar in men and women, several early studies suggested that women may be more susceptible to tobacco carcinogens [6–12]. Further supporting this hypothesis, several studies have found higher levels of tobacco carcinogen induced DNA adducts in lung tumors from women smokers in comparison to male smokers despite lower levels of cigarette exposures [13–15]. Despite this biologic evidence and early case–control studies which suggested an increased susceptibility in female smokers to tobacco carcinogens, several other studies have failed to demonstrate an excess risk for women [16–21]. Therefore, the hypothesis that female smokers are more susceptible to carcinogenic effects of smoking remains controversial.

Sex Differences in Lung Cancer Presentation

Age and Histology

Although the role of sex in lung cancer risk is unclear, a substantial body of literature exists to support the notion that the epidemiology and biology of lung cancer is distinct between the sexes including age, histology, smoking changes, molecular alterations, and the possible role of viral infection (Fig. 7.2). A series of large studies have found that women are diagnosed with lung cancer at an earlier age than men including a large Polish study which included over 20,000 lung cancer patients (age 60.02 versus age 62.18 years; p value <0.001) and a significantly higher percentage of women compared to men were diagnosed under the age of 50 [22]. Although adenocarcinoma (AC) of the lung is the most common non-small cell lung

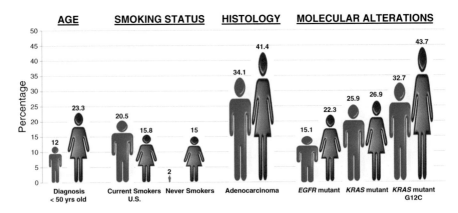

Fig. 7.2 Sex differences in the epidemiology and biology of lung cancer. Compared to men, women with lung cancer are more likely to be younger at diagnosis, never smokers, adenocarcinoma histology, and *EGFR* mutation positive. See text for details

cancer (NSCLC) histology in both men and women, AC is more common in women (41.4 %) than men (34.1 %) [22–24]. Conversely squamous cell carcinoma (SCC) is more common in men [25]. This difference in histology is attributed at least in part to the differences in tar content and filters in the cigarettes smoked by men and women which lead to more central (associated with SCC) or peripheral inhalation of cigarette smoke (associated with AC) [26, 27].

Never-Smoking Status

Although smoking is the causative factor in the majority of lung cancers, between 16,000 and 24,000 never smokers die of lung cancer each year [28]. Interestingly, the vast majority (70–80 %) of these patients are women [29]. In the United States, approximately 15 % of women compared to 2 % men with lung cancer are never smokers and these numbers rise sharply in Asian populations (reviewed in [30]). A study by Wakelee et al. which examined six large, prospective cohort studies found that the age-adjusted incidence of lung cancer was significantly higher in female versus male never smokers [31]. Remarkably, the death rate from never-smoking lung cancer is 25 % higher in men compared to women suggesting a distinct biology based on sex [32]. In addition to the differences noted above, distinct molecular alterations including targetable and untargetable oncogene drivers are more common in female lung cancer patients.

Molecular Alterations: Oncogenic Drivers and Tumor Suppressors

Over the last decade, much of the progress that has been made in lung cancer therapy has come from the recognition that lung cancer, especially lung cancer in never smokers, is driven by oncogenic drivers which in some cases can be potently targeted. *Epidermal Growth Factor Receptor* (*EGFR*) mutant lung cancer was the first oncogene driver-dependent lung cancer to be targeted successfully in the clinic. Mutations in *EGFR* occur in 21 % of metastatic AC of the lung and predict a 70 % response rate to EGFR tyrosine kinase inhibitors (TKIs) [33]. Shortly after the discovery of *EGFR* mutations in 2004 [34–36], it quickly became apparent that *EGFR* mutations were more common in AC of the lung, women (22.3 %) compared to men (15.1 %), and never smokers compared to ever smokers [37, 38]. As these mutations are predictive for response to EGFR TKIs, this may in part explain the increased survival advantage of women with lung cancer. The second most frequent observed targetable oncogene driver in AC of the lung is the anaplastic lymphoma kinase (ALK). Translocations involving the *ALK* gene result in a constitutively active fusion protein and are found in 8 % of lung ACs [33]. Similar to *EGFR* mutant disease, ALK TKIs result in a 70 % response rate in *ALK* translocation positive lung cancer [39, 40]. *ALK* translocations are also more common in AC of the lung, never smokers, and younger patients and until recently were thought to be more common in men [41]. However, a recent large meta-analysis of 17 studies and 4511 NSCLC cases has suggested that *ALK* translocations are more frequent in women than men [42]. A second larger meta-analysis in 1178 *ALK* rearranged cases from 20,541 NSCLC patients also found that *ALK* translocations were more frequent in women than men but only in Asian women [43]. Interestingly, the investigators found that in Caucasian populations, men were more likely to have *ALK* fusions than women. Regardless of ethnicity, there is clearly a significant difference in frequency of ALK translocations between men and women. Finally, the most frequent oncogene driver in AC of the lung, mutant *KRAS*, also differs according to sex. KRAS mutations are found in 25 % of ACs and portend a poor prognosis in the metastatic setting and KRAS mutant NSCLC is currently untargetable [44]. KRAS mutations were previously reported to be more common in women (26.2 %) compared to men (17.4 %) [45]. However, a more recent and larger study found that KRAS mutations were only slightly more common in women than men overall, but the frequency of distinct KRAS mutations was different in men and women. The smoking associated and most frequently observed KRAS G12C variant was significantly more common in female smokers (43.7 %) versus male smokers (32.7 %) [38]. Interestingly, this higher frequency of the KRAS G12C allele occurred despite females having a lower pack-year smoking history and younger age, suggesting an increased susceptibility to acquire smoking-induced KRAS mutations [38].

In addition to the significant differences in the observed frequency of oncogenic driver mutations, a significant difference in the frequency of mutations in the most common tumor suppressor, p53, has been observed between men and women. Several studies have demonstrated that smoking-related p53 mutations are more common in women versus men [13, 15, 46]. These findings are speculated to be related to an increased susceptibility of tobacco carcinogen-induced DNA adducts which has been observed in female smokers [13–15].

Role of HPV in Female Lung Cancer

Several epidemiologic studies have suggested a potential role of HPV in lung tumorigenesis in never-smoking women [47, 48] and reviewed in [49]. Most recently, a large meta-analysis of nine studies with a total of 1094 lung cancer cases and 484 noncancer controls found that HPV infection in lung tissue was associated with lung cancer. Similar results were found in with "high-risk" HPV16 and HPV18 positive cases. As previously reported, the association was stronger with SCC than AC of the lung [50]. Two potential mechanisms of HPV infection of the lung have been proposed. The first route of transmission is through the primary infection of the female cervix followed by hematogenous transmission to the lung. Supporting this route of transmission is the fact that women with anogenital malignancies have a higher risk of lung cancer as compared to those without anogenital malignancies [51, 52].

The second proposed route of transmission is through the high-risk sexual activity leading to infection of the oral cavity and subsequent transmission to the lungs. Although there is substantial evidence for the association between oral sex, HPV infection, and head and neck cancer, to date, little data exists to support the transmission of oral HPV infection to the lung resulting in a subsequent lung cancer [49]. The role of HPV in lung cancer and its routes of transmissions remain an unanswered question which requires further investigation.

Sex as a Prognostic Factor in Lung Cancer Outcome

Female sex has been repeatedly demonstrated to be a favorable prognostic factor for lung cancer. Women display superior lung cancer survival rates independent of other factors such as stage, histology, treatment, and smoking status, even after taking into account sex-specific life expectancy [53–55]. Multiple studies have shown better overall survival rates in women with NSCLC following surgical resection [53, 56–63]. This trend has also been observed in female patients with small cell lung cancer (SCLC) [64, 65]. Although the causes of these differences are not well defined, the etiology behind these observations may be linked to genetic or molecular factors discussed in other sections of this chapter. Nakamura et al. recently conducted a meta-analysis of 39 published studies on NSCLC survival differences between men and women which included 32,701 women and 54,099 men and reported that survival of women with NSCLC was significantly better than that for men [66]. This survival advantage was significant regardless of type of statistical analyses used, stage, histology, and smoking status. Biological behaviors, such as differential smoking habits between men and women, have been hypothesized to potentially affect such comparisons and thus a definitive conclusion about the prognostic influence of sex cannot be made. However, the death rate in female never smokers with lung cancer is 25 % lower than male never smokers suggesting a distinct biology based on sex [32].

Because lung cancer prognosis differs between males and females, the male/female ratio has been compared to clinical treatment outcome for lung cancer. Several studies have suggested that sex may be considered not only a prognostic factor but a predictive factor as well. An improved benefit from chemotherapy has been observed for women with SCLC compared to men in multiple studies [64, 67, 68]. However, the data regarding an increased benefit from chemotherapy in females with NSCLC have been conflicting with some studies showing no difference in response rates [69] while others demonstrating a survival benefit for women [70]. In addition, women have been reported to experience greater toxicity from certain chemotherapeutic drugs [67, 68]. However, the choice of chemotherapy is currently not influenced by patient's sex based on the limited data and observed modest differences in chemotherapy efficacy for lung cancer patients.

Targeted therapies also have shown differential sex outcomes, particularly for the EGFR TKIs, gefitinib and erlotinib [71–73]. As mentioned previously, EGFR mutations are more frequently observed in lung tumors from female patients and the presence of these mutations confers a response to EGFR TKIs which is thought to account for the observed female response benefit [37, 38]. It is unknown whether there is a sex difference in response rate or overall survival in patients with *EGFR* TKI sensitizing mutations. Interestingly, a recently published pooled analysis of the EGFR TKI, afatinib, versus chemotherapy in the first-line setting in patients with advanced *EGFR* mutant demonstrated for the first time an overall survival benefit for an EGFR TKI. However, there was no difference in overall survival between men and women with *EGFR* mutations (exon 19 del or L858R), suggesting that there may not be a sex difference in terms of response or survival for EGFR mutant NSCLC patients [74]. Similarly, other targetable oncogenes such as ALK also display differential sex-specific alterations; however, improved response to ALK-targeted treatment in women has not been observed [75]. Vandetanib is a TKI with dual activity against both the VEGFR and EGFR pathways that failed to demonstrate a survival improvement in NSCLC. However, a trend for greater benefit in females was found in all treatment arms containing vandetanib across different trials [76, 77]. Sex may also influence radiation treatment outcomes. A meta-analysis demonstrated that female sex is associated with better survival following radiation treatment for lung cancer with male mortality rates 1.23 times higher than the mortality rate for women [78]. This was subsequently confirmed in another study of Stage IIIB NSCLC patients treated with radiotherapy, with or without chemotherapy [79]. The variation in response rates between men and women as observed with chemotherapeutic drugs, targeted TKIs, and radiotherapy is interesting but insufficient to allow the sex of the patient to guide therapeutic choices. All large trials in lung cancer should stratify patients according to sex, and as we move forward in an era of personalized medicine, understanding how lung cancer in men and women differs will be a critical factor in therapeutic choice.

Influence of Sex-Related Genetic Factors

Tobacco Carcinogen Metabolism

While a family history of lung cancer is an independent risk factor for lung cancer, genetic factors such as germline gene variants may play a role in the observed differential lung cancer survival rates between men and women. Pro-carcinogenic tobacco smoke constituents require activation by phase I enzymes (encoded by the CYP family of genes) for conversion to highly reactive carcinogens. Conversely, the phase II enzymes, including the glutathione *S*-transferases, are then responsible for detoxifying the activated forms of these polycyclic aromatic hydrocarbons. The reactive carcinogens that are not detoxified may bind DNA to form DNA adducts capable of inducing mutations and initiating the carcinogenesis. An appropriate balance between the phase I and phase II enzymes is necessary for optimum cellular protection from carcinogens. Metabolic activity of these enzymes can be altered by genetic polymorphisms and numerous studies have been reported examining their association with lung cancer yielding variable results [80]. In addition, these genetic polymorphisms may have distinct phenotypic outcomes in men and women.

Among the carcinogen-metabolizing enzymes, the sex-specific roles of genetic polymorphism in cytochrome P450 1A1 (CYP1A1) and glutathione S-transferase M1 (GSTM1) have been the most widely studied. Several studies have suggested that polymorphisms in these genes may help explain the significantly higher level of pulmonary DNA adducts found in female lung cancer patients compared to men [13–15]. Female lung cancer patients with an isoleucine to valine substitution in exon 7 of the *CYP1A1* gene or a *GSTM1* null phenotype had an increased lung cancer risk compared to men with these variants [81, 82]. In addition, female lung cancer patients were more likely than male lung cancer patients to have both variant genotypes (*CYP1A1/GSTM1* null) and this combination resulted in an odds ratio of 6.54 for women compared to only 2.36 for men, independent of age and smoking history [81]. Clearly, regulation of carcinogen-metabolizing genes expressed in the lung is impacted by sex-related factors.

Interestingly, the *CYP1A1* and *GSTM1* genes not only are key players in tobacco carcinogen metabolism pathways but also play a role in estrogen metabolism [83]. Estrogen metabolism to the highly oxidative catechol estrogens is a known cause of DNA damage. The association of polymorphisms in estrogen and tobacco metabolism and DNA repair pathway genes was reported by Cote et al. [83, 84]. In this large population-based study, female smokers carrying at least two at-risk alleles had an increased risk of lung cancer compared to those without any of the risk alleles suggesting a complex interaction between altered estrogen biosynthesis, tobacco carcinogen metabolism, and the inability to repair DNA damage. Not only can estrogens act as substrates for the phase I enzymes and cause DNA damage by way of estrogen oxidation products, but estrogens can also stimulate lung tumor proliferation and cellular responses.

DNA Repair Capacity

Another possible explanation for the better survival outcome in women is the decreased DNA repair capacity (DRC) in women leading to lung cancers in females being more responsive to platinum-based chemotherapies. Supporting this explanation, DNA repair machinery has been shown to be more defective in women, contributing to the hypotheses that women are more susceptible to tobacco carcinogens and also more responsive to systemic chemotherapies. Suboptimal DRC has been linked to increased lung cancer risk and a lower DRC has been observed in younger female patients and in patients with a family history of lung cancer [85]. These findings were subsequently confirmed in a larger case–control study where the mean DRC was significantly lower in women compared to men [86]. This variation in DRC is most likely attributed to genetic variants in DNA repair genes and several suggestive genetic determinants affecting the DRC phenotype have been identified [87].

Clearly, further characterization of the functional relevance and sex-specific phenotypes of these genetic variations is warranted.

Recent studies have focused on identification of associations between polymorphisms in carcinogen metabolism and DNA repair genes and the development of *EGFR* and other targetable gene mutations. It has been shown that the exon 19 *EGFR* deletion is associated with polymorphisms in a number of genes related to mutagen detoxification as well as DNA repair in never-smoking lung adenocarcinoma patients [88]. Furthermore, the number of risk alleles in these genes correlated to an increase in the frequency of the *EGFR* exon 19 deletion, particularly in female lung adenocarcinoma patients.

Gastrin-Releasing Peptide Receptor

Another potential genetic factor that has been hypothesized to contribute to the increase of lung cancer in women is the *gastrin-releasing peptide receptor* (*GRPR*) gene. GRPR is activated through bombesin-like peptides to induce cell proliferation in bronchial epithelial cells which contributes to the lung carcinogenic process. Interestingly, *GRPR* is found on the X chromosome and is known to escape X inactivation so that women have two actively transcribed alleles [89]. Shriver et al. reported that *GRPR* mRNA expression in bronchial tissue was associated with an increased risk of lung cancer in female never smokers compared to male never smokers in a study of 78 subjects [90]. However, in a more recent larger case–control study which included 331 subjects, *GRPR* was reported to be increased in normal bronchial epithelia in lung cancer cases compared to cancer-free controls and this association was most profound in never smokers or former smokers with similar risk to both sexes [91]. While *GRPR* overexpression in normal epithelial mucosa appears to be a candidate risk factor for lung cancer with limited tobacco exposure, this genetic factor does not likely contribute to sex-related lung cancer biology as originally hypothesized.

Role of Estrogen in Lung Cancer Risk

Hormone Replacement Therapy and Lung Cancer Risk

The observations of sex differences in lung cancer presentation and survival suggest a role of estrogens in lung cancer. Support for a role for estrogens in lung cancer comes from several population studies which examined the use of hormone replacement therapy (HRT) and risk of lung cancer incidence and death. The link between HRT use and increased lung cancer risk was first suggested in the late 1980s in a small population-based case–control study of 672 women [92] followed by a larger population study of 23,244 women [93]. Additional evidence of an increase in lung cancer risk in women using HRT was a small case–control study that demonstrated a positive interaction between HRT use, smoking, and lung cancer development [94]. Ganti et al. reported a significant association with a shorter OS in lung cancer patients who received HRT around the time of diagnosis versus those who did not and the effect was most pronounced in women who smoked suggesting an interaction between estrogen and tobacco carcinogens [95]. Several studies reported either no association between HRT use and increased lung cancer risk or a protective effect [96–102]. There are many possible explanations for the inconsistencies in these studies including the type of HRT used, duration of use, time of use relative to lung cancer diagnosis, or genetic variation in study populations.

Recent studies have examined specific HRT type including combined estrogen plus progestin therapy versus estrogen alone. A randomized double-blind placebo-controlled trial in over 16,000 postmenopausal women who either received estrogen plus progestin HRT or placebo for 5 years was conducted by the Women's Health Initiative. In this study, a significant negative effect on survival was observed for the HRT group with a trend toward in increased lung cancer diagnoses compared to the placebo group [103]. The combined hormone therapy significantly increased mortality from NSCLC; however, there was no effect on deaths from SCLC ([103] and Fig. 7.3). In a separate study conducted by the same group, the use of estrogen alone did not increase lung cancer incidence or death in more than 10,000 postmenopausal women who were randomized to receive estrogen alone or placebo [104]. In the Vitamins and Lifestyle Study, a large prospective population-based cohort of 36,588 peri- and postmenopausal women, combined estrogen plus progestin HRT use was associated with increased lung cancer risk that was duration dependent with the highest risk observed with 10 or more years of HRT use [105]. Although the association of estrogen plus progestin with cancer death was not analyzed in this study, a positive association between combined HRT use and advanced stage disease was found. Estrogen use alone had no effect on lung cancer risk in this study. The biological mechanisms responsible for this association are highly complex, most likely involving genetic and environmental interactions, and warrant further investigation.

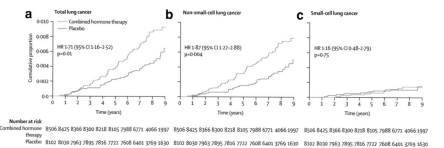

Fig. 7.3 Kaplan–Meier cumulative hazard for death from lung cancer by category, randomization group, and time in the trial. Hazard ratios (*HR*), 95 % confidence interval (*CI*), and *P*-values are from Cox proportional hazards regression models, stratified by age and dietary modification randomization group. (Reprinted with permission from Chlebowski et al. [103]

Anti-estrogens Protect Against Lung Cancer Mortality

Further evidence for a role of estrogens in lung cancer is that anti-estrogen usage may influence survival in lung cancer patients. The association of lung cancer incidence and mortality with anti-estrogen use was evaluated in 6655 women with breast cancer registered in the Geneva Cancer Registry [106]. This study reported a fivefold lower lung cancer mortality in breast cancer patients who received anti-estrogen treatment compared to the expected mortality rate in the general population while lung cancer incidence was not affected [106]. A separate retrospective population-based study using data from the Canadian Manitoba Cancer Registry reported similar results [107]. In this study of 2320 women diagnosed with NSCLC, use of anti-estrogens both before and after lung cancer diagnosis was significantly associated with a decrease in lung cancer mortality [107]. Early phase clinical trials evaluating the use of anti-estrogen therapy for lung cancer treatment are discussed below.

Estrogen Receptors and Local Estrogen Synthesis in Lung Carcinomas

Estrogen receptors (ERs) mediate the biological effects of estrogen. The two main ER isoforms, ERα and ERβ, are encoded by separate genes and have differential tissue distribution and functions [108]. Increasing evidence demonstrates that these and other steroid hormone receptors are present and functional in many tissues outside of the reproductive system, including lung. In contrast to the predominant expression of ERα in breast cancer, ERβ is the predominant ER expressed in lung tumors from both males and females [98, 109–114]. Reported expression of ERα in lung tumors is highly variable but is generally expressed less frequently compared to ERβ [110, 111, 113–116]. Furthermore, comparison of ERα and ERβ selective agonists demonstrates that the biological effects are predominantly mediated by ERβ in the lung [117]. ER expression is localized to both nuclear and cytoplasmic compartments in lung tumors and is found in tumors from both male and female patients. Expression in both cellular locations is thought to be important because estrogen exerts its effects through both genomic and non-genomic mechanisms in the lung (Fig. 7.4; Reviewed in [118]). Genomic effects of estrogen include ligand-dependent activation of nuclear ERs followed by modulation of estrogen-responsive genes including genes involved in cell proliferation. Non-genomic extranuclear estrogen signaling occurs through rapid activation of the EGFR and subsequent activation of the ERK and AKT downstream signaling pathways.

While numerous studies have examined ER tumor expression status in relation to lung cancer survival, there is still not a clear consensus. Nuclear ERβ expression in lung tumors was found to be a positive prognostic indicator in some studies [111–113, 115, 119]. In some reports, the prognostic significance of ERβ was only observed in male patients [111, 115] or was limited to a subset of lung cancer

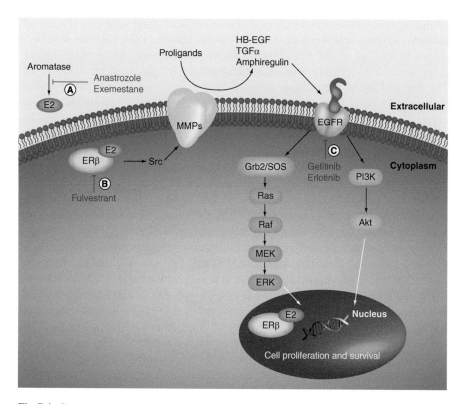

Fig. 7.4 Genomic and non-genomic estrogen signaling in lung cancer. Nuclear ERs are activated in a ligand-dependent manner by E2 binding to nuclear ERs at estrogen-responsive elements or AP-1 sites in the promoters of estrogen-regulated genes. Non-genomic estrogen action occurs through rapid activation of EGFR in the cell membrane, which occurs through activation of Src and MMP cleavage of the EGFR proligands to activate EGFR and the ERK and Akt downstream signaling pathways. Both of these mechanisms of estrogen action in lung cancer lead to cell proliferation and survival. Therapeutic approaches to target the estrogen signaling pathway include (**a**) inhibition of estrogen synthesis with aromatase inhibitors, such as anastrozole or exemestane; (**b**) downregulation of ERs using antiestrogens such as fulvestrant; and (**c**) targeting growth factor pathways that are activated by estrogens with agents such as gefitinib or erlotinib. These strategies can be used as single agents or in combination. (Reprinted with permission from Burns and Stabile [118])

patients with *EGFR* mutations [119]. The discovery of sub-isoforms and distinct cellular localizations of both ERα and ERβ has further complicated our understanding. Isoform specificity was reported in a study which demonstrated that ERβ-1, but not ERβ-2, was related to poor prognosis of female early stage lung cancer patients [120]. Furthermore, cytoplasmic ERβ-1 expression was found to be a strong negative prognostic indicator for both males and female lung cancer patients [110]. Conversely, nuclear ERβ-1 was also linked to poor survival but only in the metastatic setting [121]. Furthermore, high cytoplasmic expression of other ERβ isoforms, ERβ-2 and ERβ-5, was positively correlated with survival [122]. High

ERβ-mediated bioactivity in patient sera also predicted poor lung cancer survival; however, isoform specificity of this effect is not known [123]. ERβ has also been shown to localize to the mitochondria in lung cancer cells and a novel ligand-independent anti-apoptotic role of mitochondrial ERβ has been identified [124]. The role of ERα in lung cancer outcome is also controversial with some reports demonstrating that ERα has no effect while others report a correlation of high expression with poor prognosis [110, 112, 113]. Standardization of immunohisto-chemical procedures and criteria for positivity will be necessary to completely understand the role of ERs in lung cancer.

Lung cancer cells also have the ability to synthesize estrogen locally through the action of the aromatase enzyme which catalyzes the conversion of androgens to estrogen and β-estradiol [125, 126]. Several studies have suggested a role for intra-tumoral estrogen synthesis in lung tumorigenesis. Intratumoral estradiol levels were positively correlated with aromatase expression as well as lung tumor size and estradiol concentrations were significantly higher in lung tumor tissue compared to normal lung tissue from the same patient [125]. In a separate report, aromatase expression was higher in metastases than in the corresponding primary lung tumor [127]. Furthermore, in postmenopausal women with early stage lung cancer, high aromatase tumor expression predicted poor survival [128]. A high occurrence of co-expression of aromatase and ERβ has also been observed in lung tumors [129] and this co-expression was a strong negative lung cancer survival predictor in both men and women, especially strong in the postmenopausal female group [130]. In a separate study that included both women and men with all stages of lung cancer, aromatase expression was not predictive alone but was correlated with poor survival when combined with other hormonal markers including ERβ and progesterone receptor [110]. Interestingly, aromatase protein has been found to be localized to both the epithelial cells in lung tumors as well as in infiltrating macrophages, sug-gesting that release of estrogen might affect the microenvironment [131]. Other enzymes involved in intratumoral estrogen production and metabolism have also been investigated and 17β-hydroxysteroid dehydrogenase type 1 was identified as negative prognostic indicator of lung cancer survival [132].

Targeting the Estrogen Pathway for Lung Cancer Therapy

Preclinical Rationale for Targeting the Estrogen Pathway in Lung Cancer

A series of observations have supported a role for estrogen receptor in lung cancer tumorigenesis both in vitro and in vivo. First, NSCLC proliferation is increased with estrogen treatment both in vitro [109, 133] as well as in human NSCLC xeno-grafts [109], and in a genetically defined mouse model of lung adenocarcinoma [134]. Furthermore, pharmacologic inhibition of the estrogen pathway with either the anti-estrogen fulvestrant or aromatase inhibitors inhibited NSCLC tumor growth in vitro and in human NSCLC xenograft models [109, 126, 127]. In addition, activity has also been observed with combination therapies targeting the estrogen pathway and other growth factor receptor pathways in cancer.

The estrogen receptor through primarily non-genomic mechanisms can positively regulate the EGFR, insulin-like growth factor 1 receptor (IGFR-1), and vascular endothelial growth factor receptor (VEGFR) signaling pathways in lung cancer (reviewed in [118] and Fig. 7.4.). Several studies have demonstrated that EGFR TKIs can synergize with the anti-estrogen fulvestrant or aromatase inhibitors in vitro and in vivo [133, 135–138]. Furthermore, similar efficacy was seen with the combination of fulvestrant with IGF-1 TKIs or the multitargeted VEGFR TKI, vandetanib [127, 139, 140].

In addition to the treatment studies above, the role of anti-estrogen therapy in lung cancer prevention has also been examined [131]. In a recent study, a tobacco carcinogen-induced animal model of lung cancer was utilized to address two critical questions. First, could the combination of the aromatase inhibitor, anastrozole, and anti-estrogen, fulvestrant, inhibit precancerous changes? Second, could this combination prevent progression of precancerous lesions to lung carcinoma? Although single-agent activity was observed with either agent, the combination was superior both in reducing precancerous lesions and in preventing progression. These preclinical studies as well as the correlative and epidemiologic studies described above support a critical role for the estrogen signaling pathway in lung tumorigenesis. As such, targeting the estrogen signaling pathway may represent a novel and effective therapeutic strategy for lung cancer. Although the use of anti-estrogen therapy in lung cancer is novel, anti-estrogen therapy in cancer is not a new concept but rather a well-accepted standard of care in hormone positive breast cancer.

Clinical Trials of Anti-estrogen Therapy in Lung Cancer

The large clinical experience with anti-estrogens in breast cancer has served as a model for the current ongoing development in NSCLC. The use of anti-estrogen therapy in hormone positive breast cancer in both the adjuvant and metastatic setting is standard of care and, since the late 1980s, has led to an almost 30 % decrease in breast cancer mortality rate [141, 142]. A number of studies over several decades have led to the development of several classes of anti-estrogens which are being tested in lung cancer (Fig. 7.4.). The first class of anti-estrogens, selective estrogen receptor modulators (SERMs) such as tamoxifen, are used in both adjuvant and metastatic setting [141]. The second class of anti-estrogens, aromatase inhibitors, work through inhibition of the peripheral conversion of androgens to estrogen [143]. As such, use of AIs in the premenopausal setting without ovarian suppression is ineffective and likely detrimental. In addition to SERMs and AIs, fulvestrant represents a third class of anti-estrogen therapy which leads to the direct degradation of ER and is utilized in the second-line setting for advanced breast cancer. The use of this compound has increased significantly in recent years following the recognition that it is much more clinically efficacious at a higher dose than its original FDA-approved dose [144].

The first clinical trial examining the role of anti-estrogen therapy in lung cancer opened in 2004 and over the last decade the study of anti-estrogen therapy in lung cancer has evolved and expanded. To date, two early phase clinical trials NSCLC have been completed [145, 146] and several more are under way (NCT01556191, NCT01664754) or in the planning stages. Based on the preclinical data suggesting that dual inhibition of the estrogen and EGFR pathways led to increased efficacy, these initial trials have looked at the combination of the anti-estrogen, fulvestrant, with the EGFR TKIs, gefitinib or erlotinib, respectively.

Results of the first Phase I trial of anti-estrogen therapy in lung cancer were published in 2009 and demonstrated safety and potential efficacy [146]. This trial tested the combination of fulvestrant and the EGFR TKI, gefitinib, in postmenopausal women with advanced NSCLC regardless of histology or lines of therapy. Of the 20 patients evaluated for response, the therapy was well tolerated and three partial responses (PRs) were observed (response rate of 15 %, 95 % CI: 5–36 %). However, one of these responses was found in a patient with a TKI sensitizing *EGFR* mutation which predicts for response to gefitinib alone. The observed median progression-free survival (PFS) of 12 weeks, overall survival (OS) of 38.5 weeks, and estimated 1-year OS of 41 % (95 % CI: 20–62 %) were encouraging given that this was a heavily pretreated population. Furthermore, a preliminary biomarker analysis suggested that high ERβ nuclear staining may predict for increased survival (OS 65.5 weeks $\geq$60 % ERβ nuclear IHC staining vs. 21 weeks if <60 % ERβ nuclear IHC staining) although these results did not reach statistical significance in this small trial.

These promising results led to a follow-up trial examining at the combination of erlotinib and fulvestrant vs. erlotinib alone in the second-line advanced setting in a randomized Phase II study [145]. Two significant changes were made to the drug combination in this trial. First, erlotinib replaced gefitinib as the EGFR TKI since gefitinib was no longer available in the United States and a clinically more effective dose of fulvestrant was used (500 mg vs. previous 250 mg dose in the Phase I). Patients with advanced NSCLC were randomized 2:1 to receive the combination of erlotinib and fulvestrant (E + F Arm) vs. EGFR TKI erlotinib alone (E Arm). A total of 100 patients were evaluated and the combination was well tolerated and adverse events well balanced between arms. In the intent to treat to population there was no significant difference between the arms in RR, PFS, or OS, although there were trends toward improved RR (23.6 % vs. 14.8 %, p=0.35) and OS (9.4 vs. 5.7 months, HR 0.96 (0.6, 1.55)). Importantly, this trial was conducted in the era prior to routine molecular testing for *EGFR* TKI sensitizing mutations which predicts for a 70 % response to erlotinib alone. Therefore, a retrospective analysis was performed on the 69 patients who had archival material for *EGFR* mutation testing and whose mutational status was successfully determined. As expected, this analysis confirmed that *EGFR* mutations strongly predicted for response in both arms, PFS and OS ($p$$\leq$0.0002 for each). Interestingly, in EGFR wild-type population (n=52), three PRs were observed in the combination arm versus no responses with erlotinib alone. Furthermore, there was a statistically significant improvement in clinical benefit rate [CBR (RR + stable disease): 54.8 % vs. 8.3 %, p=0.0056] in the *EGFR* wild-type population. In addition, trends toward improvement in PFS and OS were observed as well. Of note, a preplanned tumor and serum biomarker analysis is under way which will be critical to identify which if any NSCLC subtypes may benefit from the combination. In the interim, the French thoracic intergroup has already begun accrual to a larger confirmatory randomized phase II trial in women with advanced non-squamous lung cancer examining the combination of fulvestrant and an EGFR TKI (erlotinib or gefitinib) vs. an EGFR TKI alone (erlotinib or gefitinib) (NCT01556191).

Finally, trials looking at the aromatase inhibitors in combination with chemotherapy or as monotherapy are currently ongoing or being planned. In the first-line metastatic setting, the combination of a standard platinum doublet in combination with exemestane is being examined (NCT01664754) [147]. In addition, phase II trials examining the role of exemestane monotherapy in both the adjuvant and second-line metastatic setting are currently in the planning stage (Burns and Stabile, personal communication).

Conclusions

While lung cancer remains the leading cause of cancer death for both men and women, there are emerging clear sex-specific distinctions in lung cancer presentation and biology. In addition, differences in lung cancer outcome and treatment responses have been observed between men and women. These differences are the result of highly complex interactions involving alterations in molecular, genetic, and hormonal factors. Both exogenous and endogenous estrogens play important roles in the biology and survival outcomes for lung cancer which has led to clinical testing of anti-estrogen therapy for this disease. Because tumors from both male and female lung cancer patients express ERs and aromatase and because estrogen may also be produced in inflammatory cells, therapies targeting the estrogen pathway may potentially benefit all patients, not just women. Sex should be considered as an important variable for future lung cancer studies and clinical trial design. Further studies to better understand the biological basis of these sex-specific differences in lung cancer pathogenesis are necessary.

References

1. Siegel R, Ma J, Zou Z, Jemal A. Cancer statistics, 2014. CA Cancer J Clin. 2014;64(1):9–29. Epub 2014/01/09.
2. Jemal A, Thun MJ, Ries LAG, Howe HL, Weir HK, Center MM, et al. Annual Report to the Nation on the Status of Cancer, 1975–2005, featuring trends in lung cancer, tobacco use, and tobacco control. J Natl Cancer Inst. 2008;100(23):1672–94.
3. Kosmidis P, Mylonakis N, Skarlos D, Samantas E, Dimopoulos M, Papadimitriou C, et al. Paclitaxel (175 mg/m2) plus carboplatin (6 AUC) versus paclitaxel (225 mg/m^2) plus carboplatin (6 AUC) in advanced non-small-cell lung cancer (NSCLC): a multicenter randomized

trial. Hellenic Cooperative Oncology Group (HeCOG). Ann Oncol. 2000;11(7):799–805. Epub 2000/09/21.
4. Giovino GA. Epidemiology of tobacco use in the United States. Oncogene. 2002;21(48): 7326–40. Epub 2002/10/16.
5. Thun MJ, Carter BD, Feskanich D, Freedman ND, Prentice R, Lopez AD, et al. 50-year trends in smoking-related mortality in the United States. N Engl J Med. 2013;368(4):351–64.
6. Brownson RC, Chang JC, Davis JR. Gender and histologic type variations in smoking-related risk of lung cancer. Epidemiology. 1992;3(1):61–4. Epub 1992/01/01.
7. Harris RE, Zang EA, Anderson JI, Wynder EL. Race and sex differences in lung cancer risk associated with cigarette smoking. Int J Epidemiol. 1993;22(4):592–9. Epub 1993/08/01.
8. McDuffie HH, Klaassen DJ, Dosman JA. Female–male differences in patients with primary lung cancer. Cancer. 1987;59(10):1825–30. Epub 1987/05/15.
9. Osann KE, Anton-Culver H, Kurosaki T, Taylor T. Sex differences in lung-cancer risk associated with cigarette smoking. Int J Cancer (Journal international du cancer). 1993;54(1):44–8. Epub 1993/04/22.
10. Risch HA, Howe GR, Jain M, Burch JD, Holowaty EJ, Miller AB. Are female smokers at higher risk for lung cancer than male smokers? A case–control analysis by histologic type. Am J Epidemiol. 1993;138(5):281–93. Epub 1993/09/01.
11. Schoenberg JB, Wilcox HB, Mason TJ, Bill J, Stemhagen A. Variation in smoking-related lung cancer risk among New Jersey women. Am J Epidemiol. 1989;130(4):688–95. Epub 1989/10/01.
12. Zang EA, Wynder EL. Differences in lung cancer risk between men and women: examination of the evidence. J Natl Cancer Inst. 1996;88(3–4):183–92. Epub 1996/02/21.
13. Kure EH, Ryberg D, Hewer A, Phillips DH, Skaug V, Bæera R, et al. p53mutations in lung tumours: relationship to gender and lung DNA adduct levels. Carcinogenesis. 1996; 17(10):2201–5.
14. Guinee DG, Travis WD, Trivers GE, Benedetti VMGD, Cawley H, Welsh JA, et al. Gender comparisons in human lung cancer: analysis of p53 mutations, anti-p53 serum antibodies and C-erbB-2 expression. Carcinogenesis. 1995;16(5):993–1002.
15. Toyooka S, Tsuda T, Gazdar AF. The TP53 gene, tobacco exposure, and lung cancer. Hum Mutat. 2003;21(3):229–39.
16. Bach PB, Kattan MW, Thornquist MD, Kris MG, Tate RC, Barnett MJ, et al. Variations in lung cancer risk among smokers. J Natl Cancer Inst. 2003;95(6):470–8. Epub 2003/03/20.
17. Bain C, Feskanich D, Speizer FE, Thun M, Hertzmark E, Rosner BA, et al. Lung cancer rates in men and women with comparable histories of smoking. J Natl Cancer Inst. 2004;96(11):826–34. Epub 2004/06/03.
18. De Matteis S, Consonni D, Pesatori AC, Bergen AW, Bertazzi PA, Caporaso NE, et al. Are women who smoke at higher risk for lung cancer than men who smoke? Am J Epidemiol. 2013;177(7):601–12. Epub 2013/02/22.
19. Halpern MT, Gillespie BW, Warner KE. Patterns of absolute risk of lung cancer mortality in former smokers. J Natl Cancer Inst. 1993;85(6):457–64. Epub 1993/03/17.
20. Kreuzer M, Boffetta P, Whitley E, Ahrens W, Gaborieau V, Heinrich J, et al. Gender differences in lung cancer risk by smoking: a multicentre case–control study in Germany and Italy. Br J Cancer. 2000;82(1):227–33. Epub 2000/01/19.
21. Prescott E, Osler M, Hein HO, Borch-Johnsen K, Lange P, Schnohr P, et al. Gender and smoking-related risk of lung cancer. The Copenhagen Center for Prospective Population Studies. Epidemiology. 1998;9(1):79–83. Epub 1998/01/16.
22. Radzikowska E, Głaz P, Roszkowski K. Lung cancer in women: age, smoking, histology, performance status, stage, initial treatment and survival. Population-based study of 20 561 cases. Ann Oncol. 2002;13(7):1087–93.
23. Egleston BL, Meireles SI, Flieder DB, Clapper ML. Population-based trends in lung cancer incidence in women. Semin Oncol. 2009;36(6):506–15. Epub 2009/12/10.
24. Kligerman S, White C. Epidemiology of lung cancer in women: risk factors, survival, and screening. AJR Am J Roentgenol. 2011;196(2):287–95. Epub 2011/01/25.

25. Lewis DR, Check DP, Caporaso NE, Travis WD, Devesa SS. US lung cancer trends by histologic type. Cancer. 2014;120(18):2883–92.
26. Thun MJ, Lally CA, Flannery JT, Calle EE, Flanders WD, Heath Jr CW. Cigarette smoking and changes in the histopathology of lung cancer. J Natl Cancer Inst. 1997;89(21):1580–6. Epub 1997/11/15.
27. Stellman SD, Muscat JE, Thompson S, Hoffmann D, Wynder EL. Risk of squamous cell carcinoma and adenocarcinoma of the lung in relation to lifetime filter cigarette smoking. Cancer. 1997;80(3):382–8. Epub 1997/08/01.
28. Samet JM, Avila-Tang E, Boffetta P, Hannan LM, Olivo-Marston S, Thun MJ, et al. Lung cancer in never smokers: clinical epidemiology and environmental risk factors. Clin Cancer Res. 2009;15(18):5626–45. Epub 2009/09/17.
29. Gorlova OY, Zhang Y, Schabath MB, Lei L, Zhang Q, Amos CI, et al. Never smokers and lung cancer risk: a case–control study of epidemiological factors. Int J Cancer (Journal international du cancer). 2006;118(7):1798–804. Epub 2005/10/12.
30. Sun S, Schiller JH, Gazdar AF. Lung cancer in never smokers—a different disease. Nat Rev Cancer. 2007;7(10):778–90. Epub 2007/09/21.
31. Wakelee HA, Chang ET, Gomez SL, Keegan TH, Feskanich D, Clarke CA, et al. Lung cancer incidence in never smokers. J Clin Oncol. 2007;25(5):472–8. Epub 2007/02/10.
32. Thun MJ, Henley SJ, Burns D, Jemal A, Shanks TG, Calle EE. Lung cancer death rates in lifelong nonsmokers. J Natl Cancer Inst. 2006;98(10):691–9.
33. Kris MG, Johnson BE, Berry LD, Kwiatkowski DJ, Iafrate AJ, Wistuba II, et al. Using multiplexed assays of oncogenic drivers in lung cancers to select targeted drugs. JAMA. 2014;311(19):1998–2006.
34. Pao W, Miller V, Zakowski M, Doherty J, Politi K, Sarkaria I, et al. EGF receptor gene mutations are common in lung cancers from "never smokers" and are associated with sensitivity of tumors to gefitinib and erlotinib. Proc Natl Acad Sci U S A. 2004;101(36):13306–11. Epub 2004/08/27.
35. Paez JG, Jänne PA, Lee JC, Tracy S, Greulich H, Gabriel S, et al. EGFR mutations in lung cancer: correlation with clinical response to gefitinib therapy. Science. 2004;304(5676):1497–500.
36. Lynch TJ, Bell DW, Sordella R, Gurubhagavatula S, Okimoto RA, Brannigan BW, et al. Activating mutations in the epidermal growth factor receptor underlying responsiveness of non-small-cell lung cancer to gefitinib. N Engl J Med. 2004;350(21):2129–39.
37. Yang SH, Mechanic LE, Yang P, Landi MT, Bowman ED, Wampfler J, et al. Mutations in the tyrosine kinase domain of the epidermal growth factor receptor in non-small cell lung cancer. Clin Cancer Res. 2005;11(6):2106–10. Epub 2005/03/25.
38. Dogan S, Shen R, Ang DC, Johnson ML, D'Angelo SP, Paik PK, et al. Molecular epidemiology of EGFR and KRAS mutations in 3,026 lung adenocarcinomas: Higher susceptibility of women to smoking-related KRAS-mutant cancers. Clin Cancer Res. 2012;18(22):6169–77.
39. Camidge DR, Bang Y-J, Kwak EL, Iafrate AJ, Varella-Garcia M, Fox SB, et al. Activity and safety of crizotinib in patients with ALK-positive non-small-cell lung cancer: updated results from a phase 1 study. Lancet Oncol. 2012;13(10):1011–9.
40. Kwak EL, Bang Y-J, Camidge DR, Shaw AT, Solomon B, Maki RG, et al. Anaplastic lymphoma kinase inhibition in non-small-cell lung cancer. N Engl J Med. 2010;363(18):1693–703.
41. Shaw AT, Yeap BY, Mino-Kenudson M, Digumarthy SR, Costa DB, Heist RS, et al. Clinical features and outcome of patients with non-small-cell lung cancer who harbor EML4-ALK. J Clin Oncol. 2009;27(26):4247–53. Epub 2009/08/12.
42. Wang Y, Wang S, Xu S, Qu J, Liu B. Clinicopathologic features of patients with non-small cell lung cancer harboring the EML4-ALK fusion gene: a meta-analysis. PLoS One. 2014;9(10), e110617. Epub 2014/11/02.
43. Fan L, Feng Y, Wan H, Shi G, Niu W. Clinicopathological and demographical characteristics of non-small cell lung cancer patients with ALK rearrangements: a systematic review and meta-analysis. PLoS One. 2014;9(6), e100866. Epub 2014/06/25.
44. Riely GJ, Marks J, Pao W. KRAS mutations in non-small cell lung cancer. Proc Am Thorac Soc. 2009;6(2):201–5.

45. Lung ML, Wong M, Lam WK, Lau KS, Kwan S, Fu KH, et al. Incidence of ras oncogene activation in lung carcinomas in Hong Kong. Cancer. 1992;70(4):760–3. Epub 1992/08/15.
46. Spitz MR, Wei Q, Li G, Wu X. Genetic susceptibility to tobacco carcinogenesis. Cancer Invest. 1999;17(8):645–59. Epub 1999/12/11.
47. Cheng YW, Chiou HL, Sheu GT, Hsieh LL, Chen JT, Chen CY, et al. The association of human papillomavirus 16/18 infection with lung cancer among nonsmoking Taiwanese women. Cancer Res. 2001;61(7):2799–803. Epub 2001/04/18.
48. Syrjänen KJ. HPV infections and lung cancer. J Clin Pathol. 2002;55(12):885–91.
49. Li YJ, Tsai YC, Chen YC, Christiani DC. Human papilloma virus and female lung adenocarcinoma. Semin Oncol. 2009;36(6):542–52. Epub 2009/12/10.
50. Zhai K, Ding J, Shi H-Z. HPV and lung cancer risk: a meta-analysis. J Clin Virol. 2015;63:84–90.
51. Frisch M, Melbye M. Risk of lung cancer in pre- and post-menopausal women with anogenital malignancies. Int J Cancer. 1995;62(5):508–11.
52. Smith EM, Ritchie JM, Summersgill KF, Klussmann JP, Lee JH, Wang D, et al. Age, sexual behavior and human papillomavirus infection in oral cavity and oropharyngeal cancers. Int J Cancer. 2004;108(5):766–72.
53. Fu JB, Kau TY, Severson RK, Kalemkerian GP. Lung cancer in women: analysis of the national Surveillance, Epidemiology, and End Results database. Chest. 2005;127(3):768–77. Epub 2005/03/15.
54. Thomas L, Doyle LA, Edelman MJ. Lung cancer in women: emerging differences in epidemiology, biology, and therapy. Chest. 2005;128(1):370–81. Epub 2005/07/09.
55. Ramalingam S, Pawlish K, Gadgeel S, Demers R, Kalemkerian GP. Lung cancer in young patients: analysis of a Surveillance, Epidemiology, and End Results database. J Clin Oncol. 1998;16(2):651–7. Epub 1998/02/20.
56. de Perrot M, Licker M, Bouchardy C, Usel M, Robert J, Spiliopoulos A. Sex differences in presentation, management, and prognosis of patients with non-small cell lung carcinoma. J Thorac Cardiovasc Surg. 2000;119(1):21–6. Epub 1999/12/29.
57. Baldini EH, Strauss GM. Women and lung cancer: waiting to exhale. Chest. 1997;112(4 Suppl):229s–34s. Epub 1997/10/23.
58. Minami H, Yoshimura M, Miyamoto Y, Matsuoka H, Tsubota N. Lung cancer in women: sex-associated differences in survival of patients undergoing resection for lung cancer. Chest. 2000;118(6):1603–9. Epub 2000/12/15.
59. Alexiou C, Onyeaka CV, Beggs D, Akar R, Beggs L, Salama FD, et al. Do women live longer following lung resection for carcinoma? Eur J Cardiothorac Surg. 2002;21(2):319–25. Epub 2002/02/05.
60. Ferguson MK, Wang J, Hoffman PC, Haraf DJ, Olak J, Masters GA, et al. Sex-associated differences in survival of patients undergoing resection for lung cancer. Ann Thorac Surg. 2000;69(1):245–9. discussion 9–50. Epub 2000/02/02.
61. Yoshino I, Baba H, Fukuyama S, Kameyama T, Shikada Y, Tomiyasu M, et al. A time trend of profile and surgical results in 1123 patients with non-small cell lung cancer. Surgery. 2002;131(1 Suppl):S242–8. Epub 2002/02/01.
62. Ouellette D, Desbiens G, Emond C, Beauchamp G. Lung cancer in women compared with men: stage, treatment, and survival. Ann Thorac Surg. 1998;66(4):1140–3. discussion 3–4. Epub 1998/11/04.
63. Rena O, Massera F, Boldorini R, Papalia E, Turello D, Davoli F, et al. Non-small cell lung cancer in surgically treated women. Tumori. 2013;99(6):661–6. Epub 2014/02/08.
64. Spiegelman D, Maurer LH, Ware JH, Perry MC, Chahinian AP, Comis R, et al. Prognostic factors in small-cell carcinoma of the lung: an analysis of 1,521 patients. J Clin Oncol. 1989;7(3):344–54. Epub 1989/03/01.
65. Osterlind K, Andersen PK. Prognostic factors in small cell lung cancer: multivariate model based on 778 patients treated with chemotherapy with or without irradiation. Cancer Res. 1986;46(8):4189–94. Epub 1986/08/01.

66. Nakamura H, Ando K, Shinmyo T, Morita K, Mochizuki A, Kurimoto N, et al. Female gender is an independent prognostic factor in non-small-cell lung cancer: a meta-analysis. Ann Thorac Cardiovasc Surg. 2011;17(5):469–80. Epub 2011/09/02.
67. Singh S, Parulekar W, Murray N, Feld R, Evans WK, Tu D, et al. Influence of sex on toxicity and treatment outcome in small-cell lung cancer. J Clin Oncol. 2005;23(4):850–6. Epub 2005/02/01.
68. Paesmans M, Sculier JP, Lecomte J, Thiriaux J, Libert P, Sergysels R, et al. Prognostic factors for patients with small cell lung carcinoma: analysis of a series of 763 patients included in 4 consecutive prospective trials with a minimum follow-up of 5 years. Cancer. 2000;89(3):523–33. Epub 2000/08/10.
69. Wakelee HA, Wang W, Schiller JH, Langer CJ, Sandler AB, Belani CP, et al. Survival differences by sex for patients with advanced non-small cell lung cancer on Eastern Cooperative Oncology Group trial 1594. J Thorac oncol. 2006;1(5):441–6. Epub 2007/04/06.
70. Scagliotti GV, Parikh P, von Pawel J, Biesma B, Vansteenkiste J, Manegold C, et al. Phase III study comparing cisplatin plus gemcitabine with cisplatin plus pemetrexed in chemotherapy-naive patients with advanced-stage non-small-cell lung cancer. J Clin Oncol. 2008;26(21):3543–51. Epub 2008/05/29.
71. Kris MG, Natale RB, Herbst RS, Lynch Jr TJ, Prager D, Belani CP, et al. Efficacy of gefitinib, an inhibitor of the epidermal growth factor receptor tyrosine kinase, in symptomatic patients with non-small cell lung cancer: a randomized trial. JAMA. 2003;290(16):2149–58. Epub 2003/10/23.
72. Fukuoka M, Yano S, Giaccone G, Tamura T, Nakagawa K, Douillard JY, et al. Multi-institutional randomized phase II trial of gefitinib for previously treated patients with advanced non-small-cell lung cancer (The IDEAL 1 Trial) [corrected]. J Clin Oncol. 2003;21(12):2237–46. Epub 2003/05/16.
73. Shepherd FA, Rodrigues Pereira J, Ciuleanu T, Tan EH, Hirsh V, Thongprasert S, et al. Erlotinib in previously treated non-small-cell lung cancer. N Engl J Med. 2005;353(2):123–32. Epub 2005/07/15.
74. Yang JC, Wu YL, Schuler M, Sebastian M, Popat S, Yamamoto N, et al. Afatinib versus cisplatin-based chemotherapy for EGFR mutation-positive lung adenocarcinoma (LUX-Lung 3 and LUX-Lung 6): analysis of overall survival data from two randomised, phase 3 trials. Lancet Oncol. 2015;16:141–51. Epub 2015/01/16.
75. Solomon BJ, Mok T, Kim D-W, Wu Y-L, Nakagawa K, Mekhail T, et al. First-line crizotinib versus chemotherapy in ALK-positive lung cancer. N Engl J Med. 2014;371(23):2167–77.
76. Heymach JV, Johnson BE, Prager D, Csada E, Roubec J, Pesek M, et al. Randomized, placebo-controlled phase II study of vandetanib plus docetaxel in previously treated non small-cell lung cancer. J Clin Oncol. 2007;25(27):4270–7. Epub 2007/09/20.
77. Heymach JV, Paz-Ares L, De Braud F, Sebastian M, Stewart DJ, Eberhardt WE, et al. Randomized phase II study of vandetanib alone or with paclitaxel and carboplatin as first-line treatment for advanced non-small-cell lung cancer. J Clin Oncol. 2008;26(33):5407–15. Epub 2008/10/22.
78. Siddiqui F, Bae K, Langer CJ, Coyne JC, Gamerman V, Komaki R, et al. The influence of gender, race, and marital status on survival in lung cancer patients: analysis of Radiation Therapy Oncology Group trials. J Thorac Oncol. 2010;5(5):631–9. Epub 2010/05/01.
79. Russell K, Healy B, Pantarotto J, Laurie SA, MacRae R, Sabri E, et al. Prognostic factors in the radical nonsurgical treatment of stage IIIB non-small-cell lung cancer. Clin Lung Cancer. 2014;15(3):237–43. Epub 2014/01/28.
80. Hecht SS. Tobacco smoke carcinogens and lung cancer. J Natl Cancer Inst. 1999;91(14):1194–210. Epub 1999/07/21.
81. Dresler CM, Fratelli C, Babb J, Everley L, Evans AA, Clapper ML. Gender differences in genetic susceptibility for lung cancer. Lung Cancer. 2000;30(3):153–60. Epub 2001/01/04.
82. Tang DL, Rundle A, Warburton D, Santella RM, Tsai WY, Chiamprasert S, et al. Associations between both genetic and environmental biomarkers and lung cancer: evidence of a greater

risk of lung cancer in women smokers. Carcinogenesis. 1998;19(11):1949–53. Epub 1998/12/17.

83. Spivack SD, Hurteau GJ, Fasco MJ, Kaminsky LS. Phase I and II carcinogen metabolism gene expression in human lung tissue and tumors. Clin Cancer Res. 2003;9(16 Pt 1):6002–11. Epub 2003/12/17.

84. Cote ML, Yoo W, Wenzlaff AS, Prysak GM, Santer SK, Claeys GB, et al. Tobacco and estrogen metabolic polymorphisms and risk of non-small cell lung cancer in women. Carcinogenesis. 2009;30(4):626–35. Epub 2009/01/29.

85. Wei Q, Cheng L, Amos CI, Wang LE, Guo Z, Hong WK, et al. Repair of tobacco carcinogen-induced DNA adducts and lung cancer risk: a molecular epidemiologic study. J Natl Cancer Inst. 2000;92(21):1764–72. Epub 2000/11/04.

86. Spitz MR, Wei Q, Dong Q, Amos CI, Wu X. Genetic susceptibility to lung cancer: the role of DNA damage and repair. Cancer Epidemiol Biomarkers Prev. 2003;12(8):689–98. Epub 2003/08/15.

87. Wang LE, Gorlova OY, Ying J, Qiao Y, Weng SF, Lee AT, et al. Genome-wide association study reveals novel genetic determinants of DNA repair capacity in lung cancer. Cancer Res. 2013;73(1):256–64. Epub 2012/10/31.

88. Yang SY, Yang TY, Li YJ, Chen KC, Liao KM, Hsu KH, et al. EGFR exon 19 in-frame deletion and polymorphisms of DNA repair genes in never-smoking female lung adenocarcinoma patients. Int J Cancer (Journal international du cancer). 2013;132(2):449–58. Epub 2012/05/11.

89. Ishikawa-Brush Y, Powell JF, Bolton P, Miller AP, Francis F, Willard HF, et al. Autism and multiple exostoses associated with an X;8 translocation occurring within the GRPR gene and 3' to the SDC2 gene. Hum Mol Genet. 1997;6(8):1241–50.

90. Shriver SP, Bourdeau HA, Gubish CT, Tirpak DL, Davis AL, Luketich JD, et al. Sex-specific expression of gastrin-releasing peptide receptor: relationship to smoking history and risk of lung cancer. J Natl Cancer Inst. 2000;92(1):24–33. Epub 2000/01/06.

91. Egloff AM, Gaither Davis A, Shuai Y, Land S, Pilewski JM, Luketich JD, et al. Gastrin-releasing peptide receptor expression in non-cancerous bronchial epithelia is associated with lung cancer: a case–control study. Respir Res. 2012;13:9. Epub 2012/02/03.

92. Wu AH, Yu MC, Thomas DC, Pike MC, Henderson BE. Personal and family history of lung disease as risk factors for adenocarcinoma of the lung. Cancer Res. 1988;48(24 Pt 1):7279–84. Epub 1988/12/15.

93. Adami HO, Persson I, Hoover R, Schairer C, Bergkvist L. Risk of cancer in women receiving hormone replacement therapy. Int J Cancer (Journal international du cancer). 1989;44(5):833–9. Epub 1989/11/15.

94. Taioli E, Wynder EL. Re: Endocrine factors and adenocarcinoma of the lung in women. J Natl Cancer Inst. 1994;86(11):869–70. Epub 1994/06/01.

95. Ganti AK, Sahmoun AE, Panwalkar AW, Tendulkar KK, Potti A. Hormone replacement therapy is associated with decreased survival in women with lung cancer. J Clin Oncol. 2006;24(1):59–63. Epub 2005/11/30.

96. Rodriguez C, Spencer Feigelson H, Deka A, Patel AV, Jacobs EJ, Thun MJ, et al. Postmenopausal hormone therapy and lung cancer risk in the cancer prevention study II nutrition cohort. Cancer Epidemiol Biomarkers Prev. 2008;17(3):655–60. Epub 2008/03/20.

97. Mahabir S, Spitz MR, Barrera SL, Dong YQ, Eastham C, Forman MR. Dietary boron and hormone replacement therapy as risk factors for lung cancer in women. Am J Epidemiol. 2008;167(9):1070–80. Epub 2008/03/18.

98. Schwartz AG, Wenzlaff AS, Prysak GM, Murphy V, Cote ML, Brooks SC, et al. Reproductive factors, hormone use, estrogen receptor expression and risk of non small-cell lung cancer in women. J Clin Oncol. 2007;25(36):5785–92. Epub 2007/12/20.

99. Schabath MB, Wu X, Vassilopoulou-Sellin R, Vaporciyan AA, Spitz MR. Hormone replacement therapy and lung cancer risk: a case–control analysis. Clin Cancer Res. 2004;10(1 Pt 1):113–23. Epub 2004/01/22.

100. Ramnath N, Menezes RJ, Loewen G, Dua P, Eid F, Alkhaddo J, et al. Hormone replacement therapy as a risk factor for non-small cell lung cancer: results of a case–control study. Oncology. 2007;73(5–6):305–10. Epub 2008/05/22.
101. Kreuzer M, Gerken M, Heinrich J, Kreienbrock L, Wichmann HE. Hormonal factors and risk of lung cancer among women? Int J Epidemiol. 2003;32(2):263–71. Epub 2003/04/26.
102. Pesatori AC, Carugno M, Consonni D, Hung RJ, Papadoupolos A, Landi MT, et al. Hormone use and risk for lung cancer: a pooled analysis from the International Lung Cancer Consortium (ILCCO). Br J Cancer. 2013;109(7):1954–64. Epub 2013/09/05.
103. Chlebowski RT, Schwartz AG, Wakelee H, Anderson GL, Stefanick ML, Manson JE, et al. Oestrogen plus progestin and lung cancer in postmenopausal women (Women's Health Initiative trial): a post-hoc analysis of a randomised controlled trial. Lancet. 2009;374(9697):1243–51. Epub 2009/09/22.
104. Chlebowski RT, Anderson GL, Manson JE, Schwartz AG, Wakelee H, Gass M, et al. Lung cancer among postmenopausal women treated with estrogen alone in the women's health initiative randomized trial. J Natl Cancer Inst. 2010;102(18):1413–21. Epub 2010/08/17.
105. Slatore CG, Chien JW, Au DH, Satia JA, White E. Lung cancer and hormone replacement therapy: association in the vitamins and lifestyle study. J Clin Oncol. 2010;28(9):1540–6. Epub 2010/02/18.
106. Bouchardy C, Benhamou S, Schaffar R, Verkooijen HM, Fioretta G, Schubert H, et al. Lung cancer mortality risk among breast cancer patients treated with anti-estrogens. Cancer. 2011;117(6):1288–95. Epub 2011/01/26.
107. Lother SA, Harding GA, Musto G, Navaratnam S, Pitz MW. Antiestrogen use and survival of women with non-small cell lung cancer in Manitoba, Canada. Horm Cancer. 2013;4(5):270–6. Epub 2013/05/30.
108. Planey SL, Kumar R, Arnott JA. Estrogen receptors (ERalpha versus ERbeta): friends or foes in human biology? J Recept Signal Transduct Res. 2014;34(1):1–5. Epub 2013/11/06.
109. Stabile LP, Davis AL, Gubish CT, Hopkins TM, Luketich JD, Christie N, et al. Human non-small cell lung tumors and cells derived from normal lung express both estrogen receptor alpha and beta and show biological responses to estrogen. Cancer Res. 2002;62(7):2141–50. Epub 2002/04/04.
110. Stabile LP, Dacic S, Land SR, Lenzner DE, Dhir R, Acquafondata M, et al. Combined analysis of estrogen receptor beta-1 and progesterone receptor expression identifies lung cancer patients with poor outcome. Clin Cancer Res. 2011;17(1):154–64. Epub 2010/11/11.
111. Skov BG, Fischer BM, Pappot H. Oestrogen receptor beta over expression in males with non-small cell lung cancer is associated with better survival. Lung Cancer. 2008;59(1):88–94. Epub 2007/10/02.
112. Wu CT, Chang YL, Shih JY, Lee YC. The significance of estrogen receptor beta in 301 surgically treated non-small cell lung cancers. J Thorac Cardiovasc Surg. 2005;130(4):979–86. Epub 2005/10/11.
113. Kawai H, Ishii A, Washiya K, Konno T, Kon H, Yamaya C, et al. Estrogen receptor alpha and beta are prognostic factors in non-small cell lung cancer. Clin Cancer Res. 2005;11(14):5084–9. Epub 2005/07/22.
114. Raso MG, Behrens C, Herynk MH, Liu S, Prudkin L, Ozburn NC, et al. Immunohistochemical expression of estrogen and progesterone receptors identifies a subset of NSCLCs and correlates with EGFR mutation. Clin Cancer Res. 2009;15(17):5359–68. Epub 2009/08/27.
115. Schwartz AG, Prysak GM, Murphy V, Lonardo F, Pass H, Schwartz J, et al. Nuclear estrogen receptor beta in lung cancer: expression and survival differences by sex. Clin Cancer Res. 2005;11(20):7280–7. Epub 2005/10/26.
116. Ishibashi H, Suzuki T, Suzuki S, Niikawa H, Lu L, Miki Y, et al. Progesterone receptor in non-small cell lung cancer—a potent prognostic factor and possible target for endocrine therapy. Cancer Res. 2005;65(14):6450–8. Epub 2005/07/19.
117. Hershberger PA, Stabile LP, Kanterewicz B, Rothstein ME, Gubish CT, Land S, et al. Estrogen receptor beta (ERbeta) subtype-specific ligands increase transcription, p44/p42

mitogen activated protein kinase (MAPK) activation and growth in human non-small cell lung cancer cells. J Steroid Biochem Mol Biol. 2009;116(1–2):102–9. Epub 2009/05/23.

118. Burns TF, Stabile LP. Targeting the estrogen pathway for the treatment and prevention of lung cancer. Lung Cancer Manag. 2014;3(1):43–52. Epub 2014/11/15.

119. Nose N, Sugio K, Oyama T, Nozoe T, Uramoto H, Iwata T, et al. Association between estrogen receptor-beta expression and epidermal growth factor receptor mutation in the postoperative prognosis of adenocarcinoma of the lung. J Clin Oncol. 2009;27(3):411–7. Epub 2008/12/10.

120. Sethi S, Coti M, Lonardo F. Expression of estrogen receptor beta 1 but not estrogen receptor beta 2 or alpha is linked to worse prognosis in stage I adenocarcinoma in women, in a large epidemiological cohort but not in a smaller, single hospital based series. US Canadian Acad Pathol. 2010; Abstract 1843.

121. Navaratnam S, Skliris G, Qing G, Banerji S, Badiani K, Tu D, et al. Differential role of estrogen receptor beta in early versus metastatic non-small cell lung cancer. Horm Cancer. 2012;3(3):93–100. Epub 2012/02/04.

122. Liu Z, Liao Y, Tang H, Chen G. The expression of estrogen receptors beta2, 5 identifies and is associated with prognosis in non-small cell lung cancer. Endocrine. 2013;44(2):517–24. Epub 2013/03/12.

123. Lim VW, Lim WY, Zhang Z, Li J, Gong Y, Seow A, et al. Serum estrogen receptor beta mediated bioactivity correlates with poor outcome in lung cancer patients. Lung Cancer. 2014;85(2):293–8. Epub 2014/06/22.

124. Zhang G, Yanamala N, Lathrop KL, Zhang L, Klein-Seetharaman J, Srinivas H. Ligand-independent antiapoptotic function of estrogen receptor-beta in lung cancer cells. Mol Endocrinol. 2010;24(9):1737–47. Epub 2010/07/28.

125. Niikawa H, Suzuki T, Miki Y, Suzuki S, Nagasaki S, Akahira J, et al. Intratumoral estrogens and estrogen receptors in human non-small cell lung carcinoma. Clin Cancer Res. 2008;14(14):4417–26. Epub 2008/06/27.

126. Weinberg OK, Marquez-Garban DC, Fishbein MC, Goodglick L, Garban HJ, Dubinett SM, et al. Aromatase inhibitors in human lung cancer therapy. Cancer Res. 2005;65(24):11287–91. Epub 2005/12/17.

127. Marquez-Garban DC, Chen HW, Goodglick L, Fishbein MC, Pietras RJ. Targeting aromatase and estrogen signaling in human non-small cell lung cancer. Ann N Y Acad Sci. 2009;1155:194–205. Epub 2009/03/03.

128. Mah V, Seligson DB, Li A, Marquez DC, Wistuba II, Elshimali Y, et al. Aromatase expression predicts survival in women with early-stage non small cell lung cancer. Cancer Res. 2007;67(21):10484–90. Epub 2007/11/03.

129. Abe K, Miki Y, Ono K, Mori M, Kakinuma H, Kou Y, et al. Highly concordant coexpression of aromatase and estrogen receptor beta in non-small cell lung cancer. Hum Pathol. 2010;41(2):190–8. Epub 2009/10/06.

130. Mah V, Marquez D, Alavi M, Maresh EL, Zhang L, Yoon N, et al. Expression levels of estrogen receptor beta in conjunction with aromatase predict survival in non-small cell lung cancer. Lung Cancer. 2011;74(2):318–25. Epub 2011/04/23.

131. Stabile LP, Rothstein ME, Cunningham DE, Land SR, Dacic S, Keohavong P, et al. Prevention of tobacco carcinogen-induced lung cancer in female mice using antiestrogens. Carcinogenesis. 2012;33(11):2181–9. Epub 2012/08/04.

132. Verma MK, Miki Y, Abe K, Suzuki T, Niikawa H, Suzuki S, et al. Intratumoral localization and activity of 17beta-hydroxysteroid dehydrogenase type 1 in non-small cell lung cancer: a potent prognostic factor. J Transl Med. 2013;11:167. Epub 2013/07/11.

133. Marquez-Garban DC, Chen HW, Fishbein MC, Goodglick L, Pietras RJ. Estrogen receptor signaling pathways in human non-small cell lung cancer. Steroids. 2007;72(2):135–43. Epub 2007/02/06.

134. Hammoud Z, Tan B, Badve S, Bigsby RM. Estrogen promotes tumor progression in a genetically defined mouse model of lung adenocarcinoma. Endocr Relat Cancer. 2008;15(2):475–83. Epub 2008/05/30.

135. Garon EB, Pietras RJ, Finn RS, Kamranpour N, Pitts S, Marquez-Garban DC, et al. Antiestrogen fulvestrant enhances the antiproliferative effects of epidermal growth factor receptor inhibitors in human non-small-cell lung cancer. J Thorac Oncol. 2013;8(3):270–8. Epub 2013/02/13.
136. Shen L, Li Z, Shen S, Niu X, Yu Y, Li Z, et al. The synergistic effect of EGFR tyrosine kinase inhibitor gefitinib in combination with aromatase inhibitor anastrozole in non-small cell lung cancer cell lines. Lung Cancer. 2012;78(3):193–200. Epub 2012/09/19.
137. Stabile LP, Lyker JS, Gubish CT, Zhang W, Grandis JR, Siegfried JM. Combined targeting of the estrogen receptor and the epidermal growth factor receptor in non-small cell lung cancer shows enhanced antiproliferative effects. Cancer Res. 2005;65(4):1459–70. Epub 2005/03/01.
138. Xu R, Shen H, Guo R, Sun J, Gao W, Shu Y. Combine therapy of gefitinib and fulvestrant enhances antitumor effects on NSCLC cell lines with acquired resistance to gefitinib. Biomed Pharmacother. 2012;66(5):384–9. Epub 2012/05/09.
139. Tang H, Liao Y, Xu L, Zhang C, Liu Z, Deng Y, et al. Estrogen and insulin-like growth factor 1 synergistically promote the development of lung adenocarcinoma in mice. Int J Cancer. 2013;133:2473–82. Epub 2013/05/08.
140. Siegfried JM, Gubish CT, Rothstein ME, Henry C, Stabile LP. Combining the multitargeted tyrosine kinase inhibitor vandetanib with the antiestrogen fulvestrant enhances its antitumor effect in non-small cell lung cancer. J Thorac Oncol. 2012;7(3):485–95. Epub 2012/01/20.
141. Sainsbury R. The development of endocrine therapy for women with breast cancer. Cancer Treat Rev. 2013;39(5):507–17.
142. Siegel R, Naishadham D, Jemal A. Cancer statistics, 2013. CA Cancer J Clin. 2013;63(1):11–30. Epub 2013/01/22.
143. Miller WR, Bartlett J, Brodie AM, Brueggemeier RW, di Salle E, Lonning PE, et al. Aromatase inhibitors: are there differences between steroidal and nonsteroidal aromatase inhibitors and do they matter? Oncologist. 2008;13(8):829–37. Epub 2008/08/13.
144. Di Leo A, Jerusalem G, Petruzelka L, Torres R, Bondarenko IN, Khasanov R, et al. Results of the CONFIRM phase III trial comparing fulvestrant 250 mg with fulvestrant 500 mg in postmenopausal women with estrogen receptor-positive advanced breast cancer. J Clin Oncol. 2010;28(30):4594–600. Epub 2010/09/22.
145. Garon EB, Siegfried JM, Dubinett SM, Elashoff RM, Park DJ, Parikh RJ, et al. Result of TORI L-03, a randomized, multicenter phase II clinical trial of erlotinib (E) or E + fulvestrant (F) in previously treated advanced non-small cell lung cancer (NSCLC) AACR Annual Meeting 2013. 2013:abstract #4664
146. Traynor AM, Schiller JH, Stabile LP, Kolesar JM, Eickhoff JC, Dacic S, et al. Pilot study of gefitinib and fulvestrant in the treatment of post-menopausal women with advanced non-small cell lung cancer. Lung cancer. 2009;64(1):51–9. Epub 2008/08/15.
147. http://clinicaltrials.gov/.

Chapter 8
Lymphangioleiomyomatosis

Jeannette Zinggeler Berg and Lisa Young

Abstract Lymphangioleiomyomatosis (LAM) is a rare progressive cystic lung disease that affects women almost exclusively, occurring in a sporadic form and in association with Tuberous Sclerosis Complex. remendous progress has been made in understanding the pathogenesis of this disorder, leading to advances in noninvasive diagnostic approaches, and a targeted therapy has now been FDA-approved for treatment of LAM (rapamycin). In LAM, progressive decline in lung function occurs as dysregulated smooth muscle-like cells (LAM cells) of uncertain origin infiltrate the lung, disrupting lymphatics and leading to parenchymal destruction and cyst formation. LAM cells have constitutive activation of the mechanistic target of rapamycin (mTOR) due to sporadic or germline mutations in tuberous sclerosis genes (TSC1 or TSC2). Inhibition of mTOR by rapamycin suppresses disease progression as was demonstrated in the Multicenter International Lymphangioleimyomatosis Efficacy of Sirolimus (MILES) trial. In animal models of LAM and in vitro cellular studies, estrogen increases cell proliferation and migration. The reason for the marked gender discrepancy remains unknown, and at this time, hormone-modulating therapies remain largely unproven or insufficiently studied in patients with LAM.

Keywords Lymphangioleiomyomatosis • LAM • Tuberous sclerosis complex • TSC • mTOR • Sirolimus • Rapamycin • VEGF-D • Cystic lung disease

J.Z. Berg, MD, PhD
Division of Pulmonary and Critical Care Medicine, Vanderbilt University School of Medicine, 1611 21st Avenue South, T-1218 Medical Center North, Nashville, TN 37232, USA
e-mail: jz.berg@vanderbilt.edu

L. Young, MD (✉)
Division of Pulmonary Medicine, Department of Pediatrics, Vanderbilt University School of Medicine, 2200 Children's Way, Nashville, TN 37232-9500, USA
e-mail: lisa.young@vanderbilt.edu

© Springer International Publishing Switzerland 2016
A.R. Hemnes (ed.), *Gender, Sex Hormones and Respiratory Disease*,
Respiratory Medicine, DOI 10.1007/978-3-319-23998-9_8

Clinical Presentation

IntroductionLymphangioleiomyomatosis (LAM) is a rare cystic lung disease with prevalence estimated at 2-5 per million women (Harknett, E. C., et al. QJM. 104.11 (2011): 971-79; Johnson, S. R. and A. E. Tattersfield. Am.J.Respir.Crit Care Med. 160.2 (1999): 628-33). Definite or probable LAM causing pulmonary symptoms has been reported in only 4 men (Miyake, M., et al. Radiat.Med. 23.7 (2005): 525-27;Schiavina, M., et al. Am.J.Respir.Crit Care Med. 176.1 (2007): 96-98; Aubry, M. C., et al. Am.J.Respir.Crit Care Med. 162.2 Pt 1 (2000): 749-52. Kim, N. R., et al. Pathol.Int. 53.4 (2003): 231-35). Dysregulated smooth muscle-like cells (LAM cells) of uncertain origin infiltrate the lung causing lymphatic disruption and congestion, cyst formation, and parenchymal destruction. The neoplastic pheno-type of LAM cells occurs as a consequence of constitutive activation of the mecha-nistic target of rapamycin (mTOR) due to loss of heterozygosity in the tuberous sclerosis genes (TSC1 or TSC2) (Henske, E. P. and F. X. McCormack. J.Clin.Invest 122.11 (2012): 3807-16. The natural history of LAM is variable but significant mor-bidity and mortality occurs (Johnson, S. R. Eur.Respir.J. 27.5 (2006): 1056-65; Ryu, J. H., et al. Am.J.Respir.Crit Care Med. 173.1 (2006): 105-11). The mTOR inhibitor sirolimus (i.e. rapamycin) is an effective suppressive therapy for LAM, though LAM cells persist and lung function decline resumes if sirolimus is discontinued McCormack, F. X., et al. N.Engl.J.Med. 364.17 (2011): 1595-606. LAM should be considered in women who present with spontaneous pneumothorax, chylous pleural effusions, unexplained dyspnea, refractory asthma-type symptoms, or incidental radiologic findings of multicystic lung disease. Other clinical manifestations can include hemoptysis, chyloptysis, chylous ascites, and chyluria. Among patients in The LAM Foundation registry, pneumothorax was reported by 66 % of respondents and 82 % had their first pneumothorax prior to diagnosis [1]. Angiomyolipoma (AMLs) may also be a presenting feature of LAM, coming to medical attention due to hematuria or retroperitoneal hemorrhage, or as an incidental radiologic finding. Several series report that delays in LAM diagnosis are common [1–3]. As discussed in more detail below, LAM is also a common pulmonary complication in women with Tuberous Sclerosis Complex (TSC), a heritable tumor suppressor syndrome.

Approach to Diagnosis

Establishing a diagnosis of LAM can be achieved by a combination of clinical char-acteristics, thin section computed tomography (CT) imaging, serum vascular endo-thelial growth factor-D (VEGF-D) levels, and/or pathology (Fig. 8.1). An appropriate index of clinical suspicion is required, as pulmonary symptoms and physiology will overlap those of more common respiratory disorders. Pulmonary function tests may be normal initially, followed by a variable rate in decline in forced vital capacity (FVC), forced expiratory volume in 1 s (FEV1), and diffusion capacity of lung for

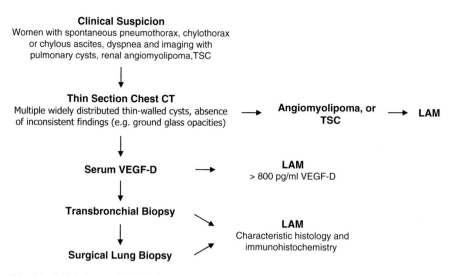

Clinical Suspicion
Women with spontaneous pneumothorax, chylothorax or chylous ascites, dyspnea and imaging with pulmonary cysts, renal angiomyolipoma,TSC

↓

Thin Section Chest CT
Multiple widely distributed thin-walled cysts, absence of inconsistent findings (e.g. ground glass opacities) → **Angiomyolipoma, or TSC** → **LAM**

↓

Serum VEGF-D → **LAM** > 800 pg/ml VEGF-D

↓

Transbronchial Biopsy

↓

Surgical Lung Biopsy → **LAM** Characteristic histology and immunohistochemistry

Fig. 8.1 LAM diagnostic algorithm. An approach to diagnosis for women in whom LAM is suspected is presented. Open lung biopsy is the historic gold standard, though it may not be necessary as outlined in the algorithm. Serum VEGF-D was approved as a clinical lab test and has been available since 2011

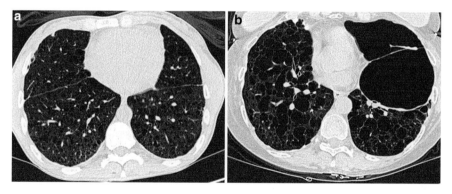

Fig. 8.2 Characteristic moderate and severe LAM CT. Numerous thin-walled cysts that are widely distributed are characteristic of LAM as seen in the CT images from LAM patients with moderate (**a**) and severe (**b**) disease

carbon monoxide (DLCO). Obstructive physiology with air-trapping may be present, or there may be a nonspecific or mixed ventilatory defect.

Chest imaging is a critical early step in the diagnostic evaluation. While chest radiographs may appear normal, multiple thin-walled cysts are seen on chest CT imaging and typically are widely distributed [4–6]. Representative CT images for moderate and severe LAM are presented in Fig. 8.2. LAM cysts vary in size from sub-cm to ~3 cm [6, 7]. An additional CT finding that aids in establishing a diagnosis is radiologic evidence for AMLs, often in the kidney [7]. Retroperitoneal or axial lymphadenopathy may also be present, but this is a nonspecific finding. Ground glass opacities are not typical in the absence of pulmonary hemorrhage or significant lymphatic congestion, and the presence of other non-cystic radiologic features should raise suspicion for alternative or additional etiologies of lung disease.

As discussed further below, radiologic findings of thin-walled lung cysts are considered sufficient for a diagnosis of LAM in women with an established diagnosis of TSC, as clinical experience from surgical biopsies and lung explants in TSC patients has revealed characteristic LAM histopathology. Additionally, in TSC, a few or many small pulmonary nodules may be present, which commonly represent multifocal micronodular pneumocyte hyperplasia (MMPH) [8, 9] and therefore are typically followed conservatively in low-risk nonsmoking individuals.

Serum VEGF-D level is a diagnostic advance that can facilitate noninvasive diagnosis of LAM. This diagnostic test became available in a Clinical Laboratory Improvement Amendments (CLIA) certified laboratory in 2011. VEGF-D is a logical pathobiologic marker in LAM, as LAM cells produce VEGF-D [10], and VEGF-D is well known to promote lymphangiogenesis, a prominent feature in LAM [11, 12]. Seyama et al. first reported serum VEGF-D levels that were three-fold higher in LAM patients versus age-matched healthy volunteers [10]. This finding has been validated by other investigators worldwide. Serum VEGF-D levels are elevated in approximately 70 % of patients with LAM, but are not elevated in women with other cystic lung diseases including emphysema, pulmonary Langerhan's cell histiocytosis, lymphoid interstitial pneumonia, Birt–Hogg–Dube syndrome, and follicular bronchiolitis [13]. When evaluated as a diagnostic test for LAM, serum VEGF-D greater than 800 pg/ml had a sensitivity of 73 % and a specificity of 100 % [13]. Importantly, in the compatible clinical and radiologic context, if serum VEGF-D is elevated above 800 pg/mL, a diagnosis of LAM is considered definite, thereby obviating the need for biopsy.

If the serum VEGF-D level is in the normal range, cytologic or tissue diagnosis should be considered for diagnostic confirmation, particularly if sirolimus therapy is being considered. Prior to lung biopsy for tissue confirmation, it is worthwhile to consider that LAM diagnosis may occasionally be confirmed by cytology of pleural fluid, ascites, or fine-needle aspirates or biopsy of lymph nodes [7], with reported yield ranging from 15 to 39 % [2].

A lung biopsy for pathology can be obtained by bronchoscopy or by video-assisted thoracoscopic surgery (VATS). Transbronchial biopsy has a reported yield of 60 % [14]. Pathologic findings of LAM include foci of smooth muscle cell infiltration of the lung parenchyma and lymphatics, and adjacent thin-walled cysts. LAM cells stain positively for α-smooth muscle actin and the melanogenesis pathway enzyme HMB-45, which has high specificity for LAM in this context [15, 16]. Histologic review by a pathologist with LAM expertise should be considered when there is clinical suspicion for LAM, as the morphology of LAM cells is sometimes confused for fibroblasts and only a minority of cells in a lesion are typically HMB-45 positive. Additional immunohistochemical markers include desmin and vimentin [15], and expression of both estrogen and progesterone receptors has been reported [17–20].

Differential Diagnosis

There are a number of other causes of multicystic lung disease that should be considered in the differential. Tobacco-associated emphysema is vastly more prevalent and may occasionally include imaging findings of cysts, particularly when chronic bronchiolitis is present, often in an apical predominant distribution. Pulmonary Langerhans Cell Histiocytosis should also be considered when the patient is a smoker, and imaging has multiple sub-centimeter nodules, irregular thick-walled cysts, and costophrenic angle sparing of cystic changes [21]. Lymphocytic interstitial pneumonitis that is idiopathic or associated with immune dysfunction or connective tissue disease has varied radiographic appearance; a serologic clue can be a polyclonal gammopathy in adults [22]. Alpha-1-antitrypsin deficiency can be diagnosed by assessing genotype and serum protein levels. Suspicion for connective tissue diseases including rheumatoid arthritis, systemic lupus erythematosus, Sjogren's, and myositis can be ascertained by history of rheumatologic symptoms, physical exam findings, and serologies including rheumatoid antigen, anti-cyclic citrullinated peptide, anti-nuclear antibody, anti-Ro/SSA, anti-La/SSB, anti-Jo-1, and anti-synthetases. Birt–Hogg–Dube (BHD) syndrome is caused by mutations in the folliculin gene with autosomal-dominant inheritance. Features of BHD include multiple pulmonary cysts, pneumothorax, skin fibrofolliculomas, and renal cell carcinoma in about 30 % of patients [23, 24]. Multiple cystic changes can also occur following prior pulmonary infection and barotrauma, and have been reported in light chain deposition disease, hyperimmunoglobulin E syndrome, and recurrent papillomatosis [2].

LAM and TSC: Clinical Association

TSC is an autosomal-dominant disorder with germline mutation in tuberous sclerosis genes, TSC1 or TSC2, that result in constitutive activation of the mTOR signaling pathway. The phenotype of TSC is multi-organ hamartomas including involvement of brain, skin, kidneys, and lungs. A subset of individuals with TSC have seizures and developmental disability. The diagnosis of TSC is not always apparent in women presenting with an LAM diagnosis, and therefore careful evaluation for TSC and genetic counseling are recommended [25].

For women, LAM is recognized as a component of the genetic syndrome TSC, occurring in about 40–80 % of women with TSC [9, 26, 27]. In a large TSC clinic, the prevalence of lung cysts was 27 % in women under age 21 among 101 women with available CT scans [26]. There are some phenotypic differences between TSC1 and TSC2 mutations, and TSC2 may confer greater susceptibility to develop LAM [27, 28]. While the natural history of LAM in women with TSC is variable, with some individuals remaining asymptomatic, some young patients do progress rapidly from minimal to severe lung disease [29]. There are limited data to inform the approach to screening from LAM in females with TSC. Currently, the European Respiratory Society guidelines recommend chest CT imaging in female TSC patients at 18 and again at 30 years of age [7]. A 2013 publication by Krueger et al. for the International Tuberous Sclerosis Consensus group recommended clinical assessment and initial CT at age 18 years, with follow-up screening imaging every 5–10 years in asymptomatic females [30].

Recent studies indicate that mild pulmonary cystic changes are seen in some men with TSC, though almost all of these cases are asymptomatic. Adriaensen et al. reviewed available chest and abdominal CT studies from 206 TSC patients and found that 42 % of females and 13 % of males had pulmonary cysts [28]. Cysts were larger in women, and extensive cystic changes were 10 times more common in women than men. In a series from the Mayo clinic, lung cysts were seen in 38 % of men with TSC, though the extent of findings was overall mild [31]. These data suggest that while TSC mutations are associated with cystic lung disease, there are marked gender differences in disease severity, with clinically significant lung disease restricted to females.

Mechanisms of mTOR Signaling and Dysregulation in TSC and LAM

Advances in the understanding of TSC biology have provided critical clues to LAM pathogenesis and treatment. Spontaneous or germline mutation of TSC is the major recognized underlying abnormality in the development of LAM. A landmark discovery was the identification of identical TSC2 mutations in DNA from LAM lesions in the lung and renal AMLs, but not in germline DNA in the blood of women with Sporadic LAM [32].

TSC1 and TSC2 proteins form a complex that inhibits signaling through the mTORC1 complex of the mTOR signaling pathway, via activation of the GTPase-activating protein Rheb. Disruption of the TSC1/TSC2 complex leads to dysregu-lated mTOR signaling, and specifically inappropriate increased signaling through mTORC1. Signaling through mTORC1 drives cell proliferation, and in fact, increased signaling through mTOR is a feature of several malignancies [33, 34]. Angiogenesis mediated by VEGF-A is regulated by TSC through mTOR signaling [35]. Sirolimus (rapamycin) is a mTOR inhibitor and in LAM it suppresses the aber-rant increased signaling that results from TSC mutations.

Natural History and Prognosis

LAM progression is variable. A favorable prognosis is associated with older age at diagnosis and the presence of a renal AML, the latter for unclear reasons [36, 37]. Oprescu et al. reported an accelerated time to transplant or death among individuals presenting with dyspnea or cough, but no increased risk of death in association with pneumothorax [37]. An obstructive pattern on pulmonary function tests and having a positive bronchodilator response portend of a worse prognosis [38, 39]. Morbidity includes recurrent pneumothorax, chylothorax, hemorrhage, hypoxemia, and pulmonary arterial hypertension. Recurrent pneumothorax is common [40, 41]. Renal AMLs occur in approximately 30 % of patients with spontaneous LAM and up to 75 % with TSC [26, 40]. Among women in the United States LAM registry, 31 % reported use of supplemental oxygen [37]. In this registry, the median age at death was 48 years and the most common cause of death was respiratory failure [37].

LAM Treatment

LAM treatment historically has focused on managing complications including pneumothorax and AMLs and providing symptomatic management and supportive therapy with bronchodilators and supplemental oxygen. Pneumothorax is frequently recurrent and therefore warrants secondary prevention. Pneumothorax recurrence occurred in 66 % of patients who had conservative management versus 27 % of 140 LAM patients treated with chemical pleurodesis, and 32 % treated with surgery [1]. Embolization is an approach to prevent hemorrhage from AMLs with prominent feeding vessels [42].

Management of LAM now includes focused pharmacologic therapy, as a disease-modifying therapy, sirolimus, was FDA approved for LAM in May 2015. The Multicenter International Lymphangioleimyomatosis Efficacy of Sirolimus (MILES) trial resulted in a momentous shift in management of LAM. This international, randomized, double-blind, placebo-controlled trial showed that sirolimus stabilized lung function and improved metrics of functional performance and quality of life in women with moderate to severe lung disease (Table 8.1) [43].

Table 8.1 MILES trial summary[a]

	Placebo $N=43$	Sirolimus $N=46$	p-value
Baseline:			
TSC Syndrome, N (%)	8 (9)	4 (9)	1.00
Age	45	46	0.74
FEV1, L (% predicted)	1.38 (48)	1.36 (49)	0.66
FVC, L (% predicted)	2.79 (80)	2.91 (81)	0.57
DLCO (% predicted)	10.4 (44)	10.1 (43)	0.52
Change at 12 months:			
Δ FEV1, ml	−134	+19	<0.001
Δ FVC, ml	−129	+97	0.001
DLCO	−0.62	−0.06	0.38
Δ VEGF-D (pg/ml)	−15	−1032	0.001

The Multicenter International Lymphangioleimyomatosis Efficacy of Sirolimus (MILES) trial demonstrated stabilization of lung function in women with LAM. Selected baseline participant characteristics and change in pulmonary function and VEGF-D at 12 months are presented
[a]Adapted from McCormack, et al. 2011, NEJM 364(17)

Serum VEGF-D levels decreased with sirolimus treatment, and patients with high baseline VEGF-D levels had incrementally greater change in pulmonary function in response to treatment [44]. Unfortunately, lung function decline resumes if patients discontinue sirolimus. While overall well tolerated, side effects of sirolimus include leukopenia, increased risk of infections, hypertension, hypercholesterolemia, diarrhea, peripheral edema, proteinuria, oral ulcers, acne, and rare others. Ongoing questions include when in the disease course to start sirolimus, and whether lower dose treatment could achieve similar efficacy with an improved safety profile. The LAM Foundation has organized a network of LAM clinics to provide improved multidisciplinary care for LAM patients and to collaborate in the development of data-driven practice guidelines.

Lung transplantation is an established option for women with severe pulmonary impairment due to LAM. Progressive decline in FEV1 and worsening dyspnea are reasons to consider an initial referral. Patients will need to maintain their functional status, i.e., walking, regardless of oxygen requirement to be eligible for transplant. The presence of a renal AML is not an exclusion factor. The risk of transplant morbidity and mortality must be weighed against risks of respiratory failure from LAM. Less than 10 % of women who receive transplants go on to have clinically significant LAM recurrence. Mortality after transplant at 5 and 10 years is 67 % and 47 %, respectively [45]. Sirolimus has typically been stopped prior to transplantation due to concern that it may impair healing at the implant anastomosis. Complications that can occur following transplant in LAM patients include chylous pleural effusions, renal AML hemorrhage, and LAM recurrence [45, 46]. Chronic immunosuppression regimens typically include sirolimus.

Sex Hormones and LAM

The gender disparity of LAM is striking as susceptibility to LAM is almost entirely limited to women. Decades of clinical observation and research findings implicate estrogen as having disease-modifying effects. LAM cells are known to express both estrogen and progesterone receptors. Higher estrogen states have been associated with progression of disease in some cases. However, definitive evidence is lacking regarding manipulating sex hormones as a therapeutic approach.

Reproductive hormones are suspected to affect LAM as clinical presentation occurs after puberty, accelerated progression is not infrequently observed during pregnancy, and menopause is associated with attenuated progression [36, 40, 47] The average age of symptom onset among LAM patients in the USA and the UK was 37 and 34 years of age, respectively, though this varies widely [36, 37, 40]. Decline in FEV1 was −170 ml/year versus −86 ml/year for premenopausal versus postmenopausal women, respectively [36]. During pregnancy, cases of pneumothorax, chylothorax, AML hemorrhage, and precipitous decline in pulmonary function have been observed [47–50]. Pregnancy risks also include an increased risk of premature births [47]. Overall women with LAM have fewer children than women without LAM for various reasons including the decision not to become pregnant [47, 51]. Despite circumstantial and anecdotal clinical experiences, limited high-quality evidence exists to guide clinical recommendations on this controversial topic. Careful clinical assessments and counseling, in the context of individual patient preferences, are recommended.

A number of studies have evaluated the effect of hormonal therapies though small sample sizes and observational study designs have limitations. Eliasson et al. reviewed 30 reported cases and interpreted that 7 of 9 patients with oophorectomy +/− progesterone treatment and 4 of 8 patients on progesterone had "stabilization" of disease [52]. Oberstein et al. reported that women on oral contraceptive pills (OCPs) had an earlier onset of symptoms and were diagnosed at an earlier age (29 vs. 33, respectively; $p = 0.04$) [53]. A prospective observational study of 275 patients showed no difference in the decline of lung function (FEV1, DLCO) over 4 years among the 139 patients who received progesterone [54]. Case series report disease exacerbation including worsening symptoms, pneumothorax, and decline in FEV1 in conjunction with tamoxifen treatment [55, 56]. Women treated with the gonadotropin-releasing hormone (GnRH) analogue triptorelin ($n = 11$) experienced ongoing decline in FEV1 over a 3-year period that was similar or greater than declines reported in other observational studies [57]. A small trial of the aromatase inhibitor letrozole that suppresses estrogen synthesis peripherally was completed in 2015 and is expected to report soon (NCT01353209).

Histologic studies and in vitro studies of LAM cells provide evidence that these cells respond to estrogen. In explanted lung tissue from LAM patients undergoing transplant, 20 of 20 tissues had LAM cells that were positive for estrogen and pro-gesterone receptors by immunohistochemistry [18]. The LAM cell staining was also notable for a high PR to ER ratio whereas ER expression dominates in other estrogen-mediated neoplasms. A primary culture of LAM cells from an angiomyo-lipoma with a proven TSC2 mutation had increased proliferation in response to estrogen and tamoxifen [58]. Estrogen influences interaction of LAM cells with the extracellular matrix. TSC2-deficient cells treated with estrogen have increased inva-sion in a collagen invasion chamber [17]. In TSC2-deficient cells, estradiol increases metallomatrix protein 2 (MMP2) which is predicted to influence predilection for metastasis [17].

While no animal model recapitulates the cystic lung disease phenotype of LAM, preclinical models have been reliable in assessing the effects of mTOR inhibition on tumor development in TSC-deficient animals. Several models provide evidence that loss of tuberin, the protein product of TSC2, is associated with tumor development and that estrogen exposure promotes cell proliferation. One intriguing model is the Eker rat, which is heterozygous for a germline TSC2 mutation, and in addition to a predilection to develop renal tumors, the female animals develop uterine leiomyo-mas [59, 60]. TSC2 loss of heterozygosity (LOH) and/or loss of tuberin protein occurs in these tumors [59]. There is a hormonal dependence: ovariectomy at 4 months eliminates tumor development, and selective estrogen receptor modulators (i.e., tamoxifen and raloxifene) decrease tumor growth. Further, using uterine leiomyoma cells from this tuberin-deficient rat model (ELT3 cells), Finlay et al. demonstrated that tuberin interacts with ERα and that re-expressing tuberin in ELT3 cells attenuated estrogen-induced proliferation [61].

Xenograft models have also been useful to study the role of estrogen on cell migration and invasion, tumor growth, and potential anti-tumor therapeutics. When ELT3 cells were injected into ovariectomized mice, estrogen treatment resulted in higher proliferative potential assessed by Ki-67 staining [62]. Additionally, mice treated with estrogen had a greater number of pulmonary metastases than the placebo control group. [62]. Estrogen upregulated signaling through the MEK/MAPK pathway and treatment with a MEK inhibitor completely eliminated the formation of pulmonary metastatic lesions while decreasing primary tumor size by a more modest 25 % [62]. Metabolomic profiling of ELT3 cells treated with estrogen identified increased glycolysis and pentose phosphate pathway intermediates [63]. In an ELT3 xenograft model, inhibition of the pentose phosphate pathway decreased estrogen-mediated colonization of ELT3 cells in the lung. Sun et al. also observed that in AML cells derived from LAM patients, estrogen increased glucose uptake in an AKT-dependent manner which was inhibited by Wortmannin and not the mTOR inhibitor rapamycin [63]. These preclinical studies have provided evidence of how estrogen may be important in LAM.

Additional Clinical Trials and Future Directions

There are many additional potential therapeutic targets in LAM. Strategies currently or recently under investigation include additional agents to inhibit mTOR, lymphangiogenesis inhibitors, drugs that affect metallomatrix proteins, and sex hormone modulating agents. Doxycycline, due to its activity as a metalloproteinase inhibitor, was evaluated in a 2-year double-blind placebo-controlled trial ($n = 23$) in which no effect was detected on pulmonary function tests (FVC, FEV1, DLCO), walk distance, or quality of life [64]. Sirolimus does not completely inhibit mTOR and therefore other inhibitors, including active site inhibitors, are being developed, as well as strategies to target both upstream and downstream of mTOR [65–67]. The mTOR inhibitor everolimus was evaluated for renal AML treatment in TSC or LAM patients in a double-blind, randomized, controlled trial ($n = 118$), and the progression-free rate for AML was 92 % at 12 months [68]; this trial was discontinued due to superiority of everolimus to placebo. A phase 2 trial of everolimus focused on pulmonary endpoints has recently been completed (NCT01059318).

Additional clinical trials for LAM currently listed at clinicaltrials.gov include simvastatin with rapamycin (NCT02061397), rapamycin with hydroxychloroquine, an autophagy inhibitor (NCT01687179), and Saracatinib (NCT02116712).

Summary

LAM is rare progressive lung disease that almost exclusively affects women, and women with TSC are a high-risk group that can benefit from screening for LAM. Diagnosis can be made without lung biopsy in many patients based on clinical features, characteristic chest CT patterns, and serum VEGF-D levels. The major known driver of disease is inappropriate activation of mTOR that leads to the proliferation and metastasis of LAM cells causing multisystem disease including cystic lung disease, lymphatic disruption, and renal AML. While the mechanisms of sex hormones on disease have been difficult to elucidate, estrogens likely contribute to LAM cell survival and migration. Clinics specifically organized for LAM patients provide centers of expertise for management of complications, treatment guidance, and infrastructure for conducting research. The MILES trial demonstrated that mTOR inhibition stabilized FEV1 and improved FVC in women with moderate to severe lung disease, but benefit persists only while sirolimus is continued. Additional efforts are needed to understand the gender disparity of LAM, improve the approach to screening in women with TSC, and develop strategies for disease prevention and treatment.

References

1. Almoosa KF, Ryu JH, Mendez J, Huggins JT, Young LR, Sullivan EJ, et al. Management of pneumothorax in lymphangioleiomyomatosis: effects on recurrence and lung transplantation complications. Chest. 2006;129(5):1274–81.
2. Meraj R, Wikenheiser-Brokamp KA, Young LR, McCormack FX. Lymphangioleiomyomatosis: new concepts in pathogenesis, diagnosis, and treatment. Semin Respir Crit Care Med. 2012;33(5):486–97.
3. Sandrini A, Krishnan A, Yates DH. S-LAM in a man: the first case report. Am J Respir Crit Care Med. 2008;177(3):356.
4. Avila NA, Chen CC, Chu SC, Wu M, Jones EC, Neumann RD, et al. Pulmonary lymphangioleiomyomatosis: correlation of ventilation-perfusion scintigraphy, chest radiography, and CT with pulmonary function tests. Radiology. 2000;214(2):441–6.
5. Muller NL, Chiles C, Kullnig P. Pulmonary lymphangiomyomatosis: correlation of CT with radiographic and functional findings. Radiology. 1990;175(2):335–9.
6. Abbott GF, Rosado-de-Christenson ML, Frazier AA, Franks TJ, Pugatch RD, Galvin JR. From the archives of the AFIP: lymphangioleiomyomatosis: radiologic-pathologic correlation. Radiographics. 2005;25(3):803–28.
7. Johnson SR, Cordier JF, Lazor R, Cottin V, Costabel U, Harari S, et al. European Respiratory Society guidelines for the diagnosis and management of lymphangioleiomyomatosis. Eur Respir J. 2010;35(1):14–26.
8. Muzykewicz DA, Black ME, Muse V, Numis AL, Rajagopal J, Thiele EA, et al. Multifocal micronodular pneumocyte hyperplasia: computed tomographic appearance and follow-up in tuberous sclerosis complex. J Comput Assist Tomogr. 2012;36(5):518–22.
9. Franz DN, Brody A, Meyer C, Leonard J, Chuck G, Dabora S, et al. Mutational and radiographic analysis of pulmonary disease consistent with lymphangioleiomyomatosis and micronodular pneumocyte hyperplasia in women with tuberous sclerosis. Am J Respir Crit Care Med. 2001;164(4):661–8.

10. Seyama K, Kumasaka T, Souma S, Sato T, Kurihara M, Mitani K, et al. Vascular endothelial growth factor-D is increased in serum of patients with lymphangioleiomyomatosis. Lymphat Res Biol. 2006;4(3):143–52.

11. Henske EP, McCormack FX. Lymphangioleiomyomatosis—a wolf in sheep's clothing. J Clin Invest. 2012;122(11):3807–16.

12. Kumasaka T, Seyama K, Mitani K, Sato T, Souma S, Kondo T, et al. Lymphangiogenesis in lymphangioleiomyomatosis: its implication in the progression of lymphangioleiomyomatosis. Am J Surg Pathol. 2004;28(8):1007–16.

13. Young LR, Vandyke R, Gulleman PM, Inoue Y, Brown KK, Schmidt LS, et al. Serum vascular endothelial growth factor-D prospectively distinguishes lymphangioleiomyomatosis from other diseases. Chest. 2010;138(3):674–81.

14. Meraj R, Wikenheiser-Brokamp KA, Young LR, Byrnes S, McCormack FX. Utility of transbronchial biopsy in the diagnosis of lymphangioleiomyomatosis. Front Med. 2012;6(4):395–405.

15. Matsumoto Y, Horiba K, Usuki J, Chu SC, Ferrans VJ, Moss J. Markers of cell proliferation and expression of melanosomal antigen in lymphangioleiomyomatosis. Am J Respir Cell Mol Biol. 1999;21(3):327–36.

16. Tanaka H, Imada A, Morikawa T, Shibusa T, Satoh M, Sekine K, et al. Diagnosis of pulmonary lymphangioleiomyomatosis by HMB45 in surgically treated spontaneous pneumothorax. Eur Respir J. 1995;8(11):1879–82.

17. Glassberg MK, Elliot SJ, Fritz J, Catanuto P, Potier M, Donahue R, et al. Activation of the estrogen receptor contributes to the progression of pulmonary lymphangioleiomyomatosis via matrix metalloproteinase-induced cell invasiveness. J Clin Endocrinol Metab. 2008;93(5):1625–33.

18. Gao L, Yue MM, Davis J, Hyjek E, Schuger L. In pulmonary lymphangioleiomyomatosis expression of progesterone receptor is frequently higher than that of estrogen receptor. Virchows Arch. 2014;464(4):495–503.

19. Flavin RJ, Cook J, Fiorentino M, Bailey D, Brown M, Loda MF. beta-Catenin is a useful adjunct immunohistochemical marker for the diagnosis of pulmonary lymphangioleiomyomatosis. Am J Clin Pathol. 2011;135(5):776–82.

20. Grzegorek I, Lenze D, Chabowski M, Janczak D, Szolkowska M, Langfort R, et al. Immunohistochemical evaluation of pulmonary lymphangioleiomyomatosis. Anticancer Res. 2015;35(6):3353–60.

21. Kulwiec EL, Lynch DA, Aguayo SM, Schwarz MI, King Jr TE. Imaging of pulmonary histiocytosis X. Radiographics. 1992;12(3):515–26.

22. Koss MN, Hochholzer L, Langloss JM, Wehunt WD, Lazarus AA. Lymphoid interstitial pneumonia: clinicopathological and immunopathological findings in 18 cases. Pathology. 1987;19(2):178–85.

23. Pavlovich CP, Walther MM, Eyler RA, Hewitt SM, Zbar B, Linehan WM, et al. Renal tumors in the Birt-Hogg-Dube syndrome. Am J Surg Pathol. 2002;26(12):1542–52.

24. Houweling AC, Gijezen LM, Jonker MA, van Doorn MB, Oldenburg RA, van Spaendonck-Zwarts KY, et al. Renal cancer and pneumothorax risk in Birt-Hogg-Dube syndrome; an analysis of 115 FLCN mutation carriers from 35 BHD families. Br J Cancer. 2011;105(12):1912–9.

25. Northrup H, Krueger DA. Tuberous sclerosis complex diagnostic criteria update: recommendations of the 2012 International Tuberous Sclerosis Complex Consensus Conference. Pediatr Neurol. 2013;49(4):243–54.

26. Cudzilo CJ, Szczesniak RD, Brody AS, Rattan MS, Krueger DA, Bissler JJ, et al. Lymphangioleiomyomatosis screening in women with tuberous sclerosis. Chest. 2013;144(2):578–85.

27. Muzykewicz DA, Sharma A, Muse V, Numis AL, Rajagopal J, Thiele EA. TSC1 and TSC2 mutations in patients with lymphangioleiomyomatosis and tuberous sclerosis complex. J Med Genet. 2009;46(7):465–8.

28. Adriaensen ME, Schaefer-Prokop CM, Duyndam DA, Zonnenberg BA, Prokop M. Radiological evidence of lymphangioleiomyomatosis in female and male patients with tuberous sclerosis complex. Clin Radiol. 2011;66(7):625–8.

29. Taveira-DaSilva AM, Jones AM, Julien-Williams P, Yao J, Stylianou M, Moss J. Severity and outcome of cystic lung disease in women with tuberous sclerosis complex. Eur Respir J. 2015;45(1):171–80.
30. Krueger DA, Northrup H. Tuberous sclerosis complex surveillance and management: recommendations of the 2012 International Tuberous Sclerosis Complex Consensus Conference. Pediatr Neurol. 2013;49(4):255–65.
31. Ryu JH, Sykes AM, Lee AS, Burger CD. Cystic lung disease is not uncommon in men with tuberous sclerosis complex. Respir Med. 2012;106(11):1586–90.
32. Carsillo T, Astrinidis A, Henske EP. Mutations in the tuberous sclerosis complex gene TSC2 are a cause of sporadic pulmonary lymphangioleiomyomatosis. Proc Natl Acad Sci U S A. 2000;97(11):6085–90.
33. Cargnello M, Tcherkezian J, Roux PP. The expanding role of mTOR in cancer cell growth and proliferation. Mutagenesis. 2015;30(2):169–76.
34. Guertin DA, Sabatini DM. Defining the role of mTOR in cancer. Cancer Cell. 2007; 12(1):9–22.
35. El-Hashemite N, Walker V, Zhang H, Kwiatkowski DJ. Loss of Tsc1 or Tsc2 induces vascular endothelial growth factor production through mammalian target of rapamycin. Cancer Res. 2003;63(17):5173–7.
36. Johnson SR, Tattersfield AE. Decline in lung function in lymphangioleiomyomatosis: relation to menopause and progesterone treatment. Am J Respir Crit Care Med. 1999;160(2):628–33.
37. Oprescu N, McCormack FX, Byrnes S, Kinder BW. Clinical predictors of mortality and cause of death in lymphangioleiomyomatosis: a population-based registry. Lung. 2013;191(1):35–42.
38. Taveira-DaSilva AM, Steagall WK, Rabel A, Hathaway O, Harari S, Cassandro R, et al. Reversible airflow obstruction in lymphangioleiomyomatosis. Chest. 2009;136(6):1596–603.
39. Kitaichi M, Nishimura K, Itoh H, Izumi T. Pulmonary lymphangioleiomyomatosis: a report of 46 patients including a clinicopathologic study of prognostic factors. Am J Respir Crit Care Med. 1995;151(2 Pt 1):527–33.
40. Ryu JH, Moss J, Beck GJ, Lee JC, Brown KK, Chapman JT, et al. The NHLBI lymphangioleiomyomatosis registry: characteristics of 230 patients at enrollment. Am J Respir Crit Care Med. 2006;173(1):105–11.
41. Hayashida M, Seyama K, Inoue Y, Fujimoto K, Kubo K. The epidemiology of lymphangioleiomyomatosis in Japan: a nationwide cross-sectional study of presenting features and prognostic factors. Respirology. 2007;12(4):523–30.
42. Patatas K, Robinson GJ, Ettles DF, Lakshminarayan R. Patterns of renal angiomyolipoma regression post embolisation on medium- to long-term follow-up. Br J Radiol. 2013;86(1024):20120633.
43. McCormack FX, Inoue Y, Moss J, Singer LG, Strange C, Nakata K, et al. Efficacy and safety of sirolimus in lymphangioleiomyomatosis. N Engl J Med. 2011;364(17):1595–606.
44. Young L, Lee HS, Inoue Y, Moss J, Singer LG, Strange C, et al. Serum VEGF-D a concentration as a biomarker of lymphangioleiomyomatosis severity and treatment response: a prospective analysis of the Multicenter International Lymphangioleiomyomatosis Efficacy of Sirolimus (MILES) trial. Lancet Respir Med. 2013;1(6):445–52.
45. Kpodonu J, Massad MG, Chaer RA, Caines A, Evans A, Snow NJ, et al. The US experience with lung transplantation for pulmonary lymphangioleiomyomatosis. J Heart Lung Transplant. 2005;24(9):1247–53.
46. Karbowniczek M, Astrinidis A, Balsara BR, Testa JR, Lium JH, Colby TV, et al. Recurrent lymphangiomyomatosis after transplantation: genetic analyses reveal a metastatic mechanism. Am J Respir Crit Care Med. 2003;167(7):976–82.
47. Cohen MM, Freyer AM, Johnson SR. Pregnancy experiences among women with lymphangioleiomyomatosis. Respir Med. 2009;103(5):766–72.
48. Brunelli A, Catalini G, Fianchini A. Pregnancy exacerbating unsuspected mediastinal lymphangioleiomyomatosis and chylothorax. Int J Gynaecol Obstet. 1996;52(3):289–90.
49. Yeoh ZW, Navaratnam V, Bhatt R, McCafferty I, Hubbard RB, Johnson SR. Natural history of angiomyolipoma in lymphangioleiomyomatosis: implications for screening and surveillance. Orphanet J Rare Dis. 2014;9:151.

50. Warren SE, Lee D, Martin V, Messink W. Pulmonary lymphangiomyomatosis causing bilateral pneumothorax during pregnancy. Ann Thorac Surg. 1993;55(4):998–1000.
51. Wahedna I, Cooper S, Williams J, Paterson IC, Britton JR, Tattersfield AE. Relation of pulmonary lymphangio-leiomyomatosis to use of the oral contraceptive pill and fertility in the UK: a national case control study. Thorax. 1994;49(9):910–4.
52. Eliasson AH, Phillips YY, Tenholder MF. Treatment of lymphangioleiomyomatosis. A meta-analysis. Chest. 1989;96(6):1352–5.
53. Oberstein EM, Fleming LE, Gomez-Marin O, Glassberg MK. Pulmonary lymphangioleiomyomatosis (LAM): examining oral contraceptive pills and the onset of disease. J Womens Health (Larchmt). 2003;12(1):81–5.
54. Taveira-DaSilva AM, Stylianou MP, Hedin CJ, Hathaway O, Moss J. Decline in lung function in patients with lymphangioleiomyomatosis treated with or without progesterone. Chest. 2004;126(6):1867–74.
55. Tomasian A, Greenberg MS, Rumerman H. Tamoxifen for lymphangioleiomyomatosis. N Engl J Med. 1982;306(12):745–6.
56. Svendsen TL, Viskum K, Hansborg N, Thorpe SM, Nielsen NC. Pulmonary lymphangioleiomyomatosis: a case of progesterone receptor positive lymphangioleiomyomatosis treated with medroxyprogesterone, oophorectomy and tamoxifen. Br J Dis Chest. 1984;78(3):264–71.
57. Harari S, Cassandro R, Chiodini I, Taveira-DaSilva AM, Moss J. Effect of a gonadotrophin-releasing hormone analogue on lung function in lymphangioleiomyomatosis. Chest. 2008;133(2):448–54.
58. Yu J, Astrinidis A, Howard S, Henske EP. Estradiol and tamoxifen stimulate LAM-associated angiomyolipoma cell growth and activate both genomic and nongenomic signaling pathways. Am J Physiol Lung Cell Mol Physiol. 2004;286(4):L694–700.
59. Walker CL, Hunter D, Everitt JI. Uterine leiomyoma in the Eker rat: a unique model for important diseases of women. Genes Chromosomes Cancer. 2003;38(4):349–56.
60. Eker R, Mossige J, Johannessen JV, Aars H. Hereditary renal adenomas and adenocarcinomas in rats. Diagn Histopathol. 1981;4(1):99–110.
61. Finlay GA, York B, Karas RH, Fanburg BL, Zhang H, Kwiatkowski DJ, et al. Estrogen-induced smooth muscle cell growth is regulated by tuberin and associated with altered activation of platelet-derived growth factor receptor-beta and ERK-1/2. J Biol Chem. 2004;279(22):23114–22.
62. Yu JJ, Robb VA, Morrison TA, Ariazi EA, Karbowniczek M, Astrinidis A, et al. Estrogen promotes the survival and pulmonary metastasis of tuberin-null cells. Proc Natl Acad Sci U S A. 2009;106(8):2635–40.
63. Sun Y, Gu X, Zhang E, Park MA, Pereira AM, Wang S, et al. Estradiol promotes pentose phosphate pathway addiction and cell survival via reactivation of Akt in mTORC1 hyperactive cells. Cell Death Dis. 2014;5, e1231.
64. Chang WY, Cane JL, Kumaran M, Lewis S, Tattersfield AE, Johnson SR. A 2-year randomised placebo-controlled trial of doxycycline for lymphangioleiomyomatosis. Eur Respir J. 2014; 43(4):1114–23.
65. Liu Q, Kirubakaran S, Hur W, Niepel M, Westover K, Thoreen CC, et al. Kinome-wide selectivity profiling of ATP-competitive mammalian target of rapamycin (mTOR) inhibitors and characterization of their binding kinetics. J Biol Chem. 2012;287(13):9742–52.
66. Caron E, Ghosh S, Matsuoka Y, Ashton-Beaucage D, Therrien M, Lemieux S, et al. A comprehensive map of the mTOR signaling network. Mol Syst Biol. 2010;6:453.
67. Thoreen CC, Kang SA, Chang JW, Liu Q, Zhang J, Gao Y, et al. An ATP-competitive mammalian target of rapamycin inhibitor reveals rapamycin-resistant functions of mTORC1. J Biol Chem. 2009;284(12):8023–32.
68. Bissler JJ, Kingswood JC, Radzikowska E, Zonnenberg BA, Frost M, Belousova E, et al. Everolimus for angiomyolipoma associated with tuberous sclerosis complex or sporadic lymphangioleiomyomatosis (EXIST-2): a multicentre, randomised, double-blind, placebo-controlled trial. Lancet. 2013;381(9869):817–24.
69. Harknett EC, Chang WY, Byrnes S, Johnson J, Lazor R, Cohen MM, et al. Use of variability in national and regional data to estimate the prevalence of lymphangioleiomyomatosis. QJM. 2011;104(11):971–9.

70. Miyake M, Tateishi U, Maeda T, Kusumoto M, Satake M, Arai Y, et al. Pulmonary lymphangioleiomyomatosis in a male patient with tuberous sclerosis complex. Radiat Med. 2005;23(7):525–7.
71. Schiavina M, Di Scioscio V, Contini P, Cavazza A, Fabiani A, Barberis M, et al. Pulmonary lymphangioleiomyomatosis in a karyotypically normal man without tuberous sclerosis complex. Am J Respir Crit Care Med. 2007;176(1):96–8.
72. Aubry MC, Myers JL, Ryu JH, Henske EP, Logginidou H, Jalal SM, et al. Pulmonary lymphangioleiomyomatosis in a man. Am J Respir Crit Care Med. 2000;162(2 Pt 1):749–52.
73. Kim NR, Chung MP, Park CK, Lee KS, Han J. Pulmonary lymphangioleiomyomatosis and multiple hepatic angiomyolipomas in a man. Pathol Int. 2003;53(4):231–5.
74. Johnson SR. Lymphangioleiomyomatosis. Eur Respir J. 2006;27(5):1056–65.

Chapter 9
Developmental Lung Disease

Patricia Silveyra

Abstract The development of the male and female mature human lungs is a highly regulated process controlled by genetic, epigenetic, hormonal, and environmental factors. Depending on the stage of lung development these come into play, they may have a different effect in male and female lung health. Normal lung development and growth varies in males and females, and it is differentially affected by risk factors that can result in reduced lung function, and persistent physiological effects that can predispose individuals to lung disease. In this chapter, we discuss major sex differences identified at the various stages of lung development, from embryonic to adult life, in terms of lung morphology, gene expression, hormonal regulation, epigenetic control, and the influence of environmental exposures.

Keywords Fetal lung development • Gene expression—epigenetics • microRNAs • Sex hormones

List of Abbreviations

AMH	Anti-Müllerian hormone
AR	Androgen receptor
BMP	Bone morphogenetic protein
BPD	Bronchopulmonary dysplasia
DHT	Dihydrotestosterone
EGF	Epidermal growth factor
ER	Estrogen receptor
FEV1	Forced expiratory volume in 1 second
FGF	Fibroblast growth factor
GC	Glucocorticoids
IGF1	Insulin-like growth factor-1

P. Silveyra, PhD (✉)
Department of Pediatrics, The Pennsylvania State
University College of Medicine, Hershey, PA, USA
e-mail: pzs13@psu.edu

© Springer International Publishing Switzerland 2016
A.R. Hemnes (ed.), *Gender, Sex Hormones and Respiratory Disease*,
Respiratory Medicine, DOI 10.1007/978-3-319-23998-9_9

PDGF   Platelet-derived growth factor
RDS   Respiratory distress syndrome
Shh   Sonic hedgehog
TGFβ   Transforming growth factor beta
VEGF   Vascular-endothelial growth factor
Wnt   Wingless-related family

Introduction

A proper lung development is essential to provide adequate oxygenation of body tissues and maintain life [1]. Numerous factors, including genetic, epigenetic, hormonal, and environmental, can affect the normal development of the male and female lungs. Even minor alterations in lung development can have marked lung health consequences that persist later in life. In this regard, population studies have shown that the magnitude of these consequences is different for men and women, and depending on the stage of lung development in which alterations occur [2–4]. For example, prenatal factors such as low gestational age and birth weight can significantly predict the development of chronic respiratory insufficiency in preterm infants.

During the fetal period, male lung maturation is usually delayed in comparison to female maturation, and surfactant production appears later in the lungs of males [5, 6]. Consequently, male neonates are at increased risk of developing respiratory distress syndrome (RDS) and a higher risk of morbidity and mortality due to RDS compared with female neonates of the same gestational age [7, 8]. Furthermore, sex differences in overall neonatal survival and pulmonary outcomes have been described with a significantly higher incidence in males versus females [9]. One example is the high incidence observed in males for the development of bronchopulmonary dysplasia (BPD), a pulmonary pathology of the neonate for which RDS is not always an anterior event [10]. Differences in gene expression, particularly at the late developmental stages, have been shown to play significant roles in these gender-associated health outcomes [2, 11, 12].

Normal Lung Development

The development of the human lung is divided into five stages: *embryonic, pseudoglandular, canalicular, saccular,* and *alveolar* (Fig. 9.1) [13]. Each stage is characterized by specific cellular and structural events that are controlled by the expression of various genes [14, 15]. Numerous studies have documented sex differences in structural, mechanical, and functional aspects of lung development, as well as in hormonal levels and regulation throughout these stages [6, 16, 17]. These are summarized in Table 9.1.

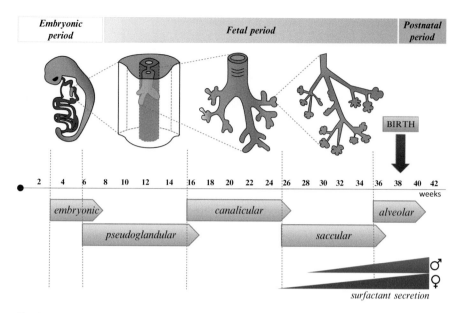

Fig. 9.1 Summary of stages of lung development from embryonic to postnatal life

The first stage is the *embryonic*, which spans from 3 to 6 weeks postconception. In this phase, the lung starts developing at around day 26 of gestation as a ventral outpouching of the foregut (Fig. 9.1). This ventral diverticulum (lung bud) will start forming the trachea and the two bronchial buds that will give rise to the left and right bronchi. The asymmetry of the main bronchi is already established at this stage: the left bud is smaller and directed laterally and the larger right bud is directed more caudally [18]. Toward the end of the embryonic stage, the bronchial buds undergo subsequent divisions, resulting in the precursor structures of the pulmonary lobes, three on the right and two on the left (Fig. 9.1), and a small pulmonary circulatory system starts developing [19, 20]. At this point, no sex differences are observed in lung development.

The embryonic stage is followed by the *pseudoglandular* stage that extends from 6 to 16 weeks of gestation and that is characterized by bronchial development and airway branching. In this stage, the bronchial tree is developed up to the terminal bronchiole, and the respiratory parenchyma and respiratory ducts are formed, together with a primitive pulmonary circulatory system [21, 22]. Lung epithelial cells begin to differentiate into precursors for bronchial smooth muscle, cartilage, and submucosal glands in a process highly dependent on epithelial and mesenchymal interactions [21, 23]. The bronchial tree is initially coated by a cubic epithelium, which is the precursor of the ciliated epithelium, and by secretory cells and immature type II cells. In this stage, sex differences begin to appear in fetal mouth movement, an indication of fetal lung maturation, showing advanced breathing in females more than in males [24].

Table 9.1 Sex differences at various lung developmental stages

Developmental stage	Main events	Airway structure development (branching status)	Sex differences
Embryonic (3–6 weeks)	Appearance of lung buds from foregut. Formation of trachea and bronchial buds.	Trachea Bronchi (2–6 generations)	–
Pseudoglandular (6–16 weeks)	Branching of airway and blood vessels. Differentiation of epithelial cells.	Bronchioles Terminal bronchioles (6–16 generations)	Fetal growth and breathing movements detected earlier in females.
Canalicular (16–26 weeks)	Subdivision of distal airways into canaliculi, vascularization. Differentiation of type I and type II cells, surfactant production.	Respiratory bronchioles (16–19 generations)	First functional differences appear. Surfactant secretion and phospholipid maturation are inhibited in males.
Saccular (26–36 weeks)	Cell differentiation, type II cell maturation, surfactant secretion. Formation of sacs. Thinning of alveolar walls, formation of primary septa and acini. Extracellular matrix components and connective tissue decrease.	Alveolar ducts (19–22 generations)	Surfactant production and phospholipid profile remain more advanced in females.
Alveolar (36 weeks—adolescence)	Alveolar multiplication (alveolarization). Alveolar enlargement and maturation. Lungs continue to grow through adolescence. Lung function (FEV1) increases with age and peaks in adolescence.	Alveolar sacs (22–23 generations)	Reduced risk for RDS and better response to surfactant therapy in girls. Faster alveolarization in females. Higher flow rate per lung volume, but smaller lung size in girls than boys. FEV1 peaks earlier in girls than boys.

The next stage is the *canalicular* phase, starting at week 16, and extending until week 26 of gestation. In this period, the basic gas-exchanging airway units are formed by further subdivisions of the distal airways (Fig. 9.1). These canaliculi are formed by branching of the terminal bronchioles, and compose the now respiratory parenchyma. The groups of air spaces that are formed from a single respiratory bronchiole form an acinus. Vascularization of the peripheral mesenchymal tissue is the foundation for the later exchange of gases at these respiratory units. The lumen of these becomes wider and the epithelial type II cells begin to secrete surfactant, and differentiate into type I cells [22]. Capillaries move into close contact with the surface epithelium, and connective tissue is reduced. The first functional sex differences are noticed at this stage, and these are attributed to hormonal influences, as well as sex differences in gene expression. At around 16 weeks of gestation, the lungs of female fetuses are usually more mature than those of males, and begin to produce surfactant lipids [5, 10, 25, 26] (Fig. 9.1).

At the end of the canalicular phase, and the beginning of the *saccular* phase, spanning from weeks 26–36 postconception, a large part of the amniotic fluid is produced by the lung epithelium. At this stage, lung maturity can be measured clinically by quantifying lipid content in the amniotic fluid (ratio of lecithin to sphingomyelin), based on the production of surfactant by type II cells [27]. As indicated, female fetuses usually show a more mature phospholipid profile at this stage, which correlates with an earlier production of surfactant components [25].

During the *saccular* phase, drastic changes occur in the morphology of the developing lung. Further subdivisions at the terminal bronchioles give rise to clusters of sacs that will later become the alveoli (Fig. 9.1). These sacculi are internally coated with type I and type II cells and the parenchyma between them contains primary septa that are composed of networks of capillaries. These contain small protrusions that will later become alveoli via delimitation by secondary septa. At the end of the saccular phase, all generations of the conducting and respiratory branches are generated, and about 1/3 of the roughly 300 million alveoli are fully developed.

The saccular phase is characterized by type II cell maturation and surfactant production, which are promoted by paracrine communications with cells of the interstitial space. Pulmonary surfactant is a lipoprotein complex (90 % lipids, 10 % proteins), responsible for preventing alveolar collapse at low lung volumes. By decreasing surface tension at the alveolus, lung surfactant promotes gas exchange and lung mechanics. Pulmonary surfactant also enhances lung innate immunity by the actions of surfactant proteins A and D (collectins). Thus, in preterm infants born at less than 30 weeks of gestational age, surfactant deficiency greatly contributes to the development of RDS, and related morbidities such as BPD, patent ductus arteriosus, arterial pulmonary hypertension, and long-term neurological disabilities [12, 28, 29]. Surfactant synthesis and secretion significantly increase after week 30 in preparation for the transition to air breathing, and the male lung begins to synthesize surfactant later in gestation than the female lung (Fig. 9.1). This delay has been attributed to androgens and other factors, as described later in the chapter [6]. Therefore, female newborns have increased airflow rates, but lower airway resistance compared with male newborns, and they are less likely to develop RDS [11, 30].

Lastly, at the postnatal *alveolar* stage, starting at birth (36 weeks postconception) and extending throughout adolescence, the number of alveoli largely increases [1]. This alveolar multiplication process (alveolarization) is very active within the first 2 years of life, although the alveolar size and number of alveoli per unit area does not change much during this period. The respiratory epithelium differentiates into a variety of cell types including ciliated, goblet, basal, and Clara cells [31]. Although maturation appears to be more advanced in female fetuses than in male fetuses, girls on average have smaller lungs and fewer respiratory bronchioles than boys at birth. Female neonates also have higher size-corrected flow rates, specific airway conductance, and a higher ratio of large airways to small airways than males, and it has been suggested that boys have more respiratory bronchioles per lung volume than girls [2, 32].

Furthermore, the growth of airways is slower than the growth of lung parenchyma in boys, whereas in girls the growth of airways is proportional to the growth of parenchyma. This "dysynaptic" growth originates in early childhood, and remains constant during growth [1, 33]. Boys in general have bigger lungs than girls of the same stature, and studies have suggested that boys have more respiratory bronchioles than girls, but no sex differences have been reported in alveolar dimensions, and in number of alveoli per unit area. In terms of lung function, studies in teenagers showed that growth in forced expiratory volume in 1 s (FEV1) increases with age, reaching a peak at ages 12–13 in girls and at age 14 in boys [34, 35]. The FEV1 was shown to increase until the age of 17 in both sexes, but the continued growth in lung function after attainment of full height is higher in boys than in girls [36]. Finally, in adult life, sex differences have also been documented in lung structure and morphology [8, 33, 37, 38]. Height-matched men have larger diameter airways, total number of alveoli, and larger lung volumes and diffusion surfaces compared with women. However, for a given lung size, women have larger airways size than men [38].

In summary, given the gender effects on lung structure and function during lung development (Table 9.1), males are at higher risk for newborn and early childhood lung complications. In postnatal and adult life, however, the lower lung capacity in females, and the influence of sex hormones, makes women more prone to the damaging effects of air pollution and pulmonary limitations during exercise [39, 40]. Additionally, by modulating circulating levels of estradiol and progesterone, the menstrual cycle can also affect pulmonary function and inflammatory lung disease outcomes in women [41–43].

Hormonal Influences During Lung Development

The developing fetal lung is exposed to circulating levels of sex hormones synthesized from both maternal and fetal adrenal steroid precursors, by the action of specific lung steroidogenic enzymes [44, 45]. As indicated above, various regulatory roles have been attributed to the effects of sex hormones throughout fetal and postnatal lung development, and associated with sex differences in lung maturation. In the stages preceding the surge of surfactant synthesis, the developing male lung is exposed to higher levels of testosterone than the female lung. In the late gestational stages, both sexes are exposed to increasing levels of estradiol synthesized by the human placenta [5]. Below we describe the main known effects of male and female hormones in fetal and postnatal lung development. These are also summarized in Table 9.2.

Female Hormones

Fetal estradiol levels appear at the beginning of the canalicular phase, at approximately week 20 of female lung development, and continue to increase throughout birth [5]. Estrogens have been found to be responsible for the sexual dimorphism

Table 9.2 Hormonal secretion and regulatory effects in lung development

Hormone	Expression and source	Functional Effects	Proposed mechanisms of sex differences	Genes regulated
Estradiol	Week 20, in males and females. Significant increase toward late development. From human placenta.	Enhances surfactant synthesis and lung maturation.	ER expression patterns and signaling in females.	VEGF PDGF
Testosterone	Week 9, in males. From testis.	Delays lung development Impairs fibroblast–type II cell communications.	TGFβ and EGF receptor signaling in males. AR expression patterns and DNA binding in males. Modulation of steroidogenic enzymes in males.	TGFβ EGF FGF Shh BMP Wnt
AMH	Week 8.5, in males. From testis.	Delays airway branching.	Enhancement of apoptosis in males.	–

observed in lung development, for alveoli formation, and for lung maintenance and regeneration [17, 46–48]. Moreover, regulation of surfactant synthesis is positively affected by estrogens, favoring lung development and maturation in the female lung [11, 49]. Sex differences observed in the expression pattern of estrogen receptors (ER) in the bronchial and alveolar epithelium suggest that these mediate signaling of estrogens, contributing to the differential pulmonary phenotype observed in males and females [48, 50, 51].

Male Hormones

In the male lung, fetal circulatory testosterone levels of testicular origin can be found as early as week 9, at the beginning of the pseudoglandular phase [5]. High levels of androgens in males have been associated with delays in fetal lung maturation [52–54]. In animal studies, maternal treatment with the androgen dihydrotestosterone (DHT) during fetal lung development inhibits surfactant phospholipid production in the female fetal lung, whereas treatment with the antiandrogen flutamide increases surfactant phospholipid production in the male fetal lung [55, 56]. Moreover, studies have shown that androgens act on the fibroblast to delay the development communications between these and type II cells, as well as surfactant production, by a mechanism involving transforming growth factor beta (TGFβ) and epidermal growth factor (EGF) receptor signaling pathways [55, 57].

The delay in the development of male fetal lungs and its response to androgens is also dependent on the expression of functional androgen receptors (AR), and by local modulation of androgen levels by steroidogenic enzymes. These are 5α-reductase (which converts testosterone into its active form DHT), 3α-hydroxysteroid dehydrogenase (which inactivates DHT into 5α-androstane-3α,17β-diol), and 17β-hydroxysteroid dehydrogenases (responsible for conversion of androstenedione into testosterone, estrone into estradiol, and dehydroepiandrosterone into androstenediol) [52, 53, 58–61].

Androgen receptors are expressed in both male and female lung epithelial cells, and they can bind to DNA sequences and regulate the expression of genes that may be involved in the control of lung cell differentiation [62]. In addition, in utero male fetuses are exposed to higher levels of anti-Müllerian hormone (AMH) than females. Anti-Müllerian hormone is a glycoprotein hormone that is detected at approximately 8.5 weeks and continues to be expressed throughout male lung development [63]. Studies showed that AMH is required for normal male reproductive tract development and delays airway branching processes in males by enhancing apoptosis [64, 65].

Glucocorticoids

Another class of steroid hormones known to affect lung development and maturation via regulation of morphological changes and surfactant synthesis are glucocorticoids (GC). The fetal lung expresses most of the genes necessary for GC local synthesis, including the enzymes 21-hydroxylase (responsible for conversion of progesterone into deoxycorticosterone) and 20α-hydroxysteroid dehydrogenase (a steroid-inactivating enzyme), and these appear to modulate lung ontogenesis through paracrine actions [66, 67].

In the developing lung, GC induce structural changes such as thinning of alveolar walls increasing lung gas volume, and stimulation of epithelial–fibroblast cell communications and type II cell differentiation [67, 68]. Glucocorticoid regulation of surfactant protein gene expression has been extensively studied and demonstrated at the transcriptional and posttranscriptional levels [69–75]. Studies in mice lacking the GC receptor showed that these fail to progress through the canalicular and saccular phases of development, and they die of respiratory failure shortly after birth, indicating that GC signaling is essential for lung development progression [76]. In addition, GC effects on lung development have been shown to be inhibited by androgens, indicating that these effects are different in males than in females [67]. In the clinic, antenatal GC is commonly administered to mothers at risk of premature delivery to reduce the risk of RDS, and sex differences have been reported in the efficiency of these treatments [77–79]. In some cases, prenatal exposure to GC has also been linked to the development of cardiovascular, metabolic, and neuroendocrine disorders, but no sex differences have been reported for these adverse events [79–81].

Gene Expression During Lung Development

During fetal lung development progression, several genes related to cell maturation, cell proliferation, surfactant protein and phospholipid synthesis, and androgen metabolism enzymes are expressed with a sexual dimorphism at different time points [59, 82]. Additionally, numerous genes are transcriptionally modulated by sex hormones in the developing lung (Table 9.2). Androgens have been shown to regulate the expression of genes related to TGFβ, EGF, fibroblast growth factor (FGF), sonic hedgehog (Shh), bone morphogenetic protein (BMP), wingless-related family (Wnt), and other signaling pathways [55]. These play important roles at different stages of lung development: TGFβ and EGF signaling are associated with inhibition of endodermal morphogenesis and cell proliferation [55, 57], FGF is mainly involved in cell proliferation, and BMP is associated with the regulation of epithelial–mesenchymal interactions and branching morphogenesis. Similarly, Shh is known to positively affect lung development during the embryonic and pseudoglandular stages, and Wnt mainly controls cell differentiation [83, 84]. Later in gestation, differential gene expression in males and females has been described for Kruppel-like factor 5 (known to regulate surfactant metabolism), glutathione peroxidase (an antioxidant enzyme), epidermal nitric oxide synthase (related to postnatal adaptation of pulmonary circulation), and Clara cell protein 16 (a major immunomodulatory protein associated with prematurity) [85–88]. Other genes differentially expressed at later stages of the developing lung are vascular-endothelial growth factor (VEGF), and platelet-derived growth factor (PDGF). The expression of these genes has been reported to be higher in the lungs of females than males, and regulated by estrogens via modulation of the ER signaling pathways.

Recent studies have also shown that epigenetic changes are also implicated in the differential expression of genes and gene networks during lung development. Epigenetic changes such as gene methylation and histone acetylation can affect the developmental timing and level of transcription of numerous genes expressed throughout development, particularly those involved in alveolarization, such as insulin-like growth factor-1 (IGF1) and PPARγ (peroxisome proliferator-activated receptor gamma) [89]. In addition, epigenetic marks imposed by exposure to nicotine or other insults during pregnancy can become permanently programmed and transferred to subsequent generations [90, 91]. MicroRNAs, a recently discovered class of noncoding RNAs that control gene expression, have also been implicated in the epigenetic regulation of lung morphogenesis and maturation [92]. In a recent study, sex differences were found in the expression of microRNAs at the canalicular and saccular stages, and associated with developmental gene expression of pathways involving retinoids, IGF1 receptor, VEGF, tumor protein p53 signaling, as well as mediators of glucose metabolism. Together these studies suggest that sex-associated differential epigenetic regulation may affect the differences observed in structural and functional lung development in males and females [93].

Environmental Exposures and Lung Development

Environmental exposures can dramatically affect lung development, and depending at which stage they occur, they can affect males and females at differential rates [41, 94–99]. For example, any insult that occurs in the pseudoglandular phase may cause developmental alterations, resulting in changes to the airway branching system. Similarly, in the saccular stage, developmental damage already affects the gas-exchange components and results in structural alterations of the later pulmonary parenchyma. In addition, impairment of the fetal airway development, for example, due to in utero exposure to toxins, may increase the risk of childhood respiratory infection and disease [100]. It has been described that in utero smoke exposure and postnatal exposure to smoke and/or air pollution may influence airway and lung development, which may lead to small airway abnormalities and asthma later in life [1, 101]. In this regard, some studies showed that maternal smoking affects lung function of female infants more than that of male infants, but others reported the opposite effect, or no effect, indicating that the damaging effects of smoke exposure may be dependent on the frequency, concentration, and time of exposure [94–96, 102–105]. Perinatal nicotine exposure affects lung growth and differentiation by altering developmental signaling pathways that are necessary for fetal lung development, resulting in the predisposition to childhood asthma [91].

Summary

Lung development is a complex process, finely regulated by hormones, gene expression, epigenetic changes, and the environment in both sexes. While at prenatal developmental stages male hormones exert mostly negative regulatory roles, the effects of female hormones are mainly stimulatory. The result is a gender disparity in lung health at birth, with males at higher risk for neonatal lung disease than females. The effects of female hormones appear to be less positive during postnatal lung development, making women more prone to suffer environmental damaging effects on lung function than men.

References

1. Boezen HM, Jansen DF, Postma DS. Sex and gender differences in lung development and their clinical significance. Clin Chest Med. 2004;25(2):237–45.
2. Becklake MR, Kauffmann F. Gender differences in airway behaviour over the human life span. Thorax. 1999;54(12):1119–38.
3. Perelman RH, Palta M, Kirby R, Farrell PM. Discordance between male and female deaths due to the respiratory distress syndrome. Pediatrics. 1986;78(2):238–44.
4. Canoy D, Pekkanen J, Elliott P, Pouta A, Laitinen J, Hartikainen AL, et al. Early growth and adult respiratory function in men and women followed from the fetal period to adulthood. Thorax. 2007;62(5):396–402.

5. Seaborn T, Simard M, Provost PR, Piedboeuf B, Tremblay Y. Sex hormone metabolism in lung development and maturation. Trends Endocrinol Metab. 2010;21(12):729–38.

6. Carey MA, Card JW, Voltz JW, Arbes SJ, Germolec DR, Korach KS, et al. It's all about sex: gender, lung development and lung disease. Trends Endocrinol Metab. 2007;18(8):308–13.

7. Ishak N, Sozo F, Harding R, De Matteo R. Does lung development differ in male and female fetuses? Exp Lung Res. 2014;40(1):30–9.

8. Thurlbeck WM. Lung growth and alveolar multiplication. Pathobiol Annu. 1975;5:1–34.

9. Henderson-Smart DJ, Hutchinson JL, Donoghue DA, Evans NJ, Simpson JM, Wright I, et al. Prenatal predictors of chronic lung disease in very preterm infants. Arch Dis Child Fetal Neonatal Ed. 2006;91(1):F40–5.

10. Provost PR, Simard M, Tremblay Y. A link between lung androgen metabolism and the emergence of mature epithelial type II cells. Am J Respir Crit Care Med. 2004;170(3):296–305.

11. Gortner L, Shen J, Tutdibi E. Sexual dimorphism of neonatal lung development. Klin Padiatr. 2013;225(2):64–9.

12. Ali K, Greenough A. Long-term respiratory outcome of babies born prematurely. Ther Adv Respir Dis. 2012;6(2):115–20.

13. DiFiore JW, Wilson JM. Lung development. Semin Pediatr Surg. 1994;3(4):221–32.

14. Warburton D, Zhao J, Berberich MA, Bernfield M. Molecular embryology of the lung: then, now, and in the future. Am J Physiol. 1999;276(5 Pt 1):L697–704.

15. Warburton D, Bellusci S. The molecular genetics of lung morphogenesis and injury repair. Paediatr Respir Rev. 2004;5(Suppl A):S283–7.

16. Carey MA, Card JW, Voltz JW, Germolec DR, Korach KS, Zeldin DC. The impact of sex and sex hormones on lung physiology and disease: lessons from animal studies. Am J Physiol Lung Cell Mol Physiol. 2007;293(2):L272–8.

17. Massaro GD, Mortola JP, Massaro D. Sexual dimorphism in the architecture of the lung's gas-exchange region. Proc Natl Acad Sci U S A. 1995;92(4):1105–7.

18. Goldin GV, Wessells NK. Mammalian lung development: the possible role of cell proliferation in the formation of supernumerary tracheal buds and in branching morphogenesis. J Exp Zool. 1979;208(3):337–46.

19. Jeffrey PK. The development of large and small airways. Am J Respir Crit Care Med. 1998;157(5 Pt 2):S174–80.

20. Kotecha S. Lung growth for beginners. Paediatr Respir Rev. 2000;1(4):308–13.

21. Kitaoka H, Burri PH, Weibel ER. Development of the human fetal airway tree: analysis of the numerical density of airway endtips. Anat Rec. 1996;244(2):207–13.

22. Kotecha S. Lung growth: implications for the newborn infant. Arch Dis Child Fetal Neonatal Ed. 2000;82(1):F69–74.

23. Masters JR. Epithelial-mesenchymal interaction during lung development: the effect of mesenchymal mass. Dev Biol. 1976;51(1):98–108.

24. Hepper PG, Shannon EA, Dornan JC. Sex differences in fetal mouth movements. Lancet. 1997;350(9094):1820.

25. Fleisher B, Kulovich MV, Hallman M, Gluck L. Lung profile: sex differences in normal pregnancy. Obstet Gynecol. 1985;66(3):327–30.

26. Torday JS, Nielsen HC. The sex difference in fetal lung surfactant production. Exp Lung Res. 1987;12(1):1–19.

27. Pryhuber GS, Hull WM, Fink I, McMahan MJ, Whitsett JA. Ontogeny of surfactant proteins A and B in human amniotic fluid as indices of fetal lung maturity. Pediatr Res. 1991;30(6):597–605.

28. Baraldi E, Filippone M. Chronic lung disease after premature birth. N Engl J Med. 2007;357(19):1946–55.

29. Bhandari A, McGrath-Morrow S. Long-term pulmonary outcomes of patients with bronchopulmonary dysplasia. Semin Perinatol. 2013;37(2):132–7.

30. Bancalari EH, Jobe AH. The respiratory course of extremely preterm infants: a dilemma for diagnosis and terminology. J Pediatr. 2012;161(4):585–8.

31. Warburton D, El-Hashash A, Carraro G, Tiozzo C, Sala F, Rogers O, et al. Lung organogenesis. Curr Top Dev Biol. 2010;90:73–158.

32. Thurlbeck WM. Pathology of chronic airflow obstruction. Chest. 1990;97(2 Suppl):6S–10S.
33. Martin TR, Feldman HA, Fredberg JJ, Castile RG, Mead J, Wohl ME. Relationship between maximal expiratory flows and lung volumes in growing humans. J Appl Physiol (1985). 1988;65(2):822–8.
34. Mashalla YJ, Masesa PC. Changing relationship between FEV1 and height during adolescence. East Afr Med J. 1992;69(5):240–3.
35. Schrader PC, Quanjer PH, van Zomeren BC, Wise ME. Changes in the FEV1-height relationship during pubertal growth. Bull Eur Physiopathol Respir. 1984;20(4):381–8.
36. Schrader PC, Quanjer PH, Olievier IC. Respiratory muscle force and ventilatory function in adolescents. Eur Respir J. 1988;1(4):368–75.
37. Hoffstein V. Relationship between lung volume, maximal expiratory flow, forced expiratory volume in one second, and tracheal area in normal men and women. Am Rev Respir Dis. 1986;134(5):956–61.
38. Hanna GM, Daniels CL, Berend N. The relationship between airway size and lung size. Br J Dis Chest. 1985;79(2):183–8.
39. Harms CA, Rosenkranz S. Sex differences in pulmonary function during exercise. Med Sci Sports Exerc. 2008;40(4):664–8.
40. Kim CS, Alexis NE, Rappold AG, Kehrl H, Hazucha MJ, Lay JC, et al. Lung function and inflammatory responses in healthy young adults exposed to 0.06 ppm ozone for 6.6 Hours. Am J Respir Crit Care Med. 2011;183(9):1215–21.
41. Cohen J, Douma WR, Ten Hacken NH, Oudkerk M, Postma DS. Physiology of the small airways: a gender difference? Respir Med. 2008;102(9):1264–71.
42. Tam A, Morrish D, Wadsworth S, Dorscheid D, Man SF, Sin DD. The role of female hormones on lung function in chronic lung diseases. BMC Womens Health. 2011;11:24.
43. Townsend EA, Miller VM, Prakash YS. Sex differences and sex steroids in lung health and disease. Endocr Rev. 2012;33(1):1–47.
44. Pasqualini JR. Enzymes involved in the formation and transformation of steroid hormones in the fetal and placental compartments. J Steroid Biochem Mol Biol. 2005;97(5):401–15.
45. Milewich L, Kaimal V, Shaw CB, Johnson AR. Androstenedione metabolism in human lung fibroblasts. J Steroid Biochem. 1986;24(4):893–7.
46. Massaro D, Massaro GD. Estrogen regulates pulmonary alveolar formation, loss, and regeneration in mice. Am J Physiol Lung Cell Mol Physiol. 2004;287(6):L1154–9.
47. Massaro D, Massaro GD, Clerch LB. Noninvasive delivery of small inhibitory RNA and other reagents to pulmonary alveoli in mice. Am J Physiol Lung Cell Mol Physiol. 2004;287(5):L1066–70.
48. Patrone C, Cassel TN, Pettersson K, Piao YS, Cheng G, Ciana P, et al. Regulation of postnatal lung development and homeostasis by estrogen receptor beta. Mol Cell Biol. 2003;23(23):8542–52.
49. Liu D, Hinshelwood MM, Giguère V, Mendelson CR. Estrogen related receptor-alpha enhances surfactant protein-A gene expression in fetal lung type II cells. Endocrinology. 2006;147(11):5187–95.
50. Carvalho O, Gonçalves C. Expression of oestrogen receptors in foetal lung tissue of mice. Anat Histol Embryol. 2012;41(1):1–6.
51. Morani A, Warner M, Gustafsson JA. Biological functions and clinical implications of oestrogen receptors alfa and beta in epithelial tissues. J Intern Med. 2008;264(2):128–42.
52. Dammann CE, Ramadurai SM, McCants DD, Pham LD, Nielsen HC. Androgen regulation of signaling pathways in late fetal mouse lung development. Endocrinology. 2000;141(8): 2923–9.
53. Kimura Y, Suzuki T, Kaneko C, Darnel AD, Akahira J, Ebina M, et al. Expression of androgen receptor and 5alpha-reductase types 1 and 2 in early gestation fetal lung: a possible correlation with branching morphogenesis. Clin Sci (Lond). 2003;105(6):709–13.
54. Volpe MV, Ramadurai SM, Mujahid S, Vong T, Brandao M, Wang KT, et al. Regulatory interactions between androgens, Hoxb5, and TGF β signaling in murine lung development. Biomed Res Int. 2013;2013:320249.

55. Bresson E, Seaborn T, Côté M, Cormier G, Provost PR, Piedboeuf B, et al. Gene expression profile of androgen modulated genes in the murine fetal developing lung. Reprod Biol Endocrinol. 2010;8:2.

56. Card JW, Zeldin DC. Hormonal influences on lung function and response to environmental agents: lessons from animal models of respiratory disease. Proc Am Thorac Soc. 2009;6(7):588–95.

57. Bhaskaran M, Kolliputi N, Wang Y, Gou D, Chintagari NR, Liu L. Trans-differentiation of alveolar epithelial type II cells to type I cells involves autocrine signaling by transforming growth factor beta 1 through the Smad pathway. J Biol Chem. 2007;282(6):3968–76.

58. Boucher E, Provost PR, Plante J, Tremblay Y. Androgen receptor and 17beta-HSD type 2 regulation in neonatal mouse lung development. Mol Cell Endocrinol. 2009;311(1–2):109–19.

59. Plante J, Simard M, Rantakari P, Côté M, Provost PR, Poutanen M, et al. Epithelial cells are the major site of hydroxysteroid (17beta) dehydrogenase 2 and androgen receptor expression in fetal mouse lungs during the period overlapping the surge of surfactant. J Steroid Biochem Mol Biol. 2009;117(4–5):139–45.

60. Tremblay Y, Provost PR. 17Beta-HSD type 5 expression and the emergence of differentiated epithelial Type II cells in fetal lung: a novel role for androgen during the surge of surfactant. Mol Cell Endocrinol. 2006;248(1–2):118–25.

61. Tremblay Y, Provost PR. Major enzymes controlling the androgenic pressure in the developing lung. J Steroid Biochem Mol Biol. 2013;137:93–8.

62. Boucher E, Provost PR, Devillers A, Tremblay Y. Levels of dihydrotestosterone, testosterone, androstenedione, and estradiol in canalicular, saccular, and alveolar mouse lungs. Lung. 2010;188(3):229–33.

63. Rajpert-De Meyts E, Jørgensen N, Graem N, Müller J, Cate RL, Skakkebaek NE. Expression of anti-Müllerian hormone during normal and pathological gonadal development: association with differentiation of Sertoli and granulosa cells. J Clin Endocrinol Metab. 1999;84(10):3836–44.

64. Catlin EA, Powell SM, Manganaro TF, Hudson PL, Ragin RC, Epstein J, et al. Sex-specific fetal lung development and müllerian inhibiting substance. Am Rev Respir Dis. 1990;141(2):466–70.

65. Catlin EA, Tonnu VC, Ebb RG, Pacheco BA, Manganaro TF, Ezzell RM, et al. Müllerian inhibiting substance inhibits branching morphogenesis and induces apoptosis in fetal rat lung. Endocrinology. 1997;138(2):790–6.

66. Boucher E, Provost PR, Tremblay Y. Ontogeny of adrenal-like glucocorticoid synthesis pathway and of 20α-hydroxysteroid dehydrogenase in the mouse lung. BMC Res Notes. 2014;7:119.

67. Provost PR, Boucher E, Tremblay Y. Glucocorticoid metabolism in the developing lung: adrenal-like synthesis pathway. J Steroid Biochem Mol Biol. 2013;138:72–80.

68. Lee HJ, Kim BI, Choi ES, Choi CW, Kim EK, Kim HS, et al. Effects of postnatal dexamethasone or hydrocortisone in a rat model of antenatal lipopolysaccharide and neonatal hyperoxia exposure. J Korean Med Sci. 2012;27(4):395–401.

69. Alcorn JL, Gao E, Chen Q, Smith ME, Gerard RD, Mendelson CR. Genomic elements involved in transcriptional regulation of the rabbit surfactant protein-A gene. Mol Endocrinol. 1993;7(8):1072–85.

70. Boggaram V, Smith M, Mendelson C. Posttranscriptional regulation of surfactant protein-A messenger RNA in human fetal lung in vitro by glucocorticoids. Mol Endocrinol. 1991;5(3):414–23.

71. Karinch AM, Deiter G, Ballard PL, Floros J. Regulation of expression of human SP-A1 and SP-A2 genes in fetal lung explant culture. Biochim Biophys Acta. 1998;1398(2):192–202.

72. Liley HG, White RT, Benson BJ, Ballard PL. Glucocorticoids both stimulate and inhibit production of pulmonary surfactant protein A in fetal human lung. Proc Natl Acad Sci U S A. 1988;85(23):9096–100.

73. Mendelson CR. Role of transcription factors in fetal lung development and surfactant protein gene expression. Annu Rev Physiol. 2000;62:875–915.

74. Rooney SA, Young SL, Mendelson CR. Molecular and cellular processing of lung surfactant. FASEB J. 1994;8(12):957–67.
75. Wang G, Guo X, Floros J. Human SP-A 3′-UTR variants mediate differential gene expression in basal levels and in response to dexamethasone. Am J Physiol Lung Cell Mol Physiol. 2003;284(5):L738–48.
76. Manwani N, Gagnon S, Post M, Joza S, Muglia L, Cornejo S, et al. Reduced viability of mice with lung epithelial-specific knockout of glucocorticoid receptor. Am J Respir Cell Mol Biol. 2010;43(5):599–606.
77. Pérez Pérez G, Navarro MM. [Bronchopulmonary dysplasia and prematurity. Short-and long-term respiratory changes]. An Pediatr (Barc). 2010;72(1):79e1–16.
78. Berger TM, Bachmann II, Adams M, Schubiger G. Impact of improved survival of very low-birth-weight infants on incidence and severity of bronchopulmonary dysplasia. Biol Neonate. 2004;86(2):124–30.
79. Wapner RJ. Antenatal corticosteroids for periviable birth. Semin Perinatol. 2013;37(6):410–3.
80. Saizou C, Sachs P, Benhayoun M, Beaufils F. [Antenatal corticosteroids: benefits and risks]. J Gynecol Obstet Biol Reprod (Paris). 2005;34(1 Suppl):S111–7.
81. Tam EW, Chau V, Ferriero DM, Barkovich AJ, Poskitt KJ, Studholme C, et al. Preterm cerebellar growth impairment after postnatal exposure to glucocorticoids. Sci Transl Med. 2011;3(105):105ra.
82. Provost PR, Boucher E, Tremblay Y. Apolipoprotein A-I, A-II, C-II, and H expression in the developing lung and sex difference in surfactant lipids. J Endocrinol. 2009; 200(3):321–30.
83. Pongracz JE, Stockley RA. Wnt signalling in lung development and diseases. Respir Res. 2006;7:15.
84. Chuong CM, Patel N, Lin J, Jung HS, Widelitz RB. Sonic hedgehog signaling pathway in vertebrate epithelial appendage morphogenesis: perspectives in development and evolution. Cell Mol Life Sci. 2000;57(12):1672–81.
85. Tondreau MY, Boucher E, Simard M, Tremblay Y, Bilodeau JF. Sex-specific perinatal expression of glutathione peroxidases during mouse lung development. Mol Cell Endocrinol. 2012;355(1):87–95.
86. Miller AA, Hislop AA, Vallance PJ, Haworth SG. Deletion of the eNOS gene has a greater impact on the pulmonary circulation of male than female mice. Am J Physiol Lung Cell Mol Physiol. 2005;289(2):L299–306.
87. Miller AA, De Silva TM, Jackman KA, Sobey CG. Effect of gender and sex hormones on vascular oxidative stress. Clin Exp Pharmacol Physiol. 2007;34(10):1037–43.
88. Perni SC, Vardhana S, Kalish R, Chasen S, Witkin SS. Clara cell protein 16 concentration in mid-trimester amniotic fluid: association with fetal gender, fetal G>A +38 CC16 gene polymorphism and pregnancy outcome. J Reprod Immunol. 2005;68(1–2):85–90.
89. Joss-Moore LA, Albertine KH, Lane RH. Epigenetics and the developmental origins of lung disease. Mol Genet Metab. 2011;104(1–2):61–6.
90. Dasgupta C, Xiao D, Xu Z, Yang S, Zhang L. Developmental nicotine exposure results in programming of alveolar simplification and interstitial pulmonary fibrosis in adult male rats. Reprod Toxicol. 2012;34(3):370–7.
91. Rehan VK, Liu J, Naeem E, Tian J, Sakurai R, Kwong K, et al. Perinatal nicotine exposure induces asthma in second generation offspring. BMC Med. 2012;10:129.
92. Sayed D, Abdellatif M. MicroRNAs in development and disease. Physiol Rev. 2011;91(3):827–87.
93. Mujahid S, Logvinenko T, Volpe MV, Nielsen HC. miRNA regulated pathways in late stage murine lung development. BMC Dev Biol. 2013;13:13.
94. Brown RW, Hanrahan JP, Castile RG, Tager IB. Effect of maternal smoking during pregnancy on passive respiratory mechanics in early infancy. Pediatr Pulmonol. 1995;19(1):23–8.
95. Tager IB, Hanrahan JP, Tosteson TD, Castile RG, Brown RW, Weiss ST, et al. Lung function, pre- and post-natal smoke exposure, and wheezing in the first year of life. Am Rev Respir Dis. 1993;147(4):811–7.

96. Tager IB, Ngo L, Hanrahan JP. Maternal smoking during pregnancy. Effects on lung function during the first 18 months of life. Am J Respir Crit Care Med. 1995;152(3):977–83.

97. Almqvist C, Worm M, Leynaert B. Impact of gender on asthma in childhood and adolescence: a GA2LEN review. Allergy. 2008;63(1):47–57.

98. Bjornson CL, Mitchell I. Gender differences in asthma in childhood and adolescence. J Gend Specif Med. 2000;3(8):57–61.

99. Ooi GC, Khong PL, Chan-Yeung M, Ho JC, Chan PK, Lee JC, et al. High-resolution CT quantification of bronchiectasis: clinical and functional correlation. Radiology. 2002;225(3):663–72.

100. Gilliland FD, Berhane K, Li YF, Rappaport EB, Peters JM. Effects of early onset asthma and in utero exposure to maternal smoking on childhood lung function. Am J Respir Crit Care Med. 2003;167(6):917–24.

101. Jedrychowski WA, Perera FP, Maugeri U, Mroz E, Klimaszewska-Rembiasz M, Flak E, et al. Effect of prenatal exposure to fine particulate matter on ventilatory lung function of preschool children of non-smoking mothers. Paediatr Perinat Epidemiol. 2010;24(5):492–501.

102. Li YF, Gilliland FD, Berhane K, McConnell R, Gauderman WJ, Rappaport EB, et al. Effects of in utero and environmental tobacco smoke exposure on lung function in boys and girls with and without asthma. Am J Respir Crit Care Med. 2000;162(6):2097–104.

103. Young S, Arnott J, O'Keeffe PT, Le Souef PN, Landau LI. The association between early life lung function and wheezing during the first 2 yrs of life. Eur Respir J. 2000;15(1):151–7.

104. Cook DG, Strachan DP, Carey IM. Health effects of passive smoking. Thorax. 1999;54(5):469.

105. Lum S, Hoo AF, Dezateux C, Goetz I, Wade A, DeRooy L, et al. The association between birthweight, sex, and airway function in infants of nonsmoking mothers. Am J Respir Crit Care Med. 2001;164(11):2078–84.

Index

Printed in the United States
By Bookmasters